Hypnotherapy

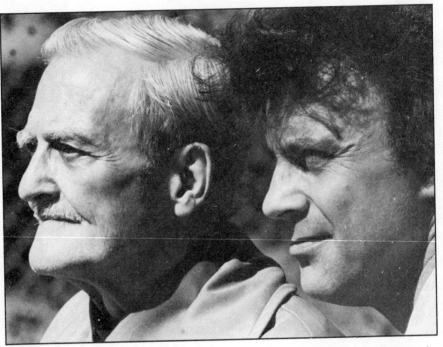

Dr. Milton Erickson and Dr. Ernest Rossi

Hypnotherapy

An Exploratory Casebook

by

Milton H. Erickson

and

Ernest L. Rossi

With a Foreword by Sidney Rosen

IRVINGTON PUBLISHERS, Inc., New York

**Halsted Press Division of
JOHN WILEY & Sons, Inc.**
New York London Toronto Sydney

The following copyrighted material is reprinted by permission:

Erickson, M. H. Concerning the nature and character of post-hypnotic behavior. *Journal of General Psychology,* 1941, *24*, 95–133 (with E. M. Erickson). Copyright © 1941.

Erickson, M. H. Hypnotic psychotherapy. *Medical Clinics of North America, New York Number,* 1948, 571–584. Copyright © 1948.

Erickson, M. H. Naturalistic techniques of hypnosis. *American Journal of Clinical Hypnosis,* 1958, *1*, 3–8. Copyright © 1958.

Erickson, M. H. Further clinical techniques of hypnosis: utilization techniques. *American Journal of Clinical Hypnosis,* 1959, *2*, 3–21. Copyright © 1959.

Erickson, M. H. An introduction to the study and application of hypnosis for pain control. In J. Lassner (Ed.), *Hypnosis and Psychosomatic Medicine: Proceedings of the International Congress for Hypnosis and Psychosomatic Medicine.* Springer Verlag, 1967. Reprinted in English and French in the *Journal of the College of General Practice of Canada,* 1967, and in French in *Cahiers d' Anesthesiologie,* 1966, *14*, 189–202. Copyright © 1966, 1967.

Distributed by HALSTED PRESS
A division of JOHN WILEY & SONS, Inc., New York

Library of Congress Cataloging in Publication Data

Erickson, Milton H.
  Hypnotherapy, an exploratory casebook.

  Includes bibliographical references.
  1. Hypnotism—Therapeutic use. I. Rossi, Ernest Lawrence, joint author. II. Title.
  RC495.E719   615'.8512   78-23839
  ISBN 0-470-26595-7

Printed in The United States of America

Contents

FOREWORD

"Speak to the wall so the door may hear"—*Sufi saying*.

Everyone who knows Milton Erickson is aware that he rarely does anything without a purpose. In fact, his goal-directedness may be the most important characteristic of his life and work.

Why is it, then, that prior to writing *Hypnotic Realities* with Ernest Rossi (Irvington, 1976) he had avoided presenting his work in book form? Why did he choose Ernest Rossi to coauthor that book and the present one? And, finally, I could not help but wonder, "Why did he ask me to write this foreword?"

Erickson has, after all, published almost 150 articles over a fifty-year period, but only two relatively minor books—*Time Distortion in Hypnosis,* written in 1954 with L. S. Cooper, and *The Practical Applications of Medical and Dental Hypnosis,* in 1961 with S. Hershman, MD and I. I. Sector, DDS. It is easy to understand that in his seventies he may well be eager to leave a legacy, a definitive summing up, a final opportunity for others to really understand and perhaps emulate him.

Rossi is an excellent choice as a coauthor. He is an experienced clinician who has trained with many giants in psychiatry—Franz Alexander, amongst others. He is a Jungian training analyst. He is a prolific author and has devoted the major part of his time over the past six years to painstaking observation, recording and discussion of Erickson's work.

Again, "Why me?" I am also a training analyst, but with a different group—the American Institute of Psychoanalysis (Karen Horney). I have been a practicing psychiatrist for almost thirty years. For almost fifteen years I have also done a great deal of work with disabled patients. I have been involved with hypnosis for over thirty-five years, since I first heard about Milton Erickson, who was then living in Eloise, Michigan.

Both Rossi and I have broad, but differing, clinical and theoretical backgrounds. Neither of us has worked primarily with "hypnosis." Therefore, neither of us has a vested interest in promoting some hypnotic theories of our own. We are genuinely devoted to the goal of presenting Erickson's theories and ideas, not only to practitioners of hypnosis, but to the community of psychotherapists and psychoanalysts which has had little familiarity with hypnosis. Towards this end, Rossi assumes the posture of a rather naive student acting on behalf of the rest of us.

Margaret Mead, who also counts herself as one of his students, writes of "the originality of Milton Erickson" in the issue of *The American Journal of Clinical Hypnosis* dedicated to him on his seventy-fifth birthday (Mead, M. "The Originality of Milton Erickson," *AJCH*, Vol. 20, No. 1, July 1977, pp. 4-5). She comments that she has been interested in his originality ever since she first met him in the summer of 1940, expanding on this idea by stating, "It can be firmly said that Milton Erickson never solved a problem in an old way if he can think of a new way—and he usually can." She feels, however, that his "unquenchable, burning originality was a barrier to the transmission of much of what he knew" and that "inquiring students would become bemused with the extraordinary and unexpected quality of each different demonstration, lost between trying to imitate the intricate, idiosyncratic response and the underlying principles which he was illuminating." In *Hypnotic Realities* and in this book, Ernest Rossi takes some large steps towards elucidating these underlying principles. He does this most directly by organizing and extracting them from Erickson's case material. Even more helpfully, though, he encourages Erickson to spell out some of these principles.

Students who study this volume carefully, as I did, will find that the authors have done the best job to date in clarifying Erickson's ideas on the nature of hypnosis and hypnotic therapy, on techniques of hypnotic induction, on ways of inducing therapeutic change, and of validating this change. In the process they have also revealed a great deal of helpful data about Erickson's philosophy of life and therapy. Many therapists, both psychoanalytic and others, will find his approaches compatible with their own and far removed from their preconceptions about "hypnosis." As the authors point out, "Hypnosis does not change the person nor does it alter past experiential life. It serves to permit him to learn more about himself and to express himself more adequately. . . . Therapeutic trance helps people side-step their own learned limitations so that they can more fully explore and utilize their potentials."

Those who read Erickson's generous offering of fascinating case histories, and then attempt to emulate him, will undoubtedly find that they do not achieve results that are at all comparable to his. They may then give up, deciding that Erickson's approach is one that is unique for him. They may note that Erickson has several handicaps that have always set him apart from others, and that may certainly permit him to have a unique way of viewing and responding. He was born with color deficient vision, tone deafness, dyslexia, and lacking a sense of rhythm. He suffered two serious attacks of crippling poliomyelitis. He has been wheelchair bound for many years from the effects of the neurological damage, supplemented by arthritis and myositis. Some will not be content with the rationalization that Erickson is a therapeutic or inimitable genius. And they will find that with the help of clarifiers and facilitators, such as Ernest Rossi, there is much in his way of working that can be learned, taught and utilized by others.

Erickson himself has advised, in *Hypnotic Realities* (page 258), "In working at a problem of difficulty, you try to make an interesting design in the handling of it. That way you have an answer to the difficult problem. Become interested in the design and don't notice the back-breaking labor." In dealing with the difficult problem of analyzing and teaching Erickson's approaches, Rossi's designs can be most helpful. Whether each reader will choose to accept Rossi's suggestion that he practice the exercises recommended in this book, is an individual matter; in my experience, it has been worthwhile to practice some of them. In fact, by deliberately and planfully applying some of Erickson's approaches as underlined by Rossi, I found that I have been able to help patients experience deeper states of trance and be more open to changing as an apparent consequence of this. I found that setting up therapeutic double binds, giving indirect posthypnotic suggestions, using questions to facilitate therapeutic responsiveness, and building up compound suggestions have been particularly helpful. Erickson and Rossi's repeated emphasis on what they call the "utilization approach" is certainly justified. In this book they give many vivid and useful examples of "accepting and utilizing the patient's manifest behavior, utilizing the patient's inner realities, utilizing the patient's resistances, and utilizing the patient's negative affect and symptoms." Erickson's creative use of jokes, puns, metaphors and symbols has been analyzed by others, notably Haley and Bandler and Grinder, but the examples and discussion in this book add a great deal to our understanding.

At times, Erickson will work with a patient in a light trance, in what he calls a "common everyday trance," or no trance at all. He does not limit himself to short-term therapy. This is illustrated in his painstaking work over a nine-month period with Pietro, the flutist with the swollen lip, described in one of the dramatic case outlines in this book. His expertise, however, in working with patients in the deepest trances, often with amnesia for the therapeutic work, has always interested observers. The question of whether or not inducing deeper trances, and giving directions or suggestions indirectly rather than directly, leads to more profound or lasting clinical results is a researchable one. It has certainly been my experience that if one does not believe in, or value, deeper trances and does not strive for them, one is not likely to see them very often. My experience has also been that the achievement of deeper trances, often including phenomena such as dissociation, time distortion, amnesia, and age-regression, *does* lead to quicker and apparently more profound changes in patients' symptoms and attitudes.

Erickson emphasizes the value of helping patients to work in the mode of what he would call the "unconscious." He values the wisdom of the unconscious. In fact, he often goes to great lengths to keep the therapeutic work from being examined and potentially destroyed by the patient's conscious mind and by the patient's "learned and limited sets." His methods of doing this are more explicitly outlined in this book than in any other writings available to date.

It is true that he tends not to distinguish between induction of trance or hypnotic techniques and therapeutic techniques or maneuvers. He feels that it is a waste of time for the therapist to use meaningless, repetitious phrases in the induction of trance as this time might be more usefully employed injecting therapeutic suggestions or in preparing the patient for change. As Rossi has pointed out, both the therapy and trance induction involve, in the early stages, a "depotentiation of the patient's usual and limited mental sets." Erickson is never content with simply inducing a trance, but is always concerned with some therapeutic role.

He points out the limited effectiveness of direct suggestion, although he is certainly aware that hypnotic techniques, using direct suggestion, will frequently enhance the effectiveness of behavior modification approaches such as desensitization and cognitive retraining. He notes that "Direct suggestion . . . does not evoke the re-association and reorganization of ideas, understandings and memories so essential for an actual cure . . . Effective results in hypnotic psychotherapy . . . derive only from the patient's activities. The therapist merely stimulates the patient into activity, often not knowing what that activity may be. And then he guides the patient and exercises clinical judgment in determining the amount of work to be done to achieve the desired results" (Erickson, 1948). From this comment, and from reading the case histories in this volume and in other publications, it should be apparent that Erickson demands and evokes much less "doctrinal compliance" than do most therapists.

It is obvious that "clinical judgment" comes only as the result of many years of intensive study of dynamics, pathology and health, and from actually working with patients.

The judgment of the therapist will also be influenced by his own philosophy and goals in life. Erickson's own philosophy is manifested by his emphasis on concepts such as "growth and delight and joy". To this he adds, "Life isn't something you can give an answer to today. You should enjoy the process of waiting, the process of becoming what you are. There is nothing more delightful than planting flower seeds and not knowing what kinds of flowers are going to come up." My own experience in this regard is illustrated by my having visited him in 1970, spending a four-hour session with him, and leaving with the feeling that I had spent this time mostly in listening to stories about his family and patients. I did not see him again until the summer of 1977. Then, at 5:00 a.m. in a Phoenix motel, while I was reviewing some tapes of Erickson at work, some very important insights became vividly evident to me. They were obviously related to work begun during our session in 1970 and to self analysis I had done in the intervening seven years. Later that morning when I excitedly mentioned these insights to Erickson, he, typically, simply smiled and did not attempt to elaborate on them in any way.

When we read some of the writings on other forms of therapy, such as family therapy or Gestalt therapy, we are struck by how much they have been influenced by Erickson. This is no accident as many of the early therapists in these schools began working with hypnosis or even with Erickson himself. I hope that Rossi will trace some of these influences in his future writings. I have alluded to some of them in my article, "Recent Experiences with Encounter Gestalt and Hypnotic Techniques" (Rosen, S. *Am J. Psychoanalysis,* Vol. 32, No. 1, 1972, pp. 90-105).

In conjunction with Erickson and Rossi's first volume *Hypnotic Realities, Hypnotherapy: An Exploratory Casebook* should serve as a firm basis for courses in Ericksonian therapy or Ericksonian hypnosis. These courses may be supplemented by other books, including those written by J. Haley and by Bandler and Grinder. In addition, we are now fortunate to have available a bibliography of the 147 articles written by Erickson himself (see Gravitz, M.A. and Gravitz, R. F., "Complete Bibliography 1929-1977," *American Journal of Clinical Hypnosis,* 1977, *20*, 84-94).

Rossi has told me that in working with Erickson he has always been struck by the fact that Erickson seems to be atheoretical. I have noted that this applies to Erickson's openness but certainly not to his emphasis on growth or his humanistic or socially oriented views. Rossi and others are constantly rediscovering the fact that Erickson always works towards goals—those of his patients', not his own. This may not seem to be such a revolutionary idea today when it is the avowed intention of almost all therapists, but perhaps many of us are limited in our capacity to carry out this intent. It is significant that both intent and practice are most successfully coordinated and realized in the work of this man who is probably the world's master in clinical hypnosis, and yet hypnosis is still associated by almost everyone with manipulation and suggestion—a typical Ericksonian paradox. The master manipulator allows and stimulates the greatest freedom!

Sidney Rosen, MD
New York

Preface

The present work is the second in a series of volumes by the authors that began with the publication of *Hypnotic Realities* (Irvington, 1976). Like that first volume, the present work is essentially the record of the senior author's efforts to train the junior author in the field of clinical hypnotherapy. As such, the present work is not of an academic or scholarly nature but rather a practical study of some of the attitudes, orientations, and skills required of the modern hypnotherapist.

In the first chapter we outline the utilization approach to hypnotherapy as the basic orientation to our work. In the second chapter we essay a more systematic presentation of the indirect forms of suggestion, which were originally selected out of the case presentations of our first volume. We now believe that the *utilization approach* and the *indirect forms of suggestion* are the essence of the senior author's therapeutic innovations over the past fifty years and account for much of his unique skill as a hypnotherapist.

In Chapter Three we illustrate how the utilization approach and the indirect forms of suggestion can be integrated to facilitate the induction of therapeutic trance in a manner that simultaneously orients the patient toward therapeutic change. In our fourth chapter we illustrate the approaches to posthypnotic suggestion that the senior author has found most effective in day-to-day clinical practice.

These first four chapters outline some of the basic principles of the senior author's approach. We hope this presentation will provide other clinicians with a broad and practical perspective of the senior author's work and serve as a source of hypotheses about the nature of therapeutic trance that will be tested with more controlled experimental studies by researchers.

At the end of each of these first four chapters we have suggested a number of exercises to facilitate learning the orientation, attitudes, and skills required of anyone who wants to put some of this material into actual practice. A simple reading and understanding of the material is not enough. An extensive effort to acquire new habits of observation and interpersonal interaction are required. All the suggested exercises have been put into practice as we have sought to hone our own skills and teach others.

Each of the remaining six chapters presents case studies illustrating and further exploring the senior author's clinical work with patients. Six of these cases (cases 1, 5, 8, 10, 11, and 12) are major studies like those in our first volume, *Hypnotic Realities,* where we transcribed tape recordings of the senior author's actual words and patterns of interaction with patients. The recording equipment for these studies was provided by a research grant from the American Society of Clinical Hypnosis— Education and Research Foundation. In our commentaries on these sessions we have presented our current understanding of the dynamics of the hypnotherapeutic process and discussed a number of issues such as the facilitation of the creative process and the functions of the left and right hemispheres.

Most of the other shorter cases were drawn from the senior author's file of unpublished records of his work in private practice, some of them from long-unopened folders containing yellowed pages more than a quarter of a century old. These cases were all reviewed and re-edited with fresh commentaries and provide an appropriate perspective on the spontaneous creativity and daring required of the hypnotherapist in clinical practice. In addition, we have skimmed through many tape recordings of the senior author's lectures and workshops at the meetings of the American Society of Clinical Hypnosis. Some of these were already typed and partially edited by Florence Sharp, Ph.D., and other members of the Society. Most of these appear under the heading "Selected Shorter Cases: Exercises for Analysis." Many of them have been repeated and published so often (Haley, 1973) that they appear anecdotal, as part of the folklore of hypnosis in the past half-century. They can serve as marvelous exercises for analysis, however. At the end of each such case we have placed in italics some of the principles we feel were involved. The reader may enjoy finding others.

It is our impression that the clinical practice of hypnotherapy is currently emerging from a period of relative quiescence into an exciting time of new discoveries and fascinating possibilities. Those who know the history of hypnosis are already familiar with this cyclic pattern of excitement and quiescence that is so characteristic of the field. Some historians of science now believe this cyclic pattern is characteristic of all branches of science and art: The excitement comes with periods of new discovery, the quiescence comes as these are assimilated. As the junior author gradually put this volume together, he frequently had a subjective sense of new discovery. But was it new only for him, or would it be new for others as well? We must rely upon you, our reader, to make an independent assessment of the matter and perhaps carry the work a step further.

Milton H. Erickson, M.D.
Ernest L. Rossi, Ph.D.

Acknowledgments

This work can be recognized as a truly community effort, with many more individuals contributing to it than we can acknowledge by name. First among these are our patients, who frequently recognized and cooperated with the exploratory nature of our work with them. Their spontaneous creativity is truly the basis of all innovative therapeutic work: We simply report what they learned to do with the hope that their success may be a useful guide for others.

Many of the teachers and participants in the seminars and workshops of the *American Society of Clinical Hypnosis* have provided a continual series of insights, illustrations, and comments that have found their way into this work. Prominent among these are Leo Alexander, Ester Bartlett, Franz Baumann, Neil D. Capua, David Cheek, Sheldon Cohen, Jerry Day, T. E. A. Von Dedenroth, Roxanne and Christie Erickson, Fredericka Freytag, Melvin Gravitz, Frederick Hanley, H. Clagett Harding, Maurice McDowell, Susan Mirow, Marion Moore, Robert Pearson, Bertha Rodger, Florence Sharp, Kay Thompson, Paul Van Dyke, M. Erik Wright.

To Robert Pearson we owe a special acknowledgment for having first suggested the basic format of this work, for his continual encouragement during its gestation, and for his critical reading of our final draft. Ruth Ingham and Margaret Ryan have contributed significant editing skills that finally enabled our work to reach the press.

Finally, we wish to acknowledge the following publishers who have generously permitted the republication of five of the papers in this volume: American Society of Clinical Hypnosis, Journal Press, W. B. Saunders Company, and Springer Verlag.

CHAPTER 1

The Utilization
Approach to Hypnotherapy

We view hypnotherapy as a process whereby we help people utilize their own mental associations, memories, and life potentials to achieve their own therapeutic goals. Hypnotic suggestion can facilitate the utilization of abilities and potentials that already exist within a person but that remain unused or underdeveloped because of a lack of training or understanding. The hypnotherapist carefully explores a patient's individuality to ascertain what life learnings, experiences, and mental skills are available to deal with the problem. The therapist then facilitates an approach to trance experience wherein the patient may utilize these uniquely personal internal responses to achieve therapeutic goals.

Our approach may be viewed as a three-stage process: (1) a period of *preparation* during which the therapist explores the patients repertory of life experiences and facilitates constructive frames of reference to orient the patient toward therapeutic change; (2) an activation and utilization of the patient's own mental skills during a period of *therapeutic trance;* (3) a careful *recognition, evaluation, and ratification of the therapeutic change* that takes place. In this first chapter we will introduce some of the factors contributing to the successful experience of each of these three stages. In the chapters that follow we will illustrate and discuss them in greater detail.

1. Preparation

The initial phase of hypnotherapeutic work consists of a careful period of observation and preparation. Initially the most important factor in any therapeutic interview is to establish a sound rapport—that is, a positive feeling of understanding and mutual regard between therapist and patient. Through this rapport therapist and patient together create a new therapeutic frame of reference that will serve as the growth medium in

1

which the patient's therapeutic responses will develop. The rapport is the means by which therapist and patient secure each others' attention. Both develop a "yes set," or acceptance of each other. The therapist presumably has a well developed ability to observe and relate; the patient is learning to observe and achieve a state of *response attentiveness*, that state of extreme attentiveness in responding to the nuances of communication presented by the therapist.

In the initial interview the therapist gathers the relevant facts regarding the patient's problems and the *repertory of life experiences and learnings that will be utilized for therapeutic purposes*. Patients have problems because of learned limitations. They are caught in mental sets, frames of reference, and belief systems that do not permit them to explore and utilize their own abilities to best advantage. Human beings are still in the process of learning to use their potentials. The therapeutic transaction ideally creates a new phenomenal world in which patients can explore their potentials, freed to some extent from their learned limitations. As we shall later see, *therapeutic trance is a period during which patients are able to break out of their limited frameworks and belief systems so they can experience other patterns of functioning within themselves*. These other patterns are usually response potentials that have been learned from previous life experience but, for one reason or another, remain unavailable to the patient. The therapist can explore patients' personal histories, character, and emotional dynamics, their field of work, interests, hobbies, and so on to assess the range of life experiences and response abilities that may be available for achieving therapeutic goals. Most of the cases in this book will illustrate this process.

As the therapist explores the patient's world and facilitates rapport, it is almost inevitable that *new frames of reference and belief systems are created*. This usually happens whenever people meet and interact closely. In hypnotherapy this spontaneous opening and shifting of mental frameworks and belief systems is carefully studied, facilitated, and utilized. The therapist is in a constant process of evaluating what limitations are at the source of the patient's problem and what new horizons can be opened to help the patient outgrow those limitations. In the preparatory phase of hypnotherapeutic work mental frameworks are facilitated in a manner that will enable the patient to respond to the suggestions that will be received later during trance. Suggestions made during trance frequently function like keys turning the tumblers of a patient's associative processes within the locks of certain mental frameworks that have already been established. A number of workers (Weitzenhoffer, 1957, Schneck, 1970, 1975) have described how what is said before trance is formally induced can enhance hypnotic suggestion. We agree and emphasize that effective trance work is usually preceded by a preparatory phase during which we help patients create an optimal attitude and belief system for therapeutic responses.

A singularly important aspect of this optimal attitude is *expectancy*. Patients' expectations of therapeutic change permits them to suspend the learned limitations and negative life experiences that are at the source of their problems. A suspension of disbelief and an extraordinarily high expectation of cure has been used to account for the "miraculous" healing sometimes achieved within a religious belief system. As will be seen in our overall analysis of the dynamics of therapeutic trance in the following section, such seemingly miraculous healing can be understood as a special manifestation of the more general process we utilize to facilitate threapeutic responses in hypnotherapy.

2. Therapeutic Trance

Therapeutic trance is a period during which the limitations of one's usual frames of reference and beliefs are temporarily altered so one can be receptive to other patterns of association and modes of mental functioning that are conducive to problem-solving. We view the dynamics of trance induction and utilization as a very personal experience wherein the therapist helps patients to find their own individual ways. Trance induction is not a standardized process that can be applied in the same way to everyone. There is no method or technique that always works with everyone or even with the same person on different occasions. Because of this we speak of "approaches" to trance experience. We thereby emphasize that we have many means of facilitating, guiding, or teaching how one might be led to experience the state of receptivity that we call therapeutic trance. However, we have no universal method for effecting the same uniform trance state in everyone. Most people with problems can be guided to experience their own unique variety of therapeutic trance when they understand that it may be useful. The art of the hypnotherapist is in helping patients reach an understanding that will help them give up some of the limitations of their common everyday world view so that they can achieve a state of receptivity to the new and creative within themselves.

For didactic purposes we have conceptualized the dynamics of trance induction and suggestion as a five-stage process, outlined in Figure 1.

While we may use this paradigm as a convenient framework for analyzing many of the hypnotherapeutic approaches we will illustrate in this volume, it must be understood that the individual manifestations of the process will be just as unique and various as are the natures of the people experiencing it. We will now outline our understanding of these five stages.

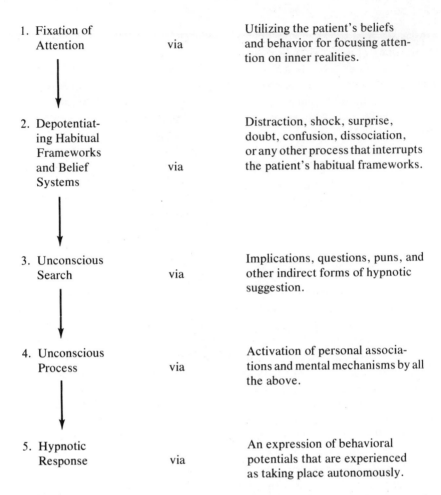

1. Fixation of Attention	via	Utilizing the patient's beliefs and behavior for focusing attention on inner realities.
2. Depotentiating Habitual Frameworks and Belief Systems	via	Distraction, shock, surprise, doubt, confusion, dissociation, or any other process that interrupts the patient's habitual frameworks.
3. Unconscious Search	via	Implications, questions, puns, and other indirect forms of hypnotic suggestion.
4. Unconscious Process	via	Activation of personal associations and mental mechanisms by all the above.
5. Hypnotic Response	via	An expression of behavioral potentials that are experienced as taking place autonomously.

Figure 1: A five-stage paradigm of the dynamics of trance induction and suggestion (from Erickson and Rossi, 1976.)

Fixation of Attention

The fixation of attention has been the classical approach for initiating therapeutic trance, or hypnosis. The therapist would ask the patient to gaze at a spot or candle flame, a bright light, a revolving mirror, the therapist's eyes, gestures, or whatever. As experience accumulated it became evident that the point of fixation could be anything that held the patient's attention. Further, the point of fixation need not be external; it is even more effective to focus attention on the patient's own body and inner experience. Thus approaches such as hand levitation and body relaxation were developed. Encouraging the patient to focus on sensations or internal imagery led attention inward even more effectively. Many of these approaches have become standardized and are well

4

described in reference works on hypnosis (Weitzenhoffer, 1957; Hartland, 1966; Haley, 1967).

The beginner in hypnotherapy may well study these standardized approaches and closely follow some of them to initiate trance in a formalized manner. They are often highly impressive to the patient and very effective in inducing trance. Student therapists will be in error, however, if they attempt to utilize only one approach as the universal method and thereby blind themselves to the unique motivations and manifestiations of trance development in each person. The therapist who carefully studies the process of attention in everyday life as well as in the consulting room will soon come to recognize that an interesting story or a fascinating fact or fantasy can fixate attention just as effectively as a formal induction. Anything that fascinates and holds or absorbs a person's attention could be described as hypnotic. We have the concept of the common everyday trance for those periods in everyday life when we are so absorbed or preoccupied with one matter or another that we momentarily lose track of our outer environment.

The most effective means of focusing and fixing attention in clinical practice is to recognize and acknowledge the patient's current experience. When the therapist correctly labels the patient's ongoing here-and-now experience, the patient is usually immediately grateful and open to whatever else the therapist may have to say. Acknowledging the patient's current reality thus opens a yes set for whatever suggestions the therapist may wish to introduce. This is the basis of the utilization approach to trance induction, wherein therapists gain their patients' attention by focusing on their current behavior and experiences (Erickson, 1958, 1959). Illustrations of this utilization approach to trance induction will be presented in our third chapter.

Depotentiating Habitual Frameworks and Belief Systems

In our view one of the most useful psychological effects of fixating attention is that it tends to depotentiate patients' habitual mental sets and common everyday frames of reference. Their belief systems are more or less interrupted and suspended for a moment or two. Consciousness has been *distracted*. During that momentary suspension latent patterns of association and sensory-perceptual experience have an opportunity to assert themselves in a manner that can initiate the altered state of consciousness that has been described as trance or hypnosis.

There are many means of depotentiating habitual frames of reference. Any experience of shock or surprise momentarily fixates attention and interrupts the previous pattern of association. Any experience of the unrealistic, the unusual, or the fantastic provides an opportunity for altered modes of apprehension. The authors have described how confusion, doubt, dissociation, and disequilibrium are all means of

5

depotentiating patients' learned limitations so that they may become open and available for new means of experiencing and learning, which are the essence of therapeutic trance (Erickson, Rossi, and Rossi, 1976).

The interruption and suspension of our common everyday belief system has been described by the junior author as a *creative moment* (Rossi, 1972a):

But what is a creative moment? Such moments have been celebrated as the exciting "hunch" by scientific workers and "inspiration" by people in the arts (Barron, 1969). *A creative moment occurs when a habitual pattern of association is interrupted*; there may be a "spontaneous" lapse or relaxation of one's habitual associative process; there may be a *psychic shock*, an overwhelming sensory or emotional experience; a psychedelic drug, a toxic condition or sensory deprivation may serve as the catalyst; yoga, Zen, spiritual and meditative exercises may likewise interrupt our habitual associations and introduce a momentary void in awareness. In that fraction of a second when the habitual contents of awareness are knocked out there is a chance for pure awareness, "the pure lihgt of the void" (Evans-Wentz, 1960) to shine through. This fraction of a second may be experienced as a "mystic state," satori, a peak experience or an altered state of consciousness (Tart, 1969). It may be experienced as a moment of "fascination" or "falling in love" when the gap in one's awareness is filled by the *new* that suddenly intrudes itself.

The creative moment is thus a gap in one's habitual pattern of awareness. Bartlett (1958) has described how the genesis of original thinking can be understood as the filling in of mental gaps. *The new that appears in creative moments is thus the basic unit of original thought and insight as well as personality change.* Experiencing a creative moment may be the phenomenological correlate of a critical change in the molecular structure of proteins within the brain associated with learning (Gaito, 1972; Rossi, 1973b), or the creation of new cell assemblies and phase sequences (Hebb, 1963).

The relation between psychological shock and creative moments is apparent: a "psychic shock" interrupts a person's habitual associations so that something new may appear. Ideally psychological shock sets up the conditions for a creative moment when a new insight, attitude, or behavior change may take place in the subject. Erickson (1948) has also described hypnotic trance itself as a special psychological state which effects a similar break in the patient's conscious and habitual associations so that creative learning can take place.

In everyday life one is continually confronted with difficult and puzzling situations that mildly shock and interrupt one's usual way of thinking. Ideally these problem situations will initiate a creative moment of reflection that may provide an opportunity for something new to emerge. Psychological problems develop when people do not permit the naturally changing circumstances of life to interrupt their old and no longer useful patterns of association and experience so that new solutions and attitudes may emerge.

Unconscious Search and Unconscious Process

In everyday life there are many approaches to fixing attention, depotentiating habitual associations, and thereby initiating an *unconscious search* for a new experience or solution to a problem. In a difficult situation, for example, one may make a joke or use a pun to interrupt and reorganize the situation from a different point of view. One may use allusions or implications to intrude another way of understanding the same situation. Like metaphor and analogy (Jaynes, 1976) these are all means of momentarily arresting attention and requesting a search— essentially a search on an unconscious level—to come up with a new association or frame of reference. These are all opportunities for creative moments in everyday life wherein a necessary reorganization of one's experience takes place.

In therapeutic trance we utilize similar means of initiating a search on an unconscious level. These are what the senior author has described as the *indirect forms of suggestion* (Erickson and Rossi, 1976; Erickson, Rossi, and Rossi, 1976). In essence, an indirect suggestion initiates an unconscious search and facilitates unconscious processes within patients so that they are usually somewhat surprised by their own responses. The indirect forms of suggestion help patients bypass their learned limitations so they are able to accomplish a lot more than they are usually able to. *The indirect forms of suggestion are facilitators of mental associations and unconscious processes.* In the next chapter we will outline our current understanding of a variety of these indirect forms of suggestion.

The Hypnotic Response

The hypnotic response is the natural outcome of the unconscious search and processes initiated by the therapist. Because it is mediated primarily by unconscious processes within the patient, the hypnotic response appears to occur automatically or autonomously; it appears to take place all by itself in a manner that may seem alien or dissociated from the person's usual mode of responding on a voluntary level. Most patients typically experience a mild sense of pleasant surprise when they find themselves responding in this automatic and involuntary manner. That sense of surprise, in fact, can generally be taken as an indication of the genuinely autonomous nature of their response.

Hypnotic responses need not be initiated by the therapist, however.

Most of the classical hypnotic phenomena, in fact, were discovered quite by accident as natural manifestations of human behavior that occurred spontaneously in trance without any suggestion whatsoever. Classical hypnotic phenomena such as catalepsy, anesthesia, amnesia, hallucinations, age regression, and time distortion are all spontaneous trance phenomena that were a source of amazement and bewilderment to early investigators. It was when they later attempted to induce trance and study trance phenomena systematically that these investigators found that they could "suggest" the various hypnotic phenomena. Once they found it possible to do this, they began to use suggestibility itself as a criterion of the validity and depth of trance experience.

When the next step was taken to utilize trance experience as a form of therapy, hypnotic suggestibility was emphasized even more as the essential factor for successful work. An unfortunate side effect of this emphasis on suggestibility was in the purported power of hypnotists to control behavior with suggestion. By this time our conception of hypnotic phenomena had moved very far indeed from their original discovery as natural and spontaneous manifestations of the mind. Hypnois acquired the connotations of manipulation and control. The exploitation of naturally occurring trance phenomena as a demonstration of power, prestige, influence, and control (as it has been used in stage hypnosis) was a most unfortunate turn in the history of hypnosis.

In an effort to correct such misconceptions the senior author (Erickson, 1948) described the merits of direct and indirect suggestion in hypnotherapy as follows:

The next consideration concerns the general role of suggestion in hypnosis. Too often, the unwarranted and unsound assumption is made that, since a trance state is induced and maintained by suggestion, and since hypnotic manifestations can be elicited by suggestion, whatever develops from hypnosis must necessarily and completely be a result and primary expression of suggestion.

Contrary to such misconceptions, the hypnotized person remains the same person. Only his behavior is altered by the trance state, but even so, that altered behavior derives from the life experience of the patient and not from the therapist. At the most, the therapist can influence only the manner of self-expression. The induction and maintenance of a trance serve to provide a special psychological state in which the patient can reassociate and reorganize his inner psychological complexities and utilize his own capacities in a manner concordant with his own experiential life. Hypnosis does not change the person, nor does it alter his past experiential life. It serves to permit him to learn more about himself and to express himself more adequately.

Direct suggestion is based primarily, if unwittingly, upon the assumption that whatever develops in hypnosis derives from the suggestions given. It implies that the therapist has the miraculous power of effecting therapeutic changes in the patient, and disregards the fact that therapy results from an inner resynthesis of the patient's behavior achieved by the patient himself. It is true that direct suggestion can effect an alteration in the patient's behavior and result in a symptomatic cure, at least temporarily. However, such a "cure" is simply a response to the suggestion and does not entail that reassociation and reorganization of ideas, understandings and memories so essential for an actual cure. It is this experience of reassociating and reorganizing his own experiential life that eventuates in a cure, not the manifestation of responsive behavior which can, at best, satisfy only the observer.

For example, anesthesia of the hand may be suggested directly and a seemingly adequate response may be elicited. However, if the patient has not spontaneously interpreted the command to include a realization of the need for inner reorganization, that anesthesia will fail to meet clinical tests and will be a pseudo anesthesia.

An effective anesthesia is better induced, for example, by initiating a train of mental activity within the patient himself by suggesting that he recall the feeling of numbness experienced after a local anesthetic, or after a leg or arm went to sleep, and then suggesting that he can now experience a similar feeling in his hand. By such an indirect suggestion the patient is enabled to go through those difficult inner processes of disorganizing, reorganizing, reassociating and projecting inner real experience to meet the requirements of the suggestion. Thus, the induced anesthesia becomes a part of his experiential life, instead of a simple, superficial response.

The same principles hold true in psychotherapy. The chronic alcoholic can be induced by direct suggestion to correct his habits temporarily, but not until he goes through the inner process of reassociating and reorganizing his experiential life can effective results occur.

In other words, hypnotic psychotherapy is a learning process for the patient, a procedure of reeducation. Effective results in hypnotic psychotherapy, or hypnotherapy, derive only from the patient's activities. The therapist merely stimulates the patient into activity, often not knowing what that activity may be, and then he guides the patient and exercises clinical judgment in determining the amount of work to be done to achieve the desired results. How to guide and to judge constitute the therapist's problem while the patient's task is that of learning through his own efforts to understand his experiential life in a new way. Such reeducation is, of course, necessarily in terms of the patient's life experiences, his understandings, memories, attitudes and ideas, and it cannot be in terms of the therapist's ideas and opinions.

In our work, therefore, we prefer to emphasize how therapeutic trance helps people sidestep their own learned limitations so that they can more fully explore and utilize their potentials. The hypnotherapist makes many approaches to altered states of functioning available to the patient. Most patients really cannot direct themselves consciously in trance experience because such direction can come only from their previously learned habits of functioning which are inhibiting the full utilization of their potentials. Patients must therefore learn to allow their own unconscious response potentials to become manifest during trance. The therapist, too, must depend upon the patient's unconscious as a source of creativity for problem-solving. The therapist helps the patient find access to this creativity via that altered state we call therapeutic trance. Therapeutic trance can thus be understood as a free period of psychological exploration wherein therapist and patient cooperate in the search for those hypnotic responses that will lead to therapeutic change. We will now turn our attention to the evaluation and facilitation of that change.

3. Ratification of Therapeutic Change

The recognition and evaluation of altered patterns of functioning facilitated by therapeutic trance is one of the most subtle and important tasks of the therapist. Many patients readily recognize and admit changes that they have experienced. Others with less introspective ability need the therapist's help in evaluating the changes that have taken place. A recognition and appreciation of the trance work is necessary, lest the patient's old negative attitudes disrupt and destroy the new therapeutic responses that are still in a fragile state of development.

The Recognition and Ratification of Trance

Different individuals experience trance in different ways. The therapist's task is to recognize these individual patterns and when necessary point them out to patients to help verify or ratify their altered state of trance. Consciousness does not always recognize its own altered states. How often do we not recognize that we are actually dreaming? It is usually only after the fact that we recognize we were in a state of reverie or daydreaming. The inexperienced user of alcohol and psychedelic drugs must also learn to recognize and then "go with" the altered state in order to enhance and fully experience its effects. Since therapeutic trance is actually only a variation of the common everyday trance or reverie that everyone is familiar with but does not necessarily recognize as an altered state, some patients will not believe they have been affected in any way. For these patients, in particular, it is important to ratify trance as an altered state. Without this proof the patient's negative attitudes and beliefs can frequently undo the value of the hypnotic suggestion and abort the therapeutic process that has been initiated.

Because of this we will list in Table 1 some of the common indicators of trance experience which we have previously discussed and illustrated in some detail (Erickson, Rossi, and Rossi, 1976). Because trance experience is highly individualized, patients will manifest these indicators in varying combinations as well as in different degrees.

TABLE 1

SOME COMMON INDICATORS OF TRANCE EXPERIENCE

Autonomous Ideation and Inner
   Experience

Balanced Tonicity (Catalepsy)

Body Immobility

Body Reorientation After Trance

Changed Voice Quality

Comfort, Relaxation

Economy of Movement

Expectancy

Eye Changes and Closure

Facial Features Smooth & Relaxed

Feeling Distanced or Dissociated

Feeling Good After Trance

Literalism

Loss or Retardation of Reflexes
   Blinking

Respiration
Swallowing
Startle reflex

Objective and Impersonal Ideation

Psychosomatic Responses

Pupillary Changes

Response Attentiveness

Sensory, Muscular & Body Changes
   (Paresthesias)

Slowing Pulse

Spontaneous Hypnotic Phenomena
   Amnesia
   Anesthesia
   Body Illusions
   Catalepsy
   Regression
   Time Distortion
   etc.

Time Lag in Motor and Conceptual
   Behavior

Most of these indicators will be illustrated as they appear in the cases of this book.

We look upon the spontaneous development of hypnotic phenomena such as age regression, anesthesia, catalepsy, and so on as more genuine indicators of trance than when these same phenomena are "suggested." When they are directly suggested, we run into the difficulties imposed by the patient's conscious attitudes and belief system. When they come about spontaneously, they are the natural result of the dissociation or reorganization of the patient's usual frames of reference and general reality orientation which is characteristic of trance.

Certain investigators have selected some of these spontaneous phenomena as defining characteristics of the fundamental nature of trance. Meares (1957) and Shor (1959), for example, have taken regression as a fundamental aspect of trance. From our point of view, however, regression per se is not a fundamental characteristic of trance, although it is often present as an epiphenomenon of the early stage of trance development, when patients are learning to give up their usual frames of reference and modes of functioning. In this first stage of learning to experience an altered state, many uncontrolled things happen, including spontaneous age regression, paresthesias, anesthesias, illusions of body distortion, psychosomatic responses, time distortion, and so on. Once patients learn to stablize these unwanted side reactions, they can then allow their unconscious minds to function freely in interacting with the therapist's suggestions without some of the limitations of their usual frames of reference.

Ideomotor and Ideosensory Signaling

Since much hypnotherapeutic work does not require a dramatic experience of classical hypnotic phenomena, it is even more important that the therapist learn to recognize the minimal manifestations of trance as alterations in a patient's *sensory-perceptual, emotional,* and *cognitive* functioning. A valuable means of evaluating these changes is in the use of ideomotor and ideosensory signaling (Erickson, 1961; Cheek and Le Cron, 1968). An experience of trance as an altered state can be ratified by requesting any one of a variety of ideomotor responses as follows:

If you have experienced some moments of trance in our work today, your right hand (or one of your fingers) can lift all by itself.

If you have been in trance today without even realizing it, your head will nod "yes" (or your eyes will close) all by itself.

The existence of a therapeutic change can be signaled in a similar manner.

12

If your unconscious no longer needs to have you experience (whatever symptom), your head will nod.

Your unconscious can review the reasons for that problem, and when it has given your conscious mind its source in a manner that is comfortable for you to discuss, your right index finger can lift all by itself.

Some subjects experience ideosensory responses more easily than other subjects. They may thus experience a feeling of lightness, heaviness, coolness, or prickliness in the designated part of the body.

In requesting such responses we are presumably allowing the patient's unconscious to respond in a manner that is experienced as involuntary by the patient. This involuntary or autonomous aspect of the movement or feeling is an indication that it comes from a response system that is somewhat dissociated from the patient's habitual pattern of voluntary or intentional response. The patient and therapist thus have indication that something has happened independently of the patient's conscious will. That "something" may be trance or whatever therapeutic response was desired.

An uncritical view of ideomotor and ideosensory signaling takes such responses to be the "true voice of the unconscious." At this stage of our understanding we prefer to view them as only another response system that must be checked and crossed-validated just as any other verbal or nonverbal response system. We prefer to evoke ideomotor responses in such a manner that the patient's conscious mind may not witness them (for example, having eyes closed or averted when a finger or hand signal is given). It is very difficult, however, to establish that the conscious mind is unaware of what response is given and that the response is in fact given independently of conscious intention. Some patients feel that the ideomotor or ideosensory response is entirely on an involuntary level. Others feel they must help it or at least know ahead of time what it is to be.

A second major use of ideomotor and ideosensory signaling is to help patients restructure their belief system. Doubts about therapeutic change may persist even after an extended period of exploring and dealing with a problem in trance. These doubts can often be relieved when the patient believes in ideomotor or ideosensory responses as an independent index of the validity of therapeutic work. The therapist may proceed, for example, with suggestions as follows:

If your unconscious acknowledges that a process of therapeutic change has been initiated, your head can nod.

When you know you need no longer be bothered by that problem, your index finger can lift, or get warm [or whatever].

In such usage there is value, of course, in having the patient's conscious mind recognize the positive response. The more autonomous or involuntary the ideomotor or ideosensory response, the more convincing it is to the patient.

At the present time we have no way of distinguishing when an ideomotor or ideosensory response is (1) a reliable and valid index of something happening in the unconscious (out of the patient's immediate range of awareness), or (2) simply a means of restructuring a conscious belief system. A great deal of carefully controlled experimental work needs to be done in this area. It is still a matter of clinical judgment to determine which process, or the degree to which both processes, are operating in any individual situation.

Summary

Our utilization approach to hypnotherapy emphasizes that therapeutic trance is a means by which we help patients learn to use their mental skills and potentials to achieve their own therapeutic goals. While our approach is patient-centered and highly dependent on the momentary needs of the individual, there are three basic phases that can be outlined and discussed for didactic purposes: Preparation, Therapeutic Trance, and Ratification of Therapeutic Change.

The goal of the initial preparatory period is to establish an optimal frame of reference to orient the patient toward therapeutic change. This is facilitated by the following factors, which were discussed in this chapter and which will be illustrated in the cases of this book.

Rapport
Response Attentiveness
Assessing Abilities to Be Utilized
Facilitating Therapeutic Frames of Reference
Creating Expectancy

Therapeutic trance is a period during which the limitations of one's habitual frames of reference are temporarily altered so that one can be receptive to more adequate modes of functioning. While the experience of trance is highly variable, the overall dynamics of therapeutic trance and suggestion could be outlined as a five-stage process: (1) Fixation of attention; (2) depotentiating habitual frameworks; (3) unconscious search; (4) unconscious processes; (5) therapeutic response.

The *utilization approach* and the *indirect forms of suggestion* are the two major means of facilitating these overall dynamics of therapeutic trance and suggestion. The utilization approach emphasizes the continual involvement of each patient's unique repertory of abilities and potentials, while the indirect forms of suggestion are the means by which the therapist facilitates these involvements.

We believe that the induction and maintenance of therapeutic trance provides a special psychological state in which patients can reassociate and reorganize their inner experience so that therapy results from an inner resynthesis of their own behavior.

Ratifying the process of therapeutic change is an integral part of our approach to hypnotherapy. This frequently involves a special effort to help patients recognize and validate their altered state. The therapist must develop special skills in learning to recognize minimal manifestations of altered functioning in sensory-perceptual, emotional, and cognitive processes. Ideomotor and ideosensory signaling are of special use as an index of therapeutic change as well as a means of facilitating an alteration of the patient's belief system.

Exercises

1. New *observational skills* are the first stage in the training of the hypnotherapist. One needs to learn to recognize the momentary variations in another's mentation. These skills can be developed by training oneself to carefully observe the mental states of people in everyday life as well as in the consulting room. There are at least four levels, ranging from the most obvious to the more subtle.

    1. Role relations
    2. Frames of reference
    3. Common everyday trance behaviors
    4. Response attentiveness

1. Role relations: Carefully note the degree to which individuals in all walks of life are caught within roles, and the degrees of flexibility they have in breaking out of their roles to relate to you as a unique person. For example, to what degree are the clerks at the supermarket identified with their roles? Notice the nuances of voice and body posture that indicate their role behavior. Does their tone and manner imply that they think of themselves as an authority to manipulate you, or are they seeking to find out something about you and what you really need? Explore the same questions with police, officials of all sorts, nurses, bus drivers, teachers, etc.

2. Frames of reference: To the above study of role relations add an inquiry into the dominant frames of reference that are guiding your subject's behavior. Is the bus or taxicab driver more dominated by a safety fame of reference? Which of the store clerks is more concerned with securing his present job and which is obviously bucking for a promotion? Is the doctor more obviously operating within a financial or therapeutic frame of reference?

3. *Common everyday trance behavior:* Table 1 can be a guide as to what to look for in evaluating a person's everyday trance behavior. Even in ordinary conversation one can take careful note of those momentary pauses when the other person is quietly looking off into the distance or staring at something, as he or she apparently reflects inward. One can ignore and actually ruin these precious moments when the other is engaged in inner search and unconscious processes by talking too much and thereby distracting the person. How much better simply to remain quiet oneself and carefully observe the individual manifestations of the other's everyday trance behavior. Notice especially whether the person's eye blink slows down or stops altogether. Do the eyes actually close for a moment? Does the body not remain perfectly immobile, perhaps even with limbs apparently cataleptic, fixed in mid-gesture?

Watching for these moments and pauses is especially important in psychotherapy. The authors will themselves sometimes freeze in mid-sentence when they observe the patient going off into such inward focus. We feel what we are saying is probably less important than allowing the patient to have that inward moment. Sometimes we can facilitate the inner search by simply saying things such as:

That's right, continue just as you are.

Follow that now.

Interesting isn't it?

Perhaps you can tell me some of that later.

After a while patients become accustomed to this unusual tolerence and reinforcement of their inner moments; the pauses grow longer and become what we would call therapeutic trance. The patients then experience increasing relaxation and comfort and may prefer to respond with ideomotor signals as they give increasing recognition to their trance state.

4. *Response Attentiveness:* This is the most interesting and useful of the trance indicators. The junior author can recall that lucky day when a series of three patients seen individually on successive hours just happened to manifest a similar wide-eyed look of expectancy, staring fixedly into his eyes. They also had a similar funny little smile (or giggle) of wistfulness and mild confusion. That was it! Suddenly he recognized what the senior author had been trying to teach him for the past five years: Response attentiveness! The patients may not have realized themselves just how much they were looking to the junior author for direction at that moment. That was the moment to introduce

16

a therapeutic suggestion or frame of reference! That was the moment to introduce trance either directly or indirectly! The junior author can recall the same slight feeling of discomfort with each patient at that moment. The patient's naked look of expectancy bespoke a kind of openness and vulnerability that is surprising and a bit disconcerting when it is suddenly encountered. In everyday situations we tend to look away and distract ourselves from such delicate moments. At most we allow ourselves to enjoy them briefly with children or during loving encounters. In therapy such creative moments are the precious openers of the yes set and positive transference. Hypnotherapists allow themselves to be open to these moments and perhaps to be equally vulnerable as they offer some tentative therapeutic suggestions. More detailed exercises on the recognition and utilization of response attentiveness will be presented at the end of Chapter Three.

CHAPTER 2

The Indirect Forms of Suggestion

1. Direct and Indirect Suggestion

A direct suggestion makes an appeal to the conscious mind and succeeds in initiating behavior when we are in agreement with the suggestion and have the capacity actually to carry it out in a voluntary manner. If someone suggests, "Please close the window," I will close it if I have the physical capacity to do so, and if I agree that it's a good suggestion. If the conscious mind had a similar capacity to carry out all manner of psychological suggestions in an agreeable and voluntary manner, then psychotherapy would be a simple matter indeed. The therapist would need only suggest that the patient give up such and such a phobia or unhappiness and that would be the end of the matter.

Obviously this does not happen. Psychological problems exist precisely because the conscious mind does not know how to initiate psychological experience and behavior change to the degree that one would like. In many such situations there is some capacity for desired patterns of behavior, but they can only be carried out with the help of an unconscious process that takes place on an involuntary level. We can make a conscious effort to remember a forgotten name, for example, but if we cannot do so, we cease trying after a few moments of futile effort. Five minutes later the name may pop up spontaneously within our minds. What has happened? Obviously a search was initiated on a conscious level, but it could only be completed by an unconscious process that continued on its own even after consciousness abandoned its effort. Sternberg (1975) has reviewed experimental data supporting the view that an unconscious search continues at the rate of approximately thirty items per second even after the conscious mind has gone on to other matters.

The indirect forms of suggestion are approaches to initiating and facilitating such searches on an unconscious level. When it is found that consciousness is unable to carry out a direct suggestion, we may then make a therapeutic effort to initiate an unconscious search for a solution by indirect suggestion. The naive view of direct suggestion which emphasizes control maintains that the patient passively does whatever the therapist asks. In our use of indirect suggestion, however, we realize that suggested behavior is actually a subjective response synthesized within the patient. It is a subjective response that utilizes the patient's unique repertory of life experiences and learning. It is not what the therapist says but what the patient does with what is said that is the essence of suggestion. In hypnotherapy the words of the therapist evoke a complex series of internal responses within the patient; these internal responses are the basis of "suggestion." Indirect suggestion does not tell the patient what to do; rather, it explores and facilitates what the patient's response system can do on an autonomous level without really making a conscious effort to direct itself.

The indirect forms of suggestion are semantic environments that facilitate the experience of new response possibilities. They automatically evoke unconscious searches and processes within us independent of our conscious will.

In this chapter we shall discuss a number of indirect forms of suggestion that have been found to be of practical value in facilitating hypnotic responsiveness. Most of these indirect forms are in common usage in everyday life. Indeed, this is where the senior author usually recognized their value as he sought more effective means of facilitating hypnotic work.

Because we have already discussed most of these indirect forms from a theoretical point of view (Erickson and Rossi, 1976; Erickson, Rossi, and Rossi, 1976), our emphasis in this chapter will be on their therapeutic applications. It will be seen that many of these indirect forms are closely related to each other, that several can be used in the same phrase or sentence, and that it is sometimes difficult to distinguish one from another. Because of this, it may be of value for the reader to recognize that an "attitude" or "approach" is being presented with this material rather than a "technique" that is designed to achieve definite and predictable (though limited) results. *The indirect forms of suggestion are most useful for exploring potentialities and facilitating a patient's natural response tendencies rather than imposing control over behavior.*

2. The Interspersal Approach

The senior author has described the *interspersal* approach (Erickson, 1966; Erickson and Rossi, 1976) along with *nonrepetition* as his most important contributions to the practice of suggestion.[1] In the older, more

---

[1] In a conversation with Anisley Mears, Gordon Ambrose, and others on the evening when the senior author, at the age of seventy-four, was awarded the Benjamin Franklin gold medal for his innovative contributions to hypnosis at the 7th International Congress of Hypnosis on July 2, 1976.

traditional forms of direct suggestion the hypnotherapist usually droned on and on, repeating the same suggestion over and over. The effort was seemingly directed to programming or deeply imprinting the mind with one fixed idea. With the advent of modern psychodynamic psychology, however, we recognize that the mind is in a continual state of growth and change; creative behavior is in a continual process of development. While direct programming can obviously influence behavior (e.g., Coueism, advertising), it does not help us explore and facilitate a patient's unique potentials. The interspersal approach, on the other hand, is a suitable means of presenting suggestions in a manner that enables the patient's own unconscious to utilize them in its own unique way.

The interspersal approach can operate on many levels. We can within a single sentence intersperse a single word that facilitates the patient's associations:

You can describe those feelings as *freely* as you wish.

The interspersed word *freely* automatically associates a positive valence of freedom with feelings patients may have suppressed. It can thereby help patients to free feelings that they really want to reveal. Each patient's individuality is still respected, however, because free choice is admitted. The senior author (Erickson, 1966) has illustrated how an entire therapeutic session can be conducted by interspersing words and concepts suggestive of comfort, utilizing the patient's own frames of reference so that pain relief is achieved without the formal induction of trance. Case 1 of this volume will give another clear illustration of this approach. In the following sections we will discuss and illustrate *indirect associative focusing* and *indirect ideodynamic focusing* as two aspects of the interspersal approach.

2a. Indirect Associative Focusing

A basic form of indirect suggestion is to raise a relevant topic without directing it in any obvious manner to the patient. The senior author likes to point out that the easiest way to help patients talk about their mothers is to talk about your own mother or mothers in general. A natural indirect associative process is thereby set in motion within patients that brings up apparently spontaneous associations about their mothers. Since we do not directly ask about a patient's mother, the usual limitations of conscious sets and habitual mental frameworks (including psychological defenses) that such a direct question might evoke are bypassed. Bandler and Grinder (1975) have described this process as a transderivational phenomenon—a basic linguistic process whereby subject and object are automatically interchanged at a deep, (unconscious), structural level.

In therapy we can use a process of indirect associative focusing to help a patient recognize a problem. The senior author, for example, will frequently intersperse remarks or tell a number of stories and anecdotes in seemingly casual conversation. Even when his "stories" appear unrelated, however, they all have a common denominator or "common focused association" which he hypothesizes to be a relevant aspect of the patient's problem. Patients may wonder why the therapist is making such interesting but apparently nonrelevant conversation during the therapy hour. If the common, focused association is in fact a relevant aspect of their problem, however, patients will frequently find themselves talking about it in a surprisingly revelatory manner. If the therapist guessed wrong, nothing is lost. The patient will simply not talk about the focused association because there is no particular recognition and contribution within the patient's own associative processes to raise it to the verbal level.

A major value of this interspersal approach is that therapists can to some degree avoid imposing their own theoretical views and preoccupations upon their patients. If the focused association is of value to patients, their own unconscious processes of search and evaluation will permit them to recognize it as an aspect of their problem and utilize it in their own way to find their own solutions. Examples of this process of indirect associative focusing to help patients recognize and resolve psychodynamic problems will be presented in a number of case illustrations of this volume (e.g., particularly Case 5, a general approach to symptomatic behavior).

2b. Indirect Ideodynamic Focusing

One of the earliest theories of hypnotic responsiveness was formulated by Bernheim (1895), who described it as *"a peculiar aptitude for transforming the idea received into an act."* He believed, for example, that in the hypnotic experience of catalepsy there was *"an exaltation of the ideo-motor reflex excitability, which effects the unconscious transformation of the thought into movement, unknown to the will."* In the hypnotic experience of sensory hallucinations he theorized that the *"memory of sensation [is] resuscitated"* along with *"exultation of the ideo-sensorial reflex excitability, which effects the unconscious transformation of the thought into sensation, or into a sensory image."* This view of ideodynamic responsiveness (that ideas can be transformed into an actual experience of movements, sensations, perceptions, emotions, and so on, independently of conscious intentionality) is still tenable today. Our utilization theory of hypnotic suggestion emphasizes that "suggestion is a process of evoking and *utilizing* a patient's own mental processes in ways that are outside his usual range of ego control (Erickson and Rossi, 1976)."

Ideodynamic processes can be evoked with an interspersal approach utilizing indirect associative focusing as described in the previous section. When the senior author addressed professional groups about hypnotic phenomena, for example, he frequently interspersed interesting case histories and told "stories" about hand levitation or hallucinatory sensations. These vivid illustrations initiated a natural process of ideomotor and ideosensory responsiveness within the listeners without their being aware of it. When he then asked for volunteers from the audience for a demonstration of hypnotic behavior, they were "primed" for responsiveness by ideodynamic processes that were already taking place within them in an involuntary manner on an unconscious level. These unrecognized ideodynamic responses can frequently be measured by electronic instrumentation (Prokasy and Raskin, 1973).

In a similar manner, when confronted with a "resistant" subject we can surround him with one or more good hypnotic subjects to whom we direct our hypnotic suggestions. A process of indirect ideodynamic responsiveness takes place automatically within the resistant subject as he listens to the suggestions and observes the responses of others. He is soon surprised at how the "hypnotic atmosphere" effects him so that he becomes much more responsive than before.

Many clear illustrations of this process of interspersing indirect ideodynamic suggestion will be found in the cases of this book. In our first case, for example, the senior author talks about his friend John, who had phantom limb pain in his foot just like the patient's:

> John was marvelous. And I discussed with him the importance of having nice feelings in your wooden foot, your wooden knee. . . .
> The importance of having good feelings in the wooden foot, the wooden knee, the wooden leg. Feeling it to be warm. Cool. Rested
> . . . you can have phantom pleasure.

In the context of a number of anecdotes and stories about how others have learned to experience phantom pleasure instead of pain, interspersed indirect ideodynamic suggestions such as the above begin automatically to initiate unconscious searches and processes that will lead to the amelioration of phantom pain even without the formal induction of trance.

3. Truisms Utilizing Ideodynamic Processes

The basic unit of ideodynamic focusing is the truism: a simple statement of fact about behavior that the patient has experienced so often that it cannot be denied. In most of our case illustrations it will be found that the senior author frequently talks about certain psychophysiological processes or mental mechanisms as if he were simply describing objective facts to the patient. Actually these verbal descriptions can function as indirect suggestions when they trip off ideodynamic responses from associations and learned patterns that already exist within patients as a repository of their life experience. The "generalized reality orientation" (Shor, 1959) usually maintains these subjective responses in appropriate check when we are engaged in ordinary conversation. When attention is fixed and focused in trance so that some of the limitations of the patient's habitual mental sets are depotentiated, however, the following truisms may actually trip off a literal and concrete experience of the suggested behavior, which is printed in *italics*.

3a. Ideomotor Processes

Most people can experience *one hand as being lighter than another.*

Everyone has had the experience of *nodding their head "yes" or shaking it "no" even without realizing it.*

When we are *tired, our eyes begin to blink slowly and sometimes close* without our quite realizing it.

Sometimes as we relax or go to sleep, a muscle will twitch so that *our arm or leg makes a slight involuntary movement* (Overlade, 1976).

3b. Ideosensory Processes

You already know how to experience pleasant sensations like the *armth* of the sun *on your skin.*

Most people enjoy the *refreshing coolness* of a light breeze.

Some people can imagine their favorite food so well they can actually *taste* it.

The salt and *smell* of a light ocean breeze is pleasant to most people.

3c. Ideoaffective Processes

Some people *blush easily when they recognize certain feelings* about themselves.

Its easy to *feel anger and resentment* when we are made to feel foolish. We usually *frown when we have memories that are all too painful to remember.*

Most of us try to avoid *thoughts and memories that bring tears,* yet they frequently deal with the most important things.

We have all enjoyed noticing someone *smile at a private thought* and we frequently find ourselves *smiling at their smile*.

In formulating such ideoaffective suggestions it is helpful to include a behavioral marker (blush, frown, tears, smile) whenever possible, to provide some possible feedback to the therapist about what the patient is receiving and acting upon.

3d. Ideocognitive Processes

We know that when you are asleep your unconscious can *dream*.

You can easily *forget* that dream when you awaken.

You can sometimes *remember* one important part of that dream that interests you.

We can sometimes know a name and have it on the tip of our tongue and yet *not be able to say* the name.

4. Truisms Utilizing Time

In hypnotherapeutic work truisms utilizing time are very important because there is frequently a time lag in the execution of hypnotic responses. The stages of unconscious search and processes leading to hypnotic responses require varying lengths of time in different patients. It is usually best to permit the patient's own unconscious to determine the appropriate amount of time required for any response.

Sooner or later your hand is going to lift (eyes close, or whatever).

Your headache (or whatever) can *now* leave *as soon as* your system is ready for it to leave.

Your symptom can *now* disappear *as soon as* your unconscious knows you can handle (such and such) problem in a more constructive manner.

5. Not Knowing, Not Doing

While truisms are an excellent means of introducing suggestions in a positive manner that the conscious mind can accept, valid hypnotic experience involves the utilization of unconscious processes. A basic aspect of therapeutic trance is to arrange circumstances so that constructive mental processes are experienced in taking place by themselves without the patient making any effort to drive or direct them. When one is relaxed, as is typical of most trance experiences, the parasympathetic system physiologically predisposes one *not to do* rather than to make any active effort of doing. Similarly when we are relaxed and the unconscious takes over, we usually feel comfortable and *do not know* how the unconscious carries out its activities. Not knowing and not doing are synonymous with the unconscious or autonomous responsiveness that is the essence of trance experience. An attitude of not knowing and not doing is therefore of great value in facilitating hypnotic responsiveness. This is particularly true during the initial stages of trance induction, where the following suggestions may be appropriate.

You don't have to talk or move or make any sort of effort.

You don't even have to hold your eyes open.

You don't have to bother trying to listen to me because your unconscious can do that and respond all by itself.

People can sleep and not know they are asleep.

They can dream and not remember that dream.

You don't know just when those eyelids will close all by themselves.

You may not know just which hand will lift first.

These examples clearly illustrate how different our indirect hypnotic forms are from the direct approach, which typically begins, "Now pay close attention to my voice and do exactly what I say." The direct approach focuses conscious attention and tends to activate conscious cooperation by the patient. This can be of value in initiating some types of responsive behavior in good hypnotic subjects, but for the average patient it may activate conscious processes to the point where unconscious processes are inhibited rather than enhanced.

Not knowing and not doing are of particular value in trance work when we wish to evoke the patient's own individuality in seeking the best modality of therapeutic response.

You don't really know just how your unconscious will help you resolve that problem. But your conscious mind can be receptive to the answer when it does come.

Your conscious mind surely has many questions, but it does not really know just when the unconscious will let you give up that undesirable habit. You don't know if it will be sooner or later. You don't know if it will be all at once or slowly, by degrees. Yet you can learn to respect your own natural way of doing things.

6. Open-Ended Suggestions

Therapists as well as patients do not always know what is the best avenue for constructive processes to express themselves. Human predispositions and potentialities are so complex that we may even consider it presumptuous to assume that anyone could possibly know ahead of time just what is the most creative approach to the new that continually overtakes us. Indeed, one view of maladjustment is that we do in fact attempt to impose old views and solutions into changed life circumstances where they are no longer appropriate (Rossi, 1972). The open-ended suggestion is a means of dealing with this problem. Open-ended suggestions permit us to explore and utilize whatever response possibilities are most available to the patient. It is of value on the level of conscious choice as well as unconscious determinism. When patients are awake and consciously directing their own behavior, the open-ended suggestion permits self-determination. When patients are in trance, the open-ended suggestion permits the unconscious to select the most appropriate means of carrying out a therapeutic response.

As we have already seen, not knowing and not doing lead naturally to open-ended suggestions. The following are further illustrations.

We all have potentials we are unaware of, and we usually don't know how they will be expressed.

Your mind can review more feelings, memories, and thoughts related to that problem, but you don't know yet which will be most useful for solving the problem you are coping with.

You can find yourself ranging into the past, the present, or the future as your unconscious selects the most appropriate means of dealing with that.

He doesn't know what he is learning, but he is learning. And it isn't right for me to tell him, "You learn this or you learn that!" Let him learn whatever he wishes, in whatever order he wishes.

While giving a great deal of apparent freedom to explore and express the patient's own individuality, such open-ended suggestions carry a strong implication that a therapeutic response will be forthcoming.

7. Covering All Possibilities of a Class of Responses

While open-ended suggestions permit the widest possible latitude for the expression of a therapeutic response, suggestions covering all possibilities of a class of responses are of more value when the therapist wishes to focus the patient's responsiveness in a particular direction. In initiating trance, for example, the following might be appropriate.

Soon you will find a finger or a thumb moving a bit, perhaps by itself. It can move up or down, to the side or press down. It can be slow or quick or perhaps not move at all. *The really important thing is to sense fully whatever feelings develop.*

All possibilities of finger movement have been covered, including the possibility of not moving at all. The suggestion is thus fail-safe. The patient is successful no matter what response develops. The therapist is simply exploring the patient's initial responsiveness while initiating trance by focusing attention.

Exactly the same approach can be used when the patient has experienced therapeutic trance and is ready to deal with a problem.

Soon you will find the weight problem being dealt with by eating more or less of the right foods you can enjoy. You may first gain weight or lose it or remain the same for a while as *you learn the really important things about yourself.*

In both of these illustrations we can observe how we are distracting the patient's consciousness from the important area of responsiveness with an interesting idea in the end (in *italics*), so that the unconscious can have more opportunity to determine which of the response possibilities (not in italics) will be expressed. This is in keeping with the classical notion of hypnosis as the simultaneous focusing and distraction of attention.

8. Questions That Facilitate New Response Possibilities

Recent research (Sternberg, 1975) indicates that the human brain, when questioned, continues an exhaustive search throughout its entire memory system on an unconscious level even after it has found an answer that is apparently satisfying on a conscious level. This unconscious search and activation of mental processes on an autonomous level is the essence of our indirect approach, wherein we seek to utilize a patient's unrecognized potentials to evoke hypnotic phenomena and therapeutic responses.

This process of an unconscious search and an autonomous processing of information is evident in many phenomena of everyday life. According to one folk saying, "The morning is wiser than the evening." After we have slept on a problem, we find the solution comes more easily in the morning. Evidently an unconscious search and problem-solving process has been taking place while the consciousness was at rest. There is evidence that dreaming can be an experimental theater of the mind, where questions can be answered and new life possibilities synthesized (Ross, 1971-1973).

The Socratic method of education, whereby a teacher asks the student a series of pointed questions, is a classical illustration of using questions as initiators of mental processes. We can wonder, indeed, if consciousness could have evolved to its current level without the development and utilization of questions as a provocative syntactical form which facilitate internal processes of inquiry. In this section we will illustrate how questions can focus associations as well as suggest and reinforce new response possibilities.

8a. Questions to Focus Associations

An interesting illustration of how questions can focus different aspects of inner experience comes from research on the subjective reports of hypnotic subjects (Barber, Dalal, and Calverley, 1968). When asked, "Did you experience the hypnotic state as basically *similar* to the waking state?" most subjects (83 percent) reported affirmatively. On the other hand, when asked, "Did you experience the hypnotic state as basically *different* from the waking state?" 72 percent responded affirmatively. We could take these apparently contradictory responses as indications of the unreliability of the subjects' reports about the hypnotic experience. From another point of view, however, we can understand how such questions focused the subjects on different aspects of their experiences. The first question focused their attention on the similarities between the waking and hypnotic states; the second focused attention on the differences. Both questions could initiate valid responses about different aspects of the subjects' inner experiences; no contradiction need be implied.

In hypnotherapy it is often of value to help patients discriminate between different aspects of their inner lives or to find the common denominator in apparently different experiences. Carefully formulated questions such as the above can facilitate this process.

8b. Questions in Trance Induction

Questions are of particular value as indirect forms of suggestion when they cannot be answered by the conscious mind. Such questions activate unconscious processes and initiate autonomous responses which are the essence of trance behavior. The following are illustrations of how a series of questions may be used to initiate and deepen trance by two different approaches to induction—eye fixation and hand levitation. In each illustration the first few questions may be answered by responsive behavior that is guided by conscious choice. The next few questions may be answered by either conscious intentionality or unconscious choice. The last few can only be answered on an unconscious or autonomous level of responsiveness. These series of questions cannot be used in a fixed and rigid manner, but must always incorporate and utilize the patient's ongoing behavior. It is understood that patients need not respond in a conventional verbal manner to these questions, but only with the responsive behavior suggested. Patients usually do not recognize that a very important but subtle shift is taking place. They are no longer verbally interacting in a social manner with their typical defenses. Rather, they are focused intensely within themselves wondering about how they will respond. This implies that a dissociation is taking place between their conscious thinking (with its sense of control) and their apparently autonomous responses to the therapist's questions. The apparently autonomous nature of their behavioral responses is usually acknowledged as "hypnotic". With that the stage is set for further autonomous and unconsciously determined therapeutic responses.

Eye Fixation

1. Would you like to find a spot you can look at comfortably?
2. As you continue looking at that spot for a while, do your eyelids want to blink?
3. Will those lids begin to blink together or separately?
4. Slowly or quickly?
5. Will they close all at once or flutter all by themselves first?
6. Will those eyes close more and more as you get more and more comfortable?
7. That's fine. Can those eyes now remain closed as your comfort deepens like when you go to sleep?
8. Can that comfort continue more and more so that you'd rather not even try to open your eyes?
9. Or would you rather try and find you cannot?
10. And how soon will you forget about them altogether because your unconscious wants to dream? (Therapist can observe slight eyeball movements as the patient's closed eyes follow changes on the inner dream scene.)

This series begins with a question that requires conscious choice and volition on the part of the patient and ends with a question that can only be carried out by unconscious processes. An important feature of this approach is that it is *fail-safe* in the sense that any failure to respond can be accepted as a valid and meaningful response to a question. Another important feature is that each question suggests an *observable* response that gives the therapist important information about how well the patient is following suggestions. These observable responses are also associated with important internal aspects of trance experience and can be used as *indicators* of them.

If there is a failure to respond adequately, the therapist can go on with a few other questions at the same level until responsive behavior is again manifest, or the therapist can question patients about their inner experience to explore any unusual response patterns or difficulties they may have. It is not uncommon for some patients, for example, to open their eyes occasionally even after it is suggested that they will remain closed. This seems to be an automatic checking device that some patients use without even being aware of it. It does not interfere with therapeutic trance work. The question format thus gives each patient's own *individuality* an opportunity to respond in a therapeutically constructive manner. These features are also found in the hand-levitation approach, which we will now illustrate.

Hand Levitation

1. **Can you feel comfortable resting your hands gently on your thighs? [As therapist demonstrates] That's right, without letting them touch each other.**
2. **Can you let those hands rest ever so lightly so that the fingertips just barely touch your thighs?**
3. **That's right. As they rest ever so light, do you notice how they tend to lift up a bit all by themselves with each breath you take?**
4. **Do they begin to lift even more lightly and easily by themselves as the rest of your body relaxes more and more?**
5. **As that goes on, does one hand or the other or maybe both continue lifting even more?**
6. **And does that hand stay up and continue lifting higher and higher, bit by bit, all by itself? Does the other hand want to catch up with it, or will the other hand relax in your lap?**
7. **That's right. And does that hand continue lifting with these slight little jerking movements, or does the lifting get smoother and smoother as the hand continues upward toward your face?**
8. **Does it move more quickly or slowly as it approaches your face with deepening comfort? Does it need to pause a bit before it finally touches your face so you'll know you are going into a trance? And it won't touch until your unconscious is really ready to let you go deeper, will it?**
9. **And will your body automatically take a deeper breath when that hand**

30

touches your face as you really relax and experience yourself going deeper?

10. That's right. And will you even bother to notice the deepening comfortable feeling when that hand slowly returns to your lap all by itself? And will your unconscious be in a dream by the time that hand comes to rest?

8c. Questions Facilitating Therapeutic Responsiveness

Questions can be combined with not knowing and with open-ended suggestions to facilitate a variety of patterns of responsiveness.

And what will be the effective means of losing weight? Will it be because you simply forget to eat and have little patience with heavy meals because they prevent you from doing more interesting things? Will certain foods that put on weight no longer appeal to you for whatever reasons? Will you discover the enjoyment of new foods and new ways of preparing them and eating so that you'll be surprised that you did lose weight because you really didn't miss anything?

The last question in this series is an illustration of how compound questions can be built up with *and* and *so* to facilitate whatever tendency is most natural for the patient.

The ambiguity and "suggestive" effect of compound questions has long been recognized in jurisprudence. The use of compound questions by attorneys is therefore forbidden during their cross-examination of a witness. In a hotly contested case a judge or an opposing attorney can often be heard objecting to the "compounds" by which an unscrupulous attorney may befuddle and perhaps ensnare an unwary witness. In our therapeutic use of compound questions their very ambiguity is of value in depotentiating the patient's learned limitations so new possibilities may be experienced.

We will now turn to a more detailed examination of compound suggestions.

9. Compound Suggestions

We have already seen in many of our previous illustrations how two or more suggestions can be combined to support each other. In this section we shall take a closer look at a variety of compound suggestions that have been found to be of value in hypnotherapeutic work. At the simplest level a compound suggestion is made up of two statements joined together with a grammatical conjunction or with a slight pause that places them in close association. Traditional grammar has classified conjunctions broadly as *coordinating* and *subordinating*. The coordinating conjunctions *and, but,* and *or* join statements that are logically coordinated or equal in rank, while subordinating conjunctions such as *though, if, so, as, after, because, since,* and *until* join one expression to another that is its adjunct or subordinate. The linguistic joining and separating expressions obviously have correspondences with similar processes in mathematics and logic as well as with the psychological processes of mental association and dissociation that are of essence in hypnotherapy. George Boole (1815-1864), one of the originators of symbolic logic, felt that he was formulating the laws of thought with his equations. We know today, however, that while logic, natural language, and mental processes share some intriguing interfaces, there is no system of complete correspondence between them. While a system of logic or mathematics can be completely defined, *natural language and mental processes are perpetually in a state of creative flux.* There is in principle no fixed formula or system of logic or language that can completely determine or control mental processes. We would be deluding ourselves, therefore, if we sought a completely deterministic means of manipulating mental processes and controlling behavior with our indirect forms of suggestion. We can use them to explore and facilitate response potentials within the patient, however. In this section we will illustrate five classes of compound suggestion that have been of particular use in hypnotherapy: (a) the yes set and reinforcement, (b) contingency, (c) apposition of opposites, (d) the negative, and (e) shock, surprise, and creative moments. Other forms of indirect suggestion such as implication, binds, and double binds are so complex that we will discuss them in separate sections.

9a. The Yes Set and Reinforcement

A basic form of compound statement widely used in daily life is the simple association of a certain and obviously good notion with the suggestion of a desirable possibility.

It's such a beautiful day, let's go swimming.

It's a holiday, *so* why shouldn't I do what I want?

You have done well *and* can continue.

In each of the above an initially positive association ("beautiful day," "holiday," "done well") introduces a yes set that facilitates the acceptance of the suggestion that follows. We saw earlier how truisms are another means of opening a yes set to facilitate suggestion.

When the truism or positive and motivating association *follows* the suggestion, we have a means of reinforcing it. Thus:

Let's go swimming, it's such a beautiful day.

9b. Contingent Suggestions and Associational Networks

A useful form of compound statement occurs when we tie a suggestion to an ongoing or inevitable pattern of behavior. A hypnotic suggestion that may be difficult for a patient is easier when it is associated with behavior that is familiar. The hypnotic suggestion "hitchhikes" onto the natural and spontaneous responses that are well within the patient's normal repertory. The contingent suggestion is *italicized* in the following examples.

With each breath you take *you can become aware of the natural rhythms of your body and feelings of comfort that develop.*

As you continue sitting there, *you will find yourself becoming more relaxed and comfortable.*

As your hand lowers, *you'll find yourself going comfortably back in time to the source of that problem.*

As you mentally review the source of that problem *your unconscious can develop some tentative ways of dealing with it.*

And when your conscious mind recognizes a plausible and worthwhile solution, *your finger can lift automatically.*

When you feel ready to talk about it, *you'll find yourself awakening feeling refreshed and alert, with an appreciation of the good work you've been able to do.*

As can be seen from the last four examples, contingent suggestions can be tied together into associational networks that create a system of mutual support and momentum for initiating and carrying out a therapeutic pattern of responses. From the broadest point of view a whole therapy session—indeed, an entire course of therapy—can be conceived as a series of contingent responses wherein each successful therapeutic step evolves from all that came before. Haley (1974) has presented a number of the senior author's clinical cases that illustrate this process.

9c. Apposition of Opposites

Another indirect form of compound suggestion is what we may describe as the balance or apposition of opposites. A balance between opponent systems is a basic biological process that is built into the structure of our nervous system (Kinsbourne, 1974). Most biological systems can be conceptualized as a homeostatic balance of processes that prevents the overall system from straying outside the relatively narrow range required for optimal functioning. To account for some of the phenomena of hypnosis, it has been proposed that there are alternatives in various opponent systems, such as the sympathetic and parasympathetic system, the left and right cerebral hemispheres, cortical versus subcortical processes, the first and second signaling system (Platonov, 1959).

This balancing or apposition of opponent processes is also evident on the psychological and social levels. There is tension and relaxation, motivation and inhibition, conscious and unconscious, eros and logos, thesis and antithesis. An awareness and understanding of the dynamics of such opponent processes is of greatest significance in any form of psychotherapy. In this section we can provide only a few illustrations of how we can balance opponent processes by means of verbal suggestion. In the process of hypnotic induction, for example, we have the following:

As that fist gets tighter and *tense*, the rest of your body *relaxes*.

As your right hand *lifts*, your left hand *lowers*.

As that arm *feels lighter* and lifts, your eyelids can feel *heavier* and *lower* until they are closed.

Similar suggestions can be formulated for virtually any of the opponent processes in the sensory, perceptual, affective, and cognitive realms.

As your forehead gets *cooler*, your hands can get *warmer*.

As your jaw becomes more and more *numb and insensitive*, notice how your left hand becomes more and more *sensitive*.

You can *experience* all your feelings about something that occurred at age X without being able to *remember* just what caused those feelings.

When you next open your eyes you will have an unusually clear *memory* of all that, but without the *feelings* you had then.

As you review that, you can now experience an appropriate balance of *thinking* and *feeling* about the whole thing.

As can be seen from the last three examples, a process of dissociation can be utilized to first help the patient very thoroughly experience both sides of an opponent system before they are brought together at a more adequate level of integration.

34

9d. The Negative

Closely associated with the apposition of opposites is the senior author's emphasis on the importance of discharging the negativity or resistance that builds up whenever a patient is following a series of suggestions. In everyday life we can recognize how people who are negative or resistant usually have a history of feeling they were imposed upon too much. Because of this they now want to "have it their way!" They resist being overdirected and very often do the opposite of what they believe others want them to do. This oppositional tendency, of course, is actually a healthy compensation for their early histories. Nature apparently wants us to be individuals, and many believe that the history of man's cultural and psychological development has been an effort to achieve ever-more-encompassing degrees of free, unfettered, and genuine self-expression.

In experimental research psychologists have developed the concept of reactive inhibition to account for similar behavioral phenomena (Woodworth and Schlosberg, 1954). After repeating some task (running a maze, solving certain problems of a similar nature) the subject, whether rat or man, appears less and less willing to go on, and more easily accepts alternative pathways and other patterns of behavior. This inhibition apparently has an adaptive function in blocking previous behavior in favor of the expression of new responses that can lead to new possibilities.

In his practical work with patients, the senior author has explored various means of coping with and actually utilizing this inhibitory or oppositional tendency. He believes that the simple expression of a negative by the therapist can often serve as a lightning rod to automatically discharge any minor inhibition and resistance that has been building up within the patient. Thus he will use such phrases as the following:

And you can, can you *not?*

You can try, *can't* you?

You *can't* stop it, can you?

You will, *won't* you?

You do, *don't* you?

Why *not* let that happen?

Research has demonstrated another value in this close juxtaposition of the positive and the negative. It has been found that it is 30 percent more difficult to comprehend a negative than a positive (Donaldson,

1959). Thus the use of negatives can introduce confusion that tends to depotentiate a patient's limited conscious set so that inner work can be done.

The use of the negative is also related to another indirect form—not knowing and not doing. This use of the negative can be very usefully and casually introduced in contingent suggestions, such as the following that utilize the connective "until."

You *don't* have to go into trance *until* you are really ready.

You *won't* take a really deep breath *until* that hand touches your face.

You *won't* really know just how comfortable you can be in trance *until* that arm slowly lowers all the way down to rest on your lap.

And you really *don't* have to do [therapeutic response] *until* [Inevitable behavior in patient's near future].

You *won't* do it until your unconscious is ready.

The latter use of the negative is actually a form of the conscious-unconscious double bind we will discuss in a later section.

9e. Shock, Surprise, and Creative Moments

A most interesting form of compound suggestion is illustrated when a shock surprises patients' habitual mental frameworks so their usual conscious sets are depotentiated and there is a momentary gap in their awareness, which can then be filled with an appropriate suggestion (Rossi, 1973; Erickson and Rossi, 1976). The shock opens the possibility of a creative moment during which the patient's unconscious is engaged in an inner search for an answer or conception that can reestablish psychic equilibrium. If the patient's own unconscious processes do not provide the answer, the therapist has an opportunity to introduce a suggestion that may have the same effect.

Shock and surprise can sometimes precipitate autonomic reactions that are normally not under voluntary control. At a delicate moment in a conversation one sometimes blushes in an uncontrolled manner when unconscious emotional processes are touched upon. If a person is not blushing during such an unguarded moment, one can frequently precipitate a blushing response by simply asking, "Why are you blushing?" This *question*—as an indirect form of suggestion administered during the "delicate" (potentially creative) moment when the listener's habitual mental frameworks are in nascent flux—evokes the suggested autonomic processes easily.

In everyday life a loud noise may startle us so that we "freeze," momentarily inhibiting all body movement; we are thrown into a momentary trance as the unconscious races for a means of comprehending what is happening. The answer may flash that it was only a car backfiring, and we relax. But if in that precise moment someone yells the suggestion, "bomb!" we almost certainly will flinch, look around in panic, or fall to the ground to protect ourselves. Daily life is filled with less dramatic examples of unexpected shocks that startle and surprise and perhaps lead to a "double-take," where we have to look back or "go over that again" to comprehend what is really going on. We could theorize that foul language is actually a form of shock that has developed in most cultures to startle the listeners so they will be more available to what is being said and be more readily influenced by it.

If people have problems because of learned limitations, it can be therapeutic to momentarily depotentiate those limitations with some form of psychological shock. They can then reevaluate their situation via the automatic process of unconscious search that is initiated within them. In this case the process of shock, surprise, and creative moments is open-ended; the patient's own unconscious processes provide whatever reorganization or solution that emerges. If nothing satisfactory comes forth, the therapist may then add suggestions as further stimuli during the momentary gap, in hope that they may catalyze a therapeutic response.

Momentary shock can be generated in therapeutic dialogue by *interspersing* shock words, taboo concepts, and emotions. Words like *sex, secrets,* and *whispering* momentarily fix attention, and the listener is more receptive. A momentary pause after the shock allows an inner search to take place. It can be followed by reassurance or an appropriate suggestion.

Your *sex* life

[Pause]
just what you need to know and understand about it.

Secretly **what you want**
[Pause]
is most important to you.

You may get *divorced*
[Pause]
unless you both really learn to get what you need in the relationship.

In each of these examples the shock in italics initiates an inner search that can lead to the expression of an important response during the pause. The therapist learns to recognize and evaluate the nonverbal body reactions to such psychological shock. If there are indications that the patient has become preoccupied with the inner search, the therapist simply remains quiet until the patient comes forth with whatever material has been stimulated. If there are no indications of material coming from the patient, the therapist ends the pause with a reassurance or suggestion, as illustrated above. The most effective initiators of shock utilize the patient's own frames of reference, taboos, and needs for a break out of the old so that a creative reorganization can take place. Illustrations of this process have been published elsewhere (Rossi, 1973b), and detailed clinical examples will be found in a number of the cases in this volume.

10. Implication and the Implied Directive

Implication is a basic linguistic-psychological form that provides us with the clearest model of the dynamics of indirect suggestion. Most psychotherapists agree that it is not what the therapist says that is important but what the patient hears. That is, the words of the therapist only function as stimuli that set off many personal trains of association within the patient. It is these personal trains of association within the patient that actually function as a major vehicle for the therapeutic process. This process can be disrupted when the therapist's innocent remarks have unfortunate implications for the patient, but it can be greatly facilitated when the therapist's words carry implications that evoke latent potentials within the patient.

A great deal of communication in daily life as well as in therapy is carried out by implication in a manner that is, for the most part, not consciously planned or even recognized by the participants. We witness this in everyday life when a housewife, for example, bangs her pots a bit louder when she is displeased with her husband but may hum softly to herself when she is pleased. She may not recognize what she is doing, and her husband may not always know quite how he is getting the message, but he feels it at some level. Body language and gesture (Birdwhistell, 1952, 1971; Scheflen, 1974) are nonverbal modes of communication that usually function via implications. In such implication the message is not stated directly but is evoked by a progress of inner search and inference. This inner search engages the patient's own unconscious processes so that the response that emerges is as much a function of the patient as it is of the therapist. Like all the other indirect forms of suggestion, our psychological use of implication ideally evokes and facilitates the patient's own processes of creativity.

On the simplest level implication is formed verbally by the *If . . . then* phrase.

If you sit down *then* you can go into trance.

Now *if* you uncross your legs and place your hands comfortably on your lap, *then* you will be ready to enter trance.

Patients who follow such suggestions by actually *sitting down, uncrossing their legs,* and *placing their hands in their lap* are also accepting, perhaps without quite realizing it, the implication that they will go into trance.

What is the value of such implication? Ideally such implications bypass consciousness and automatically evoke the desired unconscious processes that will facilitate trance induction in a way that the conscious mind could not because it does not know how. We can prepare ourselves to go to sleep, but the conscious mind cannot make it happen. Thus if we directly order a naíve patient, "Sit down and go into trance,[1]" he or she may well sit down while politely protesting, "But I've never gone into trance, and I'm afraid I don't know how." Since the essence of *hypnotic* suggestion is that responses are carried out on an autonomous or unconscious level, it is usually futile to expect the conscious mind to carry them out via direct suggestion. When direct suggestions are successful, they usually involve preparation for hypnotic work in the same sense that brushing one's teeth and lying in bed are conscious, preparatory acts that set the stage for going to sleep, which is then mediated by unconscious processes. With implication and all the other indirect forms of suggestion, we are presuming to do something more: We are making an effort to evoke and facilitate the actual unconscious processes that will create the desired response.

As we reflect upon the process of implication, we gradually become aware that everything we say has implications. Even the most general conversation can be analyzed as a study in implication—how the words of one speaker can evoke all sorts of associations in the listener. In everyday life as well as in hypnotherapy it is often the *implications that are more potent as suggestions* than what is being said directly. In a public conversation the participants are frequently inhibited, and respond with associations that are nothing more than clichés. In a more personal interaction, such as hypnotherapy, the participants have license to respond with their more intimate or idiosyncratic associations. In such personal interactions we are sometimes *surprised* at what associations and feelings we experience. When our conscious mind is surprised in this manner, the therapy has been successful in facilitating an expression of our individuality that we were not previously aware of. We could say that potentials have been released or new dimensions of insight and consciousness have been synthesized.

---

[1]The reader will note that even this apparently direct suggestion actually contains an indirect hypnotic form: a compound contingent suggestion where "and go into trance" is contingent on "Sit down". For some particularly apt or experienced subjects, therefore, this statement could facilitate an effective induction.

The following are examples of the use of implication for deepening patients' involvement with their own inner realities during trance.

Your own memories, images, and feelings are now more important to you in this state.

While giving an apparently direct suggestion about memories, images, and feelings, this statement also carries the important implication that trance is different from the ordinary awake state, and in this state everything else is irrelevant (outside noises, the time of day, the office setting, etc.).

We are usually not aware of the moment when we fall asleep and sometimes are not even aware that we slept.

This statement has obvious implications for a lack of awareness about the significant aspects of trance, a lack that can further depotentiate the limiting sets of consciousness. This implication is emphasized in the following monologue, which structures a frame of reference in which automatic and unconscious behavior can be facilitated.

Now you know you do many things all day long without being aware of them. Your heart just beats along without any help or conscious direction from you. Just as you usually breathe without being aware of it. And even when you walk, your legs seem to move by themselves and take you wherever you want to go. And your hands do most of the things you want them to do without your saying "Now hands do this, now hands do that." Your hands work automatically for you, and you usually don't have to pay attention to them. Even when you speak, you do it automatically, you don't have to be consciously aware of how to pronounce each word. You can speak without even knowing it. You know how to do it automatically without even thinking about it. Also, when you see or hear things or when you touch or feel things, they work automatically without you having to be conscious of them. They work by themselves and you don't have to pay attention. They just take care of themselves without your having to be bothered about them.

10a. The Implied Directive

A special form of implication that is closely associated with contingency suggestions is what we have termed the *implied directive* (Erickson and Rossi, 1976). The implied directive is an indirect form of suggestion that is in common usage in clinical hypnosis (Cheek and LeCron, 1968) even though it has not yet received detailed psychological analysis. Like the other indirect forms of suggestion, its use has evolved out of a recognition of its value in everyday life. The implied directive has three recognizable parts:

1. a time-binding introduction;
2. the implied suggestion that takes place within the patient;
3. a behavioral response that signals when the implied suggestion has been accomplished.

Thus,

As soon as

1. the time-binding introduction

your unconscious has reached the source of that problem,

2. the implied suggestion initiating an unconscious search taking place within the patient

your finger can lift.

3. the behavioral response that signals when the implied suggestion has been accomplished.

As can be seen from this illustration, the implied directive is an indirect form of suggestion that initiates inner search and unconscious processes and then lets us know when a therapeutic response has been accomplished. It is of particular value when we need to initiate and facilitate an extensive process of inner exploration and when we are attempting to unravel the dynamics of symptom formation.

Other indirect forms of suggestion that are particularly useful for initiating an unconscious search in hypnosis are implied directives such as the following:

When you have found a feeling of relaxation and comfort, your eyes will close all by themselves.

In this example the patient must obviously make a search on an unconscious level that will ideally initiate parasympathetic responses that can be experienced as comfort and relaxation. Eye closure is a response naturally associated with such internal comfort and thus serves as an ideal signal that the internal process has taken place.

As that comfort deepens, your conscious mind can relax while your unconscious reviews the nature of the problem. And when a relevant and

interesting thought reaches your conscious mind, your eyes will open as you carefully consider it.

This example builds upon the first and initiates another unconscious search for a general exploratory approach to a problem.

As can be seen from these examples, an unconscious search initiates an unconscious process that actually solves the problem that the conscious mind could not handle. These unconscious processes are the essence of creativity and problem-solving in everyday life as well as in therapy. Hypnotherapy, in particular, depends upon the successful utilization of such unconscious processes to facilitate a therapeutic response. Cheek and LeCron (1968) have given extensive illustrations of how a series of questions in the form of implied directives can be used for both the exploration and resolution of symptoms.

11. Binds and Double Binds

Pyschological binds and double binds have been explored by a number of authors (Haley, 1963; Watzlawick et al., 1967, 1974; Erickson and Rossi, 1975) for their use in therapeutic situations. The concept of "binds" appears to have a fascinating potential that extends our quest for new therapeutic approaches into the areas of linguistics, logic, semantics, epistemology, and the philosophy of science. Since they are the vanguard of new patterns of our therapeutic consciousness, our understanding of them is as yet very incomplete. We are not always sure what binds and double binds are, or how we can best formulate and use them. Most of our knowledge about them comes from clinical studies and theoretical formulations (Bateson, 1972) with very little controlled experimental research that exactly specifies their parameters.

Because of this, we will use the terms *bind* and *double bind* only in a very special and limited sense to describe certain forms of suggestion that offer patients an opportunity for therapeutic responses. A *bind* offers a patient a free, conscious choice between two or more alternatives. Whichever choice is made, however, leads the patient in a therapeutic direction. A *double bind,* by contrast, offers possibilities of behavior that are outside the patient's usual range of conscious choice and voluntary control. The double bind arises out of the possibility of communicating on more than one level. In daily life we frequently say something verbally while commenting on it extraverbally. We may say, "Let's go to the movies." We can say it with innumerable variations of tone and intent, however, that can have many implications. These variations are all comments or *metacommunications* on our primary verbal message about going to the movies. As we shall see in the following sections, binds and double binds are very much a function of who is receiving the message. What is a bind or double bind for one

42

person may not be for another. As is the case with all the other indirect forms of suggestion, binds and double binds utilize the patient's unique repertory of associations and patterns of long learning. Most binds and double blinds cannot be applied in a mechanical or rote fashion. Therapists must understand something about how their messages are going to be received in order to make it effective.

11a. Binds Modeled on Avoidance-Avoidance and Approach-Approach Conflicts

Psychological binds are life situations in which we experience a constriction in our behavior. Typically we are caught in circumstances that allow us only unpleasant alternatives of response. We are caught between "the devil and the deep blue sea." We thus experience an *avoidance-avoidance conflict;* we have to make a choice even though we would like to avoid all the alternatives. In such circumstances we usually choose the lesser of the two "evils."

Psychological binds can also be constructed on the model of an *approach-approach conflict.* In this case one is in the bind of having to choose only one of a number of desirable courses of action and excluding all the other desirable possibilities. In common parlance, "You can't have your cake and eat it too."

Since we have all had innumerable experiences of such binds, the avoidance-avoidance and approach-approach conflicts usually exist as established processes governing our behavior. As we study patients, we learn to recognize how some are governed more by avoidance-avoidance conflicts while others, perhaps more fortunate (but not necessarily so), appear to be perpetually juggling approach-approach alternatives. The clinical art of utilizing these models of conflict is to recognize which tendency is dominant within a particular patient and then structure binds that offer only therapeutic alternatives of response. When we do not know which tendency is more predominant, we can offer general binds that are applicable to anyone, such as the following.

Would you like to enter trance now or later?

Would you like to enter trance sitting or lying down?

Would you like to go into a light, medium, or deep trance?

The patient has free, conscious choice in responding to any of the alternatives offered above. As soon as a choice is made, however, the patient is bound to enter trance. As can be seen from these examples, the question format is particularly well suited for offering binds. When using it with ideomotor signaling, we can frequently formulate an associational network of structured inquiry that can rapidly unravel the dynamics of a problem and resolve it. Cheek and LeCron (1968) have pioneered such lines of structured inquiry for many psychological and psychosomatic conditions.

An example of the therapeutic use of an avoidance-avoidance bind to resolve a symptom of insomnia was the case of a meticulous elderly gentleman who took pride in doing all his own housework—except that he hated to wax floors. After an appraisal of his personality, the senior author told the gentleman that there was an obvious solution to the insomnia problem, but he "might not like it." The gentleman politely insisted that he would do whatever was necessary to be able to sleep. The senior author continued to demur, while permitting the gentleman to commit himself further by giving a number of examples of how persistent he was in dealing with difficult problems once he determined he would. He insisted that his "word was his bond," and he was used to dealing with unpleasant matters. This clearly confirmed that this man of admirable character was, indeed, well practiced in working through avoidance-avoidance conflicts. His determination in the face of such conflicts was utilized in structuring a therapeutic avoidance-avoidance bind. He was told that if he was not asleep within fifteen minutes of going to bed, he had to get up and wax floors until he felt he could sleep. If he was still not asleep within fifteen minutes, he had to get up again and so continue this procedure until he was asleep. The gentleman later reported that he had well-waxed floors and slept remarkably well.

We may call this situation a therapeutic avoidance-avoidance *bind* because the gentleman was presented with negative alternatives over which he had conscious, voluntary choice. He could choose between the negative alternatives of insomnia or waxing floors. As we study this example a bit further, however, it begins to reveal aspects of a *double bind*. We could conceptualize the gentleman's characterological structure, which enabled him to *persist in the face of difficulties,* as well as his *"word was his bond"* as metalevels that bound him automatically to his therapeutic task. These metalevels of his character were utilized in a manner that was outside his normal range of conscious choice and control.

This example illustrates the difficulties in any exact formulation or understanding of the operation of the bind and double bind in actual clinical practice. In general, however, we can say that the more we involve the patients' own associations and learned patterns of response, the more they are likely to experience a bind, double bind, or triple bind as an effective agent in behavior change that is experienced as taking place on an autonomous (unconscious, hypnotic) level.

11b. The Conscious-Unconscious Double Bind

Some of the most fascinating and useful double binds are those that deal with the interface between conscious and unconscious processes (Erickson, 1964; Erickson and Rossi, 1975). These double binds all rest upon the fact that while we cannot control our unconscious, we can receive a message consciously that can initiate unconscious processes. The conscious-unconscious double bind is designed to bypass the limitations of our conscious understanding and abilities so that behavior can be mediated by the hidden potentials that exist on a more autonomous or unconscious level. Any response to the following, for example, requires that the patient experience an inner focus and search that initiates unconscious processes in ways that are usually beyond conscious control.

If your unconscious wants you to enter trance, your right hand will lift all by itself. Otherwise your left hand will lift.

Whether one gets a "yes" (right hand) or "no" (left hand) response to this suggestion, one has begun to induce trance, since any truly autonomous response (lifting either hand) implies that a trance exists. If the patient simply sits quietly, and no hand response is evident after a few minutes, the therapist can introduce a further double bind with the following addition.

Since you've been sitting quietly and there is yet no hand response, you can wonder if your unconscious would prefer not to make any effort at all as you go into trance. It may be more comfortable not to have to move or talk or even bother trying to keep your eyes open.

At this point the patient's eyes may close and trance become manifest. The eyes may remain open with a passive stare, and there will be continuing body immobility suggestive of the development of trance. If the patient is experiencing difficulty, on the other hand, there will be an uneasy shifting of the body, facial movements, and finally some talk about the problem.

The conscious-unconscious double bind in association with questions, implications, not knowing–not doing, and ideomotor signaling is thus an excellent means of initiating trance and exploring a patient's patterns of response.

In therapy the conscious-unconscious double bind has innumerable uses, all based on its ability to mobilize unconscious processes. The use of the *negative* as described earlier is very useful here.

You *don't* have to listen to me because your unconscious is here and can hear what it needs to, to respond in just the right way.

And it really *doesn't* matter what your conscious mind does because your unconscious can find the right means of coping with that pain [*or whatever*].

You've said you *don't* know how to solve that problem. You are uncertain and confused. Your conscious mind really *doesn't* know what to do. And yet we know that the unconscious does have access to many memories and images and experiences that it can make available to you in ways that can be most surprising for solving that problem. You *don't* know what all your possibilities are yet. Your unconscious can work on them all by itself. And how will you know when it has been solved? Will the solution come in a dream you will remember, or will you forget the dream but find that the problem is gradually resolving itself in a way that your conscious mind *cannot* understand? Will the resolution come quickly while wide-awake or in a quiet moment of reflection or daydreaming? Will you be at work or at play, shopping or driving your car, when you finally realize it? You really *don't* know, but you certainly can be happy when the solution does come.

In these examples it can be seen how the conscious-unconscious double bind in association with questions and open-ended suggestions can facilitate whatever responses are most suitable for the patient's individuality. All the major cases of this volume illustrate how this form of double bind can be applied to a variety of problems and situations. In all such situations we are depotentiating the patient's conscious, habitual, and presumably more limited patterns in favor of unconscious processes and potentials. If we are willing to identify these unconscious processes with the activity of the nondominant cerebral hemisphere (usually the right—Galin, 1974; Hoppe, 1977) and conscious self-direction and rational processes with the dominant cerebral hemisphere (usually the left), we could say that the conscious-unconscious double bind tends to depotentiate the limitations of the dominant hemisphere and thereby possibly facilitate the potentials of the nondominant. This is particularly the case with the double dissociation double bind, to which we will now turn our attention.

11c. The Double Dissociation Double Bind

Traditionally the concept of dissociation has been used as an explanation of hypnosis. Hypnotic or autonomous behavior takes place outside the patient's immediate range of consciousness and is therefore dissociated from the conscious mind. The senior author has evolved many subtle and indirect means of facilitating dissociations that appear to utilize many entirely normal but alternate pathways of behavior that lead to the same end. "All roads lead to Rome" is a cliché that expresses the intense obviousness and, therefore, usefulness of this approach. Precisely because alternate pathways to the same response are very obviously true and respectful of the patient's individuality, suggestions that utilize them are very acceptable.

The double dissociation double bind was discovered by the authors (Erickson, Rossi, and Rossi, 1976) when we analyzed the following.

You can as a person awaken, but you do not need to awaken as a body.

[Pause]

You can awaken when your body awakens but without a recognition of your body.

In the first half of this suggestion awakening as a person is dissociated from awakening as a body. In the second half awakening as a person and as a body are dissociated from a recognition of the body. Suggestions that embody such dissociations facilitate hypnotic behavior while also exploring each individual's unique response abilities. The double dissociation double blind tends to confuse a patient's conscious mind and thus depotentiate his habitual sets, biases, and learned limitations. This sets the stage for unconscious searches and processes that may mediate creative behavior. The following examples suggest the range of its application.

You can dream you're awake even though you're in trance.
[Pause]
Or you can act as if you're in trance even while awake.

You can find your hand lifting without knowing where it is going.
[Pause]
Or you may sense where it is going even though you're not really directing it.

You can make an abstract drawing without knowing what it is.
[Pause]
You can later find some meaning in it even though it does not *seem* related to you personally.

You can speak in trance even though you don't always recognize the meaning of your words.
[Pause]
Or you can remain silent as your head very slowly nods "yes" or shakes "no" all by itself in response to my questions.

As can be seen from these examples, the double dissociation double bind is often a potpourri of all sorts of indirect forms of suggestion: implications, contingencies, negatives, open-ended suggestions, apparently covering all possibilities of a class of responses, not knowing, not doing, and so on. Their common denominator is the facilitation of dissociations that tend to depotentiate a patient's habitual conscious sets so that more involuntary levels of response can be expressed. The authors (Erickson, Rossi, and Rossi, 1976) have discussed how this form of the double bind may be related to the neuropsychological concepts formulated by Luria (1973).

A detailed study and assessment of the patient's response to carefully formulated double dissociation double binds can be of great use in planning further hypnotic work. Consider the following, which can provide either an initiation into somnambulistic training or at least a validation of trance.

Now, in a moment your eyes will open but you don't need to awaken.

[Pause]

Or you can awaken when your eyes open, but without remembering what happened when they were closed.

This double dissociation double bind has a definite marker indicating that the suggestion has been received and is being acted upon: the eyes opening. When the eyes open, the therapist notes whether (1) there is a simultaneous movement of the body, indicating that the patient is awakening or (2) the patient remains immobile, indicating that trance is continuing. If the patient's body remains immobile when the eyes open, the patient will have a complete memory of all trance events, since that trance continues. The therapist can assess this condition by questioning and then requesting an ideomotor response so the patient's unconscious can firmly validate that a trance is still present (e.g., If you are still in trance your "yes" finger can lift, your head can slowly nod "yes," and so on). An affirmative ideomotor response, indicating that the patient continues to experience trance even with eyes open, is a strong indication that the patient has entered the first stages of somnambulistic training: Patients in this state can in general act as if they are awake, yet they continue to follow suggestions as if they were in a deep trance. The therapist then simply continues this somnambulistic training by proffering further suggestions to deepen their involvement and extend their range of hypnotic responsiveness (automatic talking and writing, visual and auditory hallucinations, and so on).

If, on the other hand, such patients move and speak as if they were perfectly awake when their eyes open, they are apparently acting on the second alternative, and we would assess the validity of the trance by determining the presence of an amnesia for trance events. But what if a patient awakes and there is no amnesia? Does this mean that trance was not experienced? Possibly. More likely, however, such patients will recall only one or two things of such particular significance for them during trance that they attracted conscious attention and so are recalled easily after trance. There will tend to be an amnesia for many other trance events; however, another possibility is that amnesia may be a particularly difficult response for such patients. They may have experienced a genuine trance but for some reason cannot experience the response of amnesia. To assess this possibility the therapist reintroduces trance and then, after another double dissociation double bind, uses another modality as an indication of trance. In the following, for example, body movement (or an inhibiting verbal response) is used as a trance indication instead of amnesia.

Now, in a moment your eyes will open, but you don't need to awaken.

Or you can awaken when your eyes open, but you won't feel like moving your arms for a few minutes [or won't feel like speaking for a few minutes].

Patients who accept the second alternative and awaken can validate the trance by not moving their arms (or speaking) for a few minutes. It is wise to offer trance indicators in this permissive manner. ("You *won't feel like* moving your arms") rather than as a challenge ("You *won't be able* to move your arms"), because the challenge is often taken as an affront by our modern consciousness that takes such hubris in its apparent independence and power.

12. Multiple Levels of Meaning and Communication: The Evolution of Consciousness in Jokes, Puns, Metaphor, and Symbol.

Our five-stage paradigm of the dynamics of trance induction and utilization (Figure 1) illustrates some of the essential processes in what we may call "multiple levels of meaning and communication" (Erickson and Rossi, 1976). Most literary devices are actually means of initiating unconscious searches and processes to evoke multiple levels of meaning. This is a most interesting and significant aspect of the economy of mental dynamics and the evolution of consciousness. Freud has discussed the antithetical meaning of primal words (Freud, 1910) and the relation of jokes and puns to the unconscious (Freud, 1905). Jokes are of particular value in our approach because they help patients break through their too-limited mental sets and thus initiate unconscious searches for other and perhaps new levels of meaning. Jung has discussed the concept of the *symbol* not as a simple sign of one thing for another, but rather as the best representation of something that is still in the process of becoming conscious (Jung, 1956). The significant factor in all these conceptions is the idea of the *evolution of consciousness*. If patients have problems because of learned limitations, then it is clear that therapeutic processes can be initiated by helping them develop behavioral potentials and new patterns of consciousness that bypass those limitations.

From this point of view we can understand how metaphor and analogy can be something more than artistic devices: They can evoke new patterns and dimensions of consciousness. The very derivation of the word *metaphor* (*meta*, "beyond, over"; *pherin*, "to bring, bear") suggests how new meaning developed within the unconscious is brought over to consciousness by means of metaphor. The traditional definition of metaphor is that it is a word or phrase that literally denotes one thing but by analogy suggests another (e.g., a ship *plows* the sea; a *volley* of oaths). In our psychological usage, however, such traditionally literary devices as metaphor, analogy, and simile are understood as means of facilitating the development of insight or new consciousness in the therapeutic transaction. They are essentially stimuli that initiate unconscious searches and processes leading to the creation of new meaning and dimensions of consciousness. Recently Jaynes (1976) has integrated a broad range of data from the fields of psychology, linguistics, neuropsychology, and anthropology which affirmed the hypothesis that metaphor and analogy generate new levels of consciousness.

The senior author has pioneered the use of such approaches to facilitate therapeutic processes in hypnotherapy. His gradual development of the interspersal approach has been the most significant factor in his learning to cultivate multiple levels of meaning and communication as well as enhance the evolution of consciousness. Deterministic as well as nondeterministic processes are both in evidence here. In many of the cases in this book the senior author uses these approaches to facilitate the awareness of certain dynamics that he feels to be at the core of the patient's problems. He uses multiple levels of communication in a highly deterministic way to help the patient recognize certain definite dynamics. In most of these cases, however, the patients also learn entirely new things that neither they nor the senior author could have predicted. It is the nondeterministic aspect of these approaches that is most exciting in facilitating the evolution of consciousness. Jung has formulated these dynamics in what he calls the *transcendent function:* the integration of conscious and unconscious contents in a manner that facilitates the evolution of new patterns of awareness (Jung, 1960). We presume that many of the practical approaches illustrated by the cases in this volume are actually means of facilitating the evolution of such new patterns of awareness.

Exercises

1. We have previously presented a number of exercises to facilitate the acquisition of skill with most of the indirect forms of suggestion discussed in this chapter (Erickson, Rossi, and Rossi, 1976). So multifaceted are the possibilities of the indirect approaches, however, that one can feel overwhelmed to the point where one does not attempt a systematic beginning in practicing their use. Because of this we strongly suggest that the reader learn to use only a few at a time. The *interspersal approach*, together with all forms of *questions* and *truisms*, for example, can be utilized in any therapeutic interview even without the formal induction of trance. It is highly instructive simply to observe the development of a *yes set* when these approaches are used with the patient's own vocabulary and *frames of reference*. At this level our approach might appear similar to the nondirective, client-centered approach of Rogers (1951).

2. Even without the formal induction of trance one can explore the effectiveness of *ideodynamic process* in an *open-ended* manner with the patient simply by maintaining an attitude of *expectancy* about what can be experienced. It is instructive to note how after a period of five to twenty minutes of such exercises with the eyes closed most subjects will stretch, yawn, and reorient to their bodies when they open their eyes to end the inner work—as if they had been asleep or in trance. Perhaps they have been (Erickson, 1964). We really have no independent criterion for assessing whether they were or not.

3. The next stage of competence probably involves the planned use of the varieties of *compound suggestions*. The therapist needs time and patience to carefully write out ahead of time patterns of *contingency suggestions* and *associational networks*. The use of *shock*, *surprise*, and *creative moments* can involve a careful study and retrospective analysis of how these phenomena operate spontaneously in everyday life.

4. The use of implications can be facilitated by a careful study of tape recordings of one's therapy sessions. What are the conscious and unconscious implications of both the therapist's and the patient's remarks? After a period of such study one gradually develops more of a consciousness of the implications of words just as one is uttering them. One is then in a position to begin the planned use of implications as a therapeutic approach. The *multiple levels of meaning* via *jokes, puns,* and *metaphor* now became more easily available.

5. The therapeutic binds and double binds discussed in this

chapter are fairly simple to learn, and they provide an almost infinite range of possibilities for exploring psychodynamics and facilitation of hypnotic responsiveness. The therapist newly interested in this area can spend many enjoyable hours formulating plausible *conscious-unconscious* and *double dissociation double binds* that apparently *cover all possibilities of response*, just as others might spend their time on crossword puzzles. To test one out in clinical practice is a fail-safe procedure, since at worst the patient will probably ignore it and nothing will happen at all. Other forms of the double bind discussed by Watzlawick et al. (1967), Haley (1963, 1973), and the authors (Erickson and Rossi, 1975) still only come to the junior author by happy accident. We are here in the vanguard of our understanding of understanding. Controlled experimental studies as well as interesting clinical examples very much need to be published.

6. The indirect forms of suggestion may make a contribution to the current intriguing debate about writing a computer program to do psychotherapy (Weizenbaum, 1976; Nichols, 1978). Readers with the appropriate experience might explore the possibility that a computer programmed with these hypnotic forms could generate new combinations of suggestions uniquely suitable for specific symptom complexes, personality problems, and altered states of consciousness.

CHAPTER 3

The Utilization Approach:
Trance Induction and Suggestion

The senior author (Erickson, 1958, 1959) has distinguished between the "formalized ritualistic procedures of trance induction," where the same method is applied mechanically to everyone, and the "naturalistic approach," wherein the patient's unique personality and behavior are *utilized* to facilitate trance. In this utilization approach the patient's *attention is fixed* on some important aspect of his own personality and behavior in a manner that leads to the inner focus that we define as therapeutic trance. The patient's habitual conscious sets are more or less depoteniated, and unconscious searches and processes are initiated to facilitate a therapeutic response. In this chapter we will illustrate this utilization approach to trance induction and suggestion with a variety of examples from clinical practice. We will analyze some of the typical approaches to preparing patients for trance experience along with the actual induction and ratification of the trance. In these examples we will focus on how an interaction of *the utilization approach* and the *indirect forms of suggestion* can facilitate a therapeutic outcome in virtually any situation in which the therapist and patient find themselves.

1. Accepting and Utilizing the Patients' Manifest Behavior

The initial step in the utilization approach, as in most other forms of psychotherapy, is to accept the patients' manifest behavior and to acknowledge their personal frames of reference. This openness and acceptance of the patients' worlds facilitate a corresponding openness and acceptance of the therapist by the patients. The following examples taken from the senior author's unpublished and published records (Erickson 1958, 1959) illustrate how the rapport can develop and rapidly lead to an experience of therapeutic trance.

The development of a trance state is an intrapsychic phenomenon, dependent upon internal processes, and the activity of the hypnotist serves only to create a favorable situation. As an analogy, an incubator supplies a favorable environment for the hatching of eggs, but the actual hatching derives from the development of life processes within the egg.

In trance induction, the inexperienced hypnotist often tries to direct or bend the subject's behavior to fit his conception of how the subject "should" behave. There ought to be a constant minimization of the role of the hypnotist and a constant amplification of the subject's role. An example may be cited of a volunteer subject, used later to teach hypnosis to medical students. After a general discussion of hypnosis, she expressed a willingness to go into a trance immediately. The suggestion was offered that she select the chair and position she felt would be most comfortable. When she had settled herself to her satisfaction, she remarked that she would like to smoke a cigarette. She was immediately given one, and she proceeded to smoke lazily, meditatively watching the smoke drifting upward. Casual conversational remarks were offered about the pleasure of smoking, of watching the curling smoke, the feeling of ease in lifting the cigarette to her mouth, the inner sense of satisfaction of becoming entirely absorbed just in smoking comfortably and without need to attend to any external things. Shortly, casual remarks were made about inhaling and exhaling, these words timed to fit in with her actual breathing. Others were made about the ease with which she could almost automatically lift her cigarette to her mouth and then lower her hand to the arm of the chair. These remarks were also timed to coincide with her actual behavior. Soon, the words "inhale," "exhale," "lift," and "lower" acquired a conditioning value of which she was unaware because of the seemingly conversational nature of the suggestions. Similarly, casual suggestions were offered in which the words sleep, sleepy, and sleeping were timed to her eyelid behavior.

Before she had finished the cigarette, she had developed a light trance. Then the suggestion was made that she might continue to enjoy smoking as she slept more and more soundly; that the cigarette would be looked after by the hypnotist while she absorbed herself more and more completely in deep sleep; that, as she slept, she would continue to experience the satisfying feelings and sensations of smoking. A satisfactory profound trance resulted and she was given extensive training to teach her to respond in accord with her own unconscious pattern of behavior.

In this example the initial preparation and faciliation of an optimal frame of reference occurred as the subject listened to a general discussion of hypnosis. The senior author, as a teacher, could not help but use indirect associative focusing and ideodynamic focusing in his general talk about hypnosis. As we saw in the previous chapter, all such general discussions automatically initiate ideodynamic processes that can then serve as the foundation for trance experience.

The fact that this subject volunteered is an indication that this initial preparation was particularly effective for her. One of the joys of working with volunteers from such groups is precisely this form of self-recognition of one's readiness for trance.

Her surprising desire to smoke, once she was settled for trance work, might have been experienced as a disconcerting sign of resistance by a less experienced therapist. Indeed, when this same subject was later used by students, who did not accept her wish to smoke, they were not able to induce trance. The senior author immediately accepted her behavior, however, and even gave her a cigarette. This enhanced their rapport as they were now cooperatively engaged together in her smoking. As she proceeded to smoke "lazily, meditatively," we can begin to appreciate how her apparently disruptive behavior of smoking may have been an unconsciously determined means of cooperating with the hypnotic process. For this subject smoking led to an inner meditative mood entirely in keeping with trance induction. The senior author recognized and utilized this meditative mood to facilitate trance by *fixing her attention* even more on her smoking with "casual conversational remarks." This casual conversation, of course, provides the senior author with a general context into which he can *intersperse* suggestions about "pleasure," "ease," "inner sense of satisfaction," and "*becoming entirely absorbed*" in smoking "*comfortably without need to attend to any external things.*" These interspersed suggestions tended to *depotentiate her habitual waking orientation* even further. The process of *not knowing and not doing* that takes place when we do not have to attend to external things led her to an unconscious search for some new form of direction and orientation.

This new direction was provided by the senior author with his obvious interest in her smoking behavior. He then utilized her smoking behavior for a process of unconscious conditioning; her inhaling, exhaling, lifting and lowering of her hand became conditioned to following his voice and suggestions. This unconscious conditioning was a way of assessing and reinforcing her response attentiveness. Finally the ideodynamic associative value of words like "sleep" were then associated with her actual eyelid behavior suggestive of sleep (eyelids closing, fluttering, etc.). Even though both therapist and patient fully recognize that therapeutic trance is not sleep, words evoking the idea of sleep tend to evoke associated behaviors (like comfort and not doing) that tend to facilitate trance.

The process of rapport was further enhanced as he took her cigarette and suggested she "might continue to enjoy smoking as she slept more and more soundly." A hallucinatory wish fulfillment of something she obviously enjoyed, such as smoking, was made contingent on sleeping "more and more soundly." She was given an expectancy of continued "satisfying feelings" as she went deeper into trance. This sound utilization of her smoking behavior, together with many indirect forms of suggestion that evoked her own associative processes, then led to more extensive trance training.

Our next example is a particularly vivid illustration of how a highly intellectualized frame of reference attending primarily to external things can be gradually shifted to an internal focus that is more suitable for therapeutic trance.

This patient entered the office in a most energetic fashion and declared at once that he did not know if he was hypnotizable. He was willing to go into a trance if it were at all possible, provided the writer would approach the entire matter in an intellectual fashion rather than in a mystical, ritualistic manner. He declared that he needed psychotherapy for a variety of reasons and that he had tried various schools of psychotherapy extensively without benefit. Hypnosis had been attempted on various occasions and had failed miserably because of "mysticism" and "a lack of appreciation for the intellectual approach."

Inquiry revealed that he felt an "intelligent" approach signified, not a suggestion of ideas, but questioning him concerning his own thinking and feeling in relation to reality. The writer, he declared, should recognize that he was sitting in a chair, that the chair was in front of a desk, and that these constituted absolute facts of reality. As such, they could not be overlooked, forgotten, denied or ignored. In further illustration, he pointed out that he was obviously tense, anxious, and concerned about the tension tremors of his hands, which were resting on the arms of the chair, and that he was also highly distractable, noticing everything about him.

The writer immediately seized upon this last comment as the basis for the initial cooperation with him. He was told, "Please proceed with an account of your ideas and understanding, permitting me only enough interruptions *to insure that I understand fully and that I follow along with you.* For example, you mentioned the chair but obviously you have seen my desk and have been distracted by the objects on it. Please explain fully."

He responded verbosely with a wealth of more or less connected comments about everything in sight. At every slight pause, the writer interjected a word or phrase to direct his attention anew. These interruptions, made with increasing frequency, were as follows: "And that paperweight; the filing cabinet; your foot on the rug; the ceiling light; the draperies; your right hand on the arm of the chair; the pictures on the wall; the changing focus of your eyes as you glance about; the interest of the book titles; the tension in your shoulders; the feeling of the chair; the disturbing noises and thoughts; weight of hands and feet; weight of problems, weight of desk; the stationery stand; the records of many patients; the phenomena of life, of illness, of emotion, of physical and mental behavior; the restfulness of relaxation; the need to attend to one's needs; the need to attend to one's tension while looking at the desk or the paperweight or the filing cabinet; the comfort of withdrawal from the environment; fatigue and its development; the unchanging character of the desk; the monotony of the filing cabinet; the need to take a rest; the comfort of closing one's eyes; the relaxing sensation of a deep breath; the delight of learning passively; the capacity for intellectual learning by the unconscious." Various other similar brief interjections were offered, slowly at first and then with increasing frequency.

Initially, these interjections were merely supplementary to the patient's own train of thought and utterances. At first, the effect was simply to stimulate him to further effort. As this response was made, it became possible to utilize his acceptance of stimulation of his behavior by a procedure of pausing and hesitating in the completion of an interjection. This served to effect in him an expectant dependency upon the writer for further and more complete stimulation.

As this procedure was continued, gradually and unnoticeably to the patient his attention was progressively directed to inner subjective experiential matters. It then became possible to use almost directly a simple, progressive relaxation technique of trance induction and to secure a light medium trance.

Throughout therapy, further trance inductions were basically comparable, although the procedure became progressively abbreviated.

The patient's initial statement that "he did not know if he was hypnotizable" is an important admission of his availability for trance. As we saw in the previous chapter, "not knowing and not doing" are actually an important condition for trance experience. This highly intellectualized individual is admitting there is a place where he does not know, a place where his habitual sets and frames of reference are not stable—hypnosis is a place where these habitual, and obviously in some way inadequate mental frameworks can be bypassed so that the needed psychotherapy can take place.

The patient then states his conditions for trance experience. The writer (the senior author) must eschew all mystical and ritualistic means and use an intellectual approach. The patient's intellectual orientation is obviously the ability that any sensible therapist would assess as most suitable for utilization.

The patient then describes his "distractable" state, and the senior author immediately utilizes it as a basis for the initial cooperation with him. He encourages the patient to continue with an account of his ideas "to ensure that I understand fully and that I follow along with you." This is an unrecognized interspersed suggestion that means *understanding* and *following* are important in therapy. Just as the therapist initially understands and follows the patient, so will the patient soon come to understand and follow the therapist. Rapport, response attentiveness, and an optimal attitude for creating a therapeutic frame of reference are all implied and thereby facilitated by this initial suggestion and acceptance of the patient's behavior.

The senior author's request that the patient "explain fully" is actually an unrecognized means of focusing and fixing the patient's attention onto a prominent aspect of his own behavior (distracted by objects) that he himself pointed out. Since the patient pointed out this aspect of his own behavior, it must "hold" some special interest for him and thus can serve as an ideal means of holding his attention. This is a curious situation that may involve a double bind for this particular patient: His distractibility is used to undistract, to focus his attention.

The senior author now gingerly interacts with the patient by redirecting his attention anew at every pause as a means of cooperating with him, and at the same time, enhancing his response attentiveness. By very gradual steps the senior author builds an associative network that leads the patient from the paperweight and filing cabinet to "the delight of learning passively" and "the capacity for intellectual learning by the unconscious." The shift in focus is from the outer to the inner, which is in keeping with trance work. The shift is facilitated by a continuing utilization of the patient's intellectual approach, with the emphasis on "learning passively" and the "unconscious" learning. The passivity and unconscious aspects of trance experience are thus associated with the "learning" that the patient already accepts and knows how to do; it is thus much easier for the patient to accept passivity and the unconscious when it is associated with learning. In this shift from an outer to an inner focus the senior author has a great opportunity to intersperse many forms of indirect associative focusing (e.g., "the phenomena of life, of illness, of emotion, of physical and mental behavior") and indirect ideodynamic focusing (e.g., "the restfulness of relaxation . . . the comfort of withdrawal from the environment, fatigue and its development"). This can facilitate trance induction by initiating unconscious searches and processes that could evoke partial aspects of trance experience as well as a review of the patient's problems.

As the therapist continued to utilize "the patient's own train of thought and utterances," his response attentiveness was further enhanced and a greater degree of "expectant dependency" was experienced by the patient as he now began to look to the therapist for further direction into "inner subjective experiential matters," where his psychological problems were.

A similar approach was used in the following case, which the reader should now find easy to analyze in terms of the dynamics we have presented.

Essentially the same procedure was employed with a male patient in his early 30's who entered the office and began pacing the floor. He explained repetitiously that he could not endure relating his problems sitting quietly or lying on a couch. He had repeatedly been discharged by various psychiatrists because they "accused" him of lack of cooperation. He asked that hypnotherapy be employed, if possible, since his anxieties were almost unendurable and always increased in intensity in a psychiatrist's office making it necessary for him to pace the floor constantly.

Further repetitious explanation of his need to pace the floor was finally successfully interrupted by the question, "Are you willing to cooperate with me *by continuing to pace the floor, even as you are doing now*?" His reply was a startled, "Willing? Good God, man! I've got to do it if I stay in the office."

Thereupon, he was asked to permit the writer to participate in his pacing by the measure of directing it in part. To this he agreed rather bewilderedly. He was asked to pace back and forth, to turn to the right, to the left, to walk away from the chair, and to walk toward it. At first these instructions were given in a tempo matching his step. Gradually, the tempo of the instructions was slowed and the wording changed to "Now turn to the right away from the chair in which you can sit; turn left toward the chair in which you can sit; walk away from the chair in which you can sit; walk toward the chair in which you can sit." etc. With this wording, a foundation was laid for more cooperative behavior.

The tempo was slowed still more and the instructions again varied to include the phrase, "the chair which you will soon approach as if to seat yourself comfortably." This in turn was altered to "the chair in which you will shortly find yourself sitting comfortably."

His pacing became progressively slower and more and more dependent upon the writer's verbal instructions until direct suggestions could be given that he seat himself in the chair and go deeper and deeper into a profound trance as he related his history.

Approximately 45 minutes were spent in this manner inducing a medium trance that so lessened the patient's tension and anxiety that he could cooperate readily with therapy thereafter.

The value of this type of Utilization Technique lies in its effective demonstration to the patient that he is completely acceptable and that the therapist can deal effectively with him regardless of his behavior. It *meets both the patient's presenting needs and it employs as the significant part of the induction procedure the very behavior that dominates the patient.*

The senior author's question, "Are you willing to cooperate with me *by continuing to pace the floor, even as you are doing now?"* is an unusually fecund example of the use of a number of indirect hypnotic forms in a single sentence. Being a *question*, it immediately *fixes the patient's attention* and sends him on an *inner search* for an appropriate response. It is an excellent *compound suggestion* that associates an important suggestion about cooperation with his ongoing behavior of pacing the floor. Pacing the floor constantly was the patient's own *ability that was rapidly assessed, accepted, and utilized* to facilitate a *yes set*. The question came as a bit of a *shock and surprise* that *depotentiated his dominant mental set* about his own resistance and "startled" him into a strong exclamation of his need to cooperate. *Rapport* was thus strongly established, and therapy structured as a joint endeavor. With such a strong immediate rapport, a high *expectation* was set in motion, heightening the patient's *response attentiveness* to his own internal states as well as to the therapist's further suggestions. By a gradual process of association and unconscious conditioning this response attentiveness was heightened even further, so the patient was finally able to accept suggestions to sit down and go even deeper into himself so that he could relate his history in a state of deep absorption that is described as "profound trance."

The beginning therapist who is just learning to integrate the utilization approach with the indirect forms of suggestion may initially feel a bit overwhelmed by these examples, which seem to require such quick wits and a complete command of the material. In practice, however, most patients are desperately searching for help and are very willing to cooperate if they are given an opportunity, as indicated by the following example.

Another subject, a graduate in psychology, experienced great difficulty in going into a deep trance. After several hours of intensive effort, she timidly inquired if she could advise on technique, even though she had no other experience with hypnosis. Her offer was gladly accepted, whereupon she gave counsel: "You're talking too fast on that point; you should say that very slowly and emphatically and keep repeating it. Say that very rapidly and wait awhile and then repeat it slowly; and please, pause now and then to let me rest, and please don't split your infinitives."

With her aid, a profound, almost stuporous trance was secured in less than thirty minutes. Thereafter, she was employed extensively in a great variety of experimental work and was used to teach others how to induce deep trances.

Acceptance of such help is neither an expression of ignorance nor of incompetence; rather, it is an honest recognition that deep hypnosis is a joint endeavor in which the subject does the work and the hypnotist tries to stimulate the subject to make the necessary effort. It is an acknowledgment that no person can really understand the individual patterns of learning and response of another. While this measure works best with highly intelligent, seriously interested subjects, it is also effective with others. It establishes a feeling of trust, confidence, and active participation in a joint task. Moreover, it serves to dispel misconceptions of the mystical powers of the hypnotist and to indirectly define the respective roles of the subject and the hypnotist.

This acceptance and utilization of the patient's help is the cardinal feature of our approach, which contrasts sharply with the older, authoritarian methods that are still ingrained in the imagination of the laity and the popular press. The earlier, misguided approach that makes trance experience synonmous with passive obedience is, unfortunately, still being promulgated by stage hypnotists. More than a generation ago, however, the senior author illustrated how the patient's cooperation and self-control are of essence in good hypnotic work, as can be seen in the utilization of emergency situations described in the following section.

2. Utilizing Emergency Situations

Emergency situations are invariably trance-inducing. Cheek (Cheek and LeCron, 1968; Cheek, 1959, 1966, 1969, 1974) has illustrated how many iatrogenic problems and neurotic symptoms can be learned by overhearing unfortunate remarks during emergency and stress situations when the patient had lapsed into a spontaneous trance (as a primitive protective response to danger) and was consequently in an unusually heightened state of suggestibility.

The senior author has illustrated how such emergency situations can be utilized to gradually introduce therapeutic suggestions. Two examples with his own children are as follows.

Seven-year-old Allan fell on a broken bottle and severely lacerated his leg. He came rushing into the kitchen crying loudly from pain and fright, shouting, "It's bleeding, it's bleeding!"

As he entered the kitchen, he seized a towel and began swabbing wildly to wipe up the blood. When he paused in his shouting to catch his breath, he was urgently told, "Wipe up that blood; wipe up that blood; use a bath towel; use a bath towel; use a bath towel; a bath towel, not a hand towel, a bath towel." and one was handed to him. He dropped the towel he had already used. He was immediately told urgently and repetitiously, "Now wrap it around your leg, wrap it tightly, wrap it tightly."

This he did awkwardly but sufficiently effectively. Thereupon, with continued urgency, he was told, "Now hold it tightly, hold it tightly, let's get in the car and go to the doctor's office; hold it tightly."

All the way to the surgeon's office, careful explanation was given him that his injury was really not large enough to warrant as many stitches as his sister had had at the time of her hand injury. However, he was urgently counselled and exhorted that it would be entirely his responsibility to see to it that the surgeon put in as many stitches as possible. All the way there, he was thoroughly coached on how to emphatically demand his full rights.

Without awaiting any inquiry, Allan emphatically told the nurse at the surgeon's office that he wanted 100 stitches. She merely said, "This way, sir, right to the surgery." Allan was told, as she was followed, "That's just the nurse. The doctor is in the next room. Now don't forget to tell him everything just the way you want it."

As Allan entered the room, he announced to the surgeon. "I want 100 stitches. See!" Whipping off the towel, he pointed at his leg and declared, "Right there, 100 stitches. That's a lot more than Betty Alice had. And don't put them too far apart. And don't get in my way. I want to see. I've got to count them. And I want black thread, so you can see it. Hey, I don't want a bandage. I want stiches!"

It was explained to the surgeon that Allan understood well his situation and needed no anesthesia. To Allan, the writer explained that his leg would first have to be washed. Then he was to watch the placing of the sutures carefully to make sure they were not too far apart; he was to count each one carefully and not to make any mistakes in his counting.

Allan counted the sutures and rechecked his counting while the surgeon performed his task in puzzled silence. He demanded that the sutures be placed closer together and complainingly lamented the fact that he would not have as many as his sister. His parting statement was to the effect that, with a little more effort, the surgeon could have given him more sutures.

On the way home, Allan was comforted regarding the paucity of the sutures and adequately complimented on his competence in overseeing the entire procedure so well. It was also suggested that he eat a big dinner and go to sleep right afterwards. Thus his leg could heal faster and he would not have to go to the hospital the way his sister did. Full of zeal, Allan did as suggested.

No mention of pain or anesthesia was made at any time nor were any "comforting reassurances" offered. Neither was there any formal effort to induce a trance. Instead, various aspects of the total situation were utilized to distract Allan's attention completely away from the painful considerations and to focus it upon values of importance to a seven-year-old boy in order to secure his full, active cooperation and intense participation in dealing with the entire problem adequately.

In situations such as this, the patient experiences a tremendously urgent need to have something done. Recognition of this need, and a readiness to utilize it by doing something in direct relationship to the origin of the need, constitutes a most effective type of suggestion in securing the patient's full cooperation for adequate measures.

Little Roxanna came into the house sobbing, distressed by an inconsequential (but not to her) scratch upon her knee. Adequate therapy was not assurance that the injury was too minor to warrant treatment, nor even the statement that she was mother's brave little girl and that mother would kiss her and the pain would cease and the scratch would heal. Instead, effective therapy was based upon the utilization of the personality need for something to be done in direct relationship to the injury. Hence, a kiss *to the right*, a kiss *to the left* and a kiss *right on top* of the scratch effected for Roxie an instantaneous healing of the wound and the whole incident became a part of her thrilling historical past.

This type of technique based upon the utilization of strong personality needs is effective with children and adults. It can readily be adapted to situations requiring in some way strong, active, intense responses and participation by the patient.

As can be seen from these examples, the hypnotherapist is continually utilizing the patient's own internal frames of reference even in such "outer" emergency situations. Further illustrations of this all-important use of the patient's inner realities are presented in the next section.

3. Utilizing the Patient's Inner Realities

The utilization of patients' outer manifest behaviors can be generalized to an acceptance and utilization of their inner realities—their thoughts, feelings, and life experiences. The senior author illustrates this in the following.

Another type of utilization technique is the employment of the patient's inner, as opposed to outer, behavior; that is, using his thoughts and understandings as the basis for the induction procedure. This technique has been employed experimentally and also in therapeutic situations where the patient's type of resistances made it advisable. It has also been effectively used on naive subjects. Ordinarily, good intelligence and some degree of sophistication as well as earnestness of purpose are required.

The procedure is relatively simple. The experimental or therapeutic subject is either asked or allowed to express freely his thoughts, understandings, and opinions. He is then encourged to speculate aloud more and more extensively upon what could be the possible course of his thinking and feeling if he were to develop a trance state. As the patient does this, or even if he merely protests the impossibility of such speculation, his utterances are repeated after him in their essence as if the operator were either earnestly seeking further understanding or confirming his statements. Thus, further comment by the subject is elicited and repeated in turn by the operator. In the more sophisticated subject, there tends to be greater spontaneity; but occasionally the naive, even uneducated subject may prove to be remarkably responsive.

With this technique, the patient's utterances may vary greatly from one instance to another, but the following example is given in sufficient detail to illustrate the method.

This patient, in seeking psychiatric help, declared, "I've made no progress at all in three years of psychoanalysis, and the year I spent in hypnotherapy was also a total loss. I didn't even go into a trance. I tried hard enough. I just got nowhere. I've been referred to you and I don't see much sense in it. Probably another failure. I just can't conceive of myself going into a trance. I don't even know what a trance is." These remarks, together with the information received previously from the referring physician, suggested the possbility of employing the woman's own verbalization as the induction procedure.

The writer's utterances are in italics:

You really can't concieve of what a trance is—no, I can't, what is it?—*yes, what is it?*—a psychological state, I suppose—*A psychological state you suppose, what else?*—I don't know—*you really don't know*—no, I don't—*you don't, you wonder, you think*—think what—*yes, what do you think, feel, sense?*— (pause)—I don't know—*but you can wonder*—do you go to sleep?—*no, tired, relaxed, sleepy*—really tired—*so very tired and relaxed, what else?*—I'm puzzled—*puzzles you, you wonder, you think, you feel, what do you feel?*—my eyes—*yes, your eyes, how?*—they seem blurred—*blurred, closing*—(pause)—they are closing—*closing, breathing deeper*—(pause)—*tired and relaxed, what else?*—(pause)—*sleep, tired, relaxed, sleep, breathing* *deeper—(pause)—what else—*I feel funny—*funny, so comfortable, really learning—(pause)—learning, yes, learning more and more—(pause)—eyes closed, breathing deeply, relaxed, comfortable, so very comfortable, what else?—(pause)—*I don't know—*you really don't know, but really learning to go deeper and deeper—(pause)—*too tired to talk, just sleep—*maybe a word or two—*I don't know (spoken laboriously)—*breathing deeper and you really don't know, just going deeper, sleeping soundly, more and more soundly, not caring, just learning, continuing ever deeper and deeper and learning more and more with your unconscious mind.*

From this point on it was possible to deal with her simply and directly without any special elaborations of suggestions. Subsequent trances were secured through the use of posthypnotic suggestions.

The above is simply a condensation of the type of utterances utilized to induce trance. In general, there is much more repetition, usually only of certain ideas, and these vary from patient to patient. Sometimes this technique proves to be decidedly rapid. Frequently with anxious, fearful patients, it serves to comfort them with a conviction that they are secure, that nothing is being done to them or being imposed upon them, and they feel that they can comfortably be aware of every step of the procedure. Consequently, they are able to give full cooperation which would be difficult to secure if they were to feel that a pattern of behavior was being forcibly imposed upon them.

As can be seen from the above, the patient's experience of *not knowing*, "I don't know what trance is," can be an ideal starting point for initiating trance and the exploration of inner realities. The following is a further illustration of how a patient's life experiences can be used to facilitate trance induction.

A volunteer subject at a lecture before a university group declared, "I was hypnotized once several years ago. It was a light trance, not very satisfactory, and while I would like to cooperate with you, I'm quite certain that I can't be hypnotized." "Do you recall the physical setting of that trance?" "Oh yes, it was in the psychology laboratory of the university I was then attending." "Could you, as you sit here, recall and describe to me the physical setting of that trance situation?"

He agreeably proceeded to describe in detail the laboratory room in which he had been lightly hypnotized, including a description of the chair in which he had sat, and a description of the professor who had induced the trance. This was followed by a comparable response to the writer's request that he describe in as orderly and as comprehensive a fashion as possible his recollection of the actual suggestions given him at that time and the responses he made to them.

Slowly, thoughtfully, the subject described an eye closure technique with suggestions of relaxation, fatigue, and sleep. As he progressed in verbalizing his recollections, his eyes slowly closed, his body relaxed, his speech became slower and more hesitant; he required increasingly more prompting until it became evident that he was in a trance state. Thereupon, he was asked to state where he was and who was present: He named the previous university and the former professor. Immediately, he was asked to listen carefully to what the writer had to say also, and he was then employed to demonstrate the phenomena of the deep trance.

The junior author has found that questions focusing on memories can be a reliable means of assessing the patient's availability for trance and frequently a fine means of facilitating the actual induction of trance. When one woman was asked about her earliest memory, for example, she first responded with one that was long familiar to her. When she was encouraged to explore further, she paused for a few moments, manifesting that inner focus we call the common everyday trance, and then quietly remarked how she seemed to be looking up at a bright light, with nothing else in focus. A moment later her left leg began levitating, while the rest of her body remained immobile but noticeably relaxed. She then reported that she felt a scream building up in her throat. With that she suddenly shook her head, shuffled her body, and obviously reoriented to the awake state. In her inner search for an earlier memory she had spontaneously fallen into a trance and momentarily experienced a genuine age regression to infancy, when her visual field and her body were apparently not entirely under voluntary control, and she felt herself about to cry as an infant might. That frightened her, so she spontaneously reoriented to the awake state.

Although we do not often get responses as dramatic as this, we frequently find that questions focusing patients on an inner review of their lives and activities facilitate that inner search and the unconscious processes in a manner that leads to a recognizably therapeutic trance.

4. Utilizing the Patient's Resistances

The unfortunate dominance-submission view of hypnosis is probably the basis of much of the so-called resistance to hypnosis. Because of this the senior author developed many utilization approaches and indirect forms of suggestion to cope with this resistance. His approach is essentially the same as that oulined in the earlier section, where he first recognizes and accepts the patient's manifest behavior as a foundation for establishing rapport, and then gradually focuses the patient inward.

Many times, the apparently active resistance encountered in subjects is no more than an unconscious measure of testing the hypnotist's willingness to meet them halfway instead of trying to force them to act entirely in accord with his ideas. Thus, one subject, who had been worked with unsuccessfully by several hypnotists, volunteered to act as a demonstration subject. When her offer was accepted, she seated herself on the chair facing the audience in a stiffly upright, challenging position. This apparently unpropitious behavior was met by a casual, conversational remark to the audience that hypnosis was not necessarily dependent upon complete relaxation or automatism, but that hypnosis could be induced in a willing subject if the hypnotist was willing to fully accept the subject's behavior. The subject responded to this by rising and asking if she could be hypnotized standing up. Her inquiry was countered by the suggestion, "Why not demonstrate that it can be?" A series of suggestions resulted in the rapid development of a deep trance. Inquiries by the audience revealed that she had read extensively on hypnosis and objected strenuously to the frequently encountered misconception of the hypnotized person as a passively responsive automaton, incapable of self-expression. She explained further that it should be made clear that spontaneous behavior was fully as feasible as responsive activity and that utilization of hypnosis could be effected by recognition of this fact.

It should be noted that the reply, "Why not demonstrate that it can be?" constituted an absolute acceptance of her behavior, committed her fully to the experience of being hypnotized, and ensured her full cooperation in achieving her own purposes as well as those of the hypnotist.

Throughout the demonstration, she frequently offered suggestions to the author about what he might next ask her to demonstrate, sometimes actually altering the suggested task. At other times, she was completely passive in her responses.

Again we see how an apparently simple question with a negative—"Why *not* demonstrate that it can be?"—immediately accepts and utilizes the patient's "resistance," while initiating her into an inner search that evokes partially conscious and partially unconscious processes leading to hypnotic responses. We can see that her so-called resistance is really not a resistance so much as it is a perfectly reasonable reaction against the erroneous dominance-submission view of hypnosis.

We believe that most so-called resistances have some reasonable basis within the patient's own frame of reference. *Resistance is usually an expression of the patient's individuality*! The therapist's task is to understand, accept, and utilize that individuality to help patients bypass their learned limitations to achieve their own goals. This example is a particularly clear illustration of how a patient is really in control, while the therapist is simply a provider of useful stimuli and frames of reference that help a patient experience and express new potentialities. We see how it can be perfectly appropriate for the patient to reject or modify the therapist's suggestions in order to more adequately meet the patient's needs.

In the following example the senior author makes extensive use of the indirect forms of suggestion to utilize the patient's "resistance" in order to facilitate trance and hypnotic responsiveness. It is an unusually clear illustration of that curious blend of both leading and following the patient that is so characteristic of the senior author's approach.

One often reads in the literature about subject resistance and the techniques employed to circumvent or overcome it. In the author's experience, the most satisfactory procedure is that of accepting and utilizing the resistance as well as any other type of behavior, since properly used they can all favor the development of hypnosis. This can be done by wording suggestions in such a fashion that a positive or a negative response, or an absence of response, are all defined as responsive behavior. For example, a resistive subject who is not receptive to suggestions for hand levitation can be told, "Shortly your right hand, or it may be your left hand, will begin to lift up, or it may press down, or it may not move at all, but we will wait to see just what happens. Maybe the thumb will be first, or you may feel something happening in your little finger, but the really important thing is not whether your hand lifts up or presses down or just remains still; rather, it is your ability to sense fully whatever feelings may develop in your hand."

With such wording absence of motion, lifting up, and pressing down are all covered, and any of the possibilities constitutes responsive behavior. Thus a situation is created in which the subject can express his resistance in a constructive, cooperative fashion; manifestation of resistance by a subject is best utilized by developing a situation in which resistance serves a purpose. Hypnosis cannot be resisted if there is no hypnosis attempted. The hypnotist, recognizing this, should so develop the situation that any opportunity to manifest resistance becomes contingent upon hypnotic reponses with a localization of all resistance upon irrelevant possibilities. The subject whose resistance is manifested by failure to levitate his hand can be given suggestions that his right hand will levitate, his left hand will not. To resist successfully, contrary behavior must be manifested. The result is that the subject finds himself responding to suggestion, but to his own satisfaction. In the scores of instances where this measure has been employed, less than a half dozen subjects realized that a situation had been created in which their ambivalence had been resolved. One writer on hypnosis naively employed a similar procedure in which he asked subjects to resist going into a trance in an effort to demonstrate that they could not resist hypnotic suggestion. The subjects cooperatively and willingly proved that they could readily accept suggestions to prove that they could not. The study was published in entire innocence of its actual meaning.

Whatever the behavior offered by the subject, it should be accepted and utilized to develop further responsive behavior. Any attempt to "correct" or alter the subject's behavior, or to force him to do things he is not interested in, militates against trance induction and certainly against deep trance experience. The very fact that a subject volunteers to be hypnotized and then offers resistance indicates an ambivalence which, when recognized, can be utilized to serve successfully the purposes of both the subject and the hypnotist. Such recognition of and concession to the needs of the subject and the utilization of his behavior do not constitute, as some authors have declared, an "unorthodox technique" based upon "clinical intuition;" instead, such an approach constitutes a simple recognition of existing conditions, based upon full respect for the subject as a uniquely functioning personality.

The reader will recognize the use of many indirect forms of suggestion such as covering all possibilities of a class of responses, contingency suggestions, and double binds in the above. These approaches are integrated by the senior author in the following example of a more comprehensive approach that can be adapted to practically any situation.

Another comparable Utilization Technique has been employed experimentally and clinically on both naive and experienced subjects. It has been used as a means of circumventing resistances, as a method of initial trance induction, and as a trance reinduction procedure. It is a technique based upon an immediate and direct elicitation of meaningful but unconsciously executed behavior which is separate and apart from consciously directed activity except that of interested attention. The procedure is as follows:

Depending upon the subject's educational background, a suitable casual explanation is given relating general concepts of the conscious and of the unconscious or subconscious minds. Similarly, a casual though carefully instructive explanation is given of ideomotor activity with a citing of familiar examples, including hand levitation.

Then, with utter simplicity, the subject is told to sit quietly, to rest his hands palm down on his thighs, and to listen carefully to a question that will be asked. This question, it is explained, can be answered only by his unconscious mind, not by his conscious mind. He can, it is added, offer a conscious reply, but such a reply will be only a conscious statement and not an actual reply to the question. As for the question itself, it can be any of several pertinent questions, and it is of no particular significance to the person. Its only purpose is to give the unconscious mind an opportunity to manifest itself in the answer given. The further explanation is offered that the answer to the question asked the unconscious mind will be an ideomotor response of one or the other hand lifting upward, that of the left signifying "no," and that of the right signifying "yes."

The question is then presented: "Does your unconscious mind think that you can go into a trance?" Further collaboration is offered: "Consciously you cannot know what your unconscious mind thinks or knows. But your unconscious mind can let your conscious mind discover what it thinks or understands by the simple process of causing a levitation of either the right or the left hand. Thus your unconscious mind can communicate in a visibly recognizable way with your conscious mind. Now just watch your hands and see what the answer is. Neither you nor I know what your unconscious mind thinks, but as you see one or the other of your hands lifting, you will know."

If there is much delay, additional suggestions can be given: "One of your hands is lifting. Try to notice the slightest movement, try to feel and to see it, to enjoy the sensation of its lifting and be pleased to learn what your unconscious thinks."

Regardless of which hand levitates, a trance state frequently of the somnambulistic type supervenes simultaneously. Usually, it is advisable to utilize, rather than to test, the trance immediately since the subject tends to arouse promptly. This is often best done by remarking simply and casually. "It is very pleasing to discover that your unconscious can communicate with your conscious mind in this way. There are many other things that your unconscious can learn to do. For example, now that it has learned that it can develop a trance state and to do so remarkably well, it can learn various trance phenomena. For instance, you might be interested in—." The needs of the situation can then be met.

This technique centers around the utilization of the subject's interest in his own unconscious activity. A "yes" or "no" situation is outlined concerning thinking, with action contingent upon that thinking and constituting an overt unconscious communication, a manifestation basic to, and an integral part of a hypnotic trance. In other words, it is necessary for the subject to go into a trance in order to discover the answer to the question.

Experienced subjects approached with this technique have recognized the situation immediately: How interesting! No matter which answer you give, you have to go into a trance first.''

Willing subjects disclose their unaffected interest from the beginning. Resistant subjects manifest their attitudes by difficulty in understanding the preliminary explanations, by asking repeatedly for instructions, and then by an anticipation of hand levitation by lifting the left hand voluntarily. Those subjects who object to trance induction in this manner tend to awaken at the first effort to test or to utilize the trance. Most of them, however, will readily go back into the trance when told, ''And you can go into a trance just as easily and quickly as your unconscious answered that question just by continuing to watch as your unconscious mind continues to move your hand up toward your face. As your hand moves up, your eyes will close, and you will go into a deep trance.'' In nearly all instances, the subject then develops a trance state.

An essential component of this technique is an attitude of utter expectancy, casualness, and simplicity on the part of the operator, which places the responsibility for any developments entirely upon the subjects.

The senior author begins by carefully *assessing the patient's background* and then uses concepts that fit the patient's frames of reference. He uses a process of *indirect associative focusing* as he discusses the concepts of the conscious and unconscious to lay a foundation for his later use of the *conscious-unconscious double bind*. Patients' *expectations* are then heightened as they are asked to prepare for a *question* that initiates an *inner search* for *unconscious processes* that will lead to an *ideomotor or ideosensory response*. There is an emphasis on the pleasure of learning and a continual *utilization of each patient's areas of interest*. The conscious-unconscious double bind is structured so that any response made is *contingent* on the development of trance. This first successful experience with ideomotor activity is then generalized into a recognizable trance induction with an *implied directive*, ''As your hand moves up, your eyes will close, and you will go into a deep trance.''

An example that dramatically illustrates how trance behavior can be manifest, even when the patient resists the idea of being in a trance, was recorded during a workshop of the American Society of Clinical Hypnosis in 1960. The senior author was giving a talk on the dynamics of hypnosis. During such a talk there is ample opportunity to intersperse many ideodynamic suggestions that cannot help but activate the described ideodynamic process at least partially within most members of the audience. After giving a demonstration of hand levitation, he describes the following occurrence:

"One of the subjects felt very, very strongly that she was not a good subject. As I observed that intensely rapt attention (*response attentiveness*) she was giving me, however, I could feel very strongly that she was a good subject. So I asked her to 'Give your unconscious mind the privilege of manifesting in some way that you are a good hypnotic subject but that you will not consciously recognize it. At the same time you can continue to function well at the conscious level. I might add that the manifestation might be obvious to the audience but not to you.' Even as she continued to focus closely on me and not the audience or anything else, she said, 'I'm not a good subject, and I don't believe you can convince me.

"At this point I was utilizing her resistance to let her think she was awake and not in a somnambulistic trance. But the very intensity of her absorption in watching my every move and following everything I said was a clue to her somnambulistic condition.

"I asked her again if I could put her into a trance, but she shook her head 'no,' she wouldn't cooperate. At that moment her left hand began levitating, but she did not see it because she was looking over toward me on the right.

"She laughed and joked with the doctors in the audience and said she did not like to feel she was being uncooperative, but she did feel she couldn't go into a trance. Remember, I told her to function very well at the conscious level and very well at the unconscious level. And there she was talking to me and talking to the audience in this fashion. I indicated to one of the doctors in the audience that he should come up and pinch her levitated left hand. He found that she had a total anesthesia in that left hand, that she was willing to swear to the group that she was wide awake and that she couldn't possibly be in a trance. The doctor then came around and pinched her right hand, and she said, 'Ouch, that hurts! Naturally I would feel a pinch.' She was pinched again on the left hand but did not feel it.

"What I wanted to demonstrate to the doctors there, and what I want to stress to you, is the separation of functioning that goes on all the time in the human body, separation at an intellectual level, separation at an emotional level, separation at a sensory level, just as you have forgotten the shoes on your feet at this moment and the glasses on your face."

This dramatic example illustrates the importance of the hypnotherapist's learning to recognize that state of rapt response attentiveness when the patient is, for all practical purposes, already in a trance state fixated on the therapist, no matter what may be said to the contrary. When the senior author observes this state of intense absorption on himself, he offers patients one or more forms of indirect suggestion that provides them with an opportunity for a hypnotic response. In this case he used a form of the conscious-unconscious double bind that enabled her unconscious to select a hypnotic manifestation (hand levitating that she had already been primed for by watching others), while allowing her conscious mind to keep its usual patterns of functioning. She was thus able to keep her "resistance" while manifesting good hypnotic responsiveness.

The following is another illustration wherein trance was induced even under the most resistant conditions, where the subject was a professional actor attempting to simulate hypnosis. Unknown to the senior author, at a lecture demonstration before a medical group, one of the subjects was a trained actor. He watched the other subjects carefully and then, in accord with previous secret arrangements with several people in the audience, he "simulated" hypnosis and demonstrated anesthesia, negative and positive auditory and visual hallucinations, and developed uncontrollable sneezing upon hallucinating goldenrod in bloom, at the request of one of the conspirators, relayed through the senior author. However, the senior author noted that the actor's manifestation of catalepsy was faulty, and his time relationships were wrong. Minor startle reflexes were noted, too, and the subject was observed to be controlling the involuntary tendency to turn his head toward the author when addressed from the side. Accordingly, he was asked to demonstrate hand levitation in response to carefully given suggestions. The actor did not show the usual time lag in response to suggestions of a "sudden little jerk or quiver." This served to convince the senior author that he was being hoaxed.

Accordingly, the subject was furnished with pencil and paper and instructed to do automatic writing and to do this automatic writing in the correct style of true automatic writing. The actor had never witnessed automatic writing; however, as he began writing, suggestions were offered of "writing slowly and better and better, writing automatically the sentence, '*This* is a beautiful day in June.' " The word "this" was repeated four times with strong intonations to fixate consciousness on it, while the rest of the sentence was said more softly and swiftly, so that it would tend to be missed by consciousness and fall into the unconscious. The word "this" was written in his ordinary script, but the rest of the sentence was written in the characteristic script of automatic writing. The actor subject was now beginning to experience some genuine trance behavior without realizing it. As he finished writing, the paper and pencil were removed from his sight and he was asked to "awaken *with an amnesia for trance events.*" He roused immediately and was asked to discuss hypnosis for the audience. With great satisfaction he proceeded to expose the hoax perpetrated upon the senior author to the amazement of the audience in general and the glee of the conspirators. The subject talked freely of what he had done and demonstrated his ability to sneeze at will.

After he had recounted everything except the automatic writing, this was shown to him and he was asked what he thought of it. He read the sentence aloud, stated that it was just a simple statement with no particular relevancy. Asked about the script, he observed that it appeared to be somewhat labored and juvenile. It soon became apparent to everyone that he had a total amnesia for the writing, that he was genuinely curious about the writing and why he was being questioned about it. When his amnesia had been adequately demonstrated, he was asked to "duplicate that writing exactly." He agreed readily, but as he took the pencil and set it to the paper, it was at once obvious that he had developed a trance state again (repeating trance behavior tends by association to reinduce trance). After he had written the sentence this second time, he was aroused with instructions for an amnesia for trance events. As he aroused, he resumed his mockery of the author for being so easily deceived. Again he was shown the writing. He recognized that he had seen the one sentence a few moments ago, but there was a second sentence that he had not seen before.

He was allowed to retain the amnesia for a week. In the meantime those physicians who had arranged for the hoax sought out the senior author and related the whole plan to deceive him and to determine if hypnotic phenomena could be deliberately and successfully imitated. They also stated that they had tried to convince the actor that he had done the automatic writing but had failed in their efforts. They added that they had arranged for the actor to meet the senior author again so that the hypnotic amnesia could be removed.

Their request was met to their satisfaction and to the amazement of the actor, who summarized the entire matter by the simple statement, "Well, it is obvious to me now that the best way to fake hypnosis is to go into a trance."

5. Utilizing the Patient's Negative Affects and Confusion

Most therapists are wary of a patient's negative affects, doubts, and confusion. Negative affects are usually seen as something that must be circumvented. The following is an illustration by the senior author of how negative affects can be utilized to induce trance and to facilitate therapeutic change.

A patient's misunderstandings, doubts, and uncertainties may also be utilized as the technique of induction. Exemplifying this approach are the instances of two patients, both college-trained women, one in her late 30's, the other in her early 40's. One patient expressed extreme doubt and uncertainty about the validity of hypnotic phenomena as applied to herself, but explained that her desperate need for help compelled her to try hypnosis as a remotely possible means of therapy.

The other declared her conviction that hypnosis and physiological sleep were identical and that she could not possibly go into a trance without first developing physiological sleep. This, she explained, would preclude therapy; yet she felt that hypnosis offered the only possible, however questionable, means of psychotherapy for her, provided that the hypnotherapy was so conducted as to preclude physiological sleep. That this was possible, she disbelieved completely.

Efforts at explanation were futile and served only to increase the anxiety and tension of both patients. Therefore an approach utilizing their misapprehensions was used. The technique, except for the emphasis employed, was essentially the same for both patients. Each patient was instructed that deep hypnosis would be induced. They were to cooperate in going into a deep trance by assessing, appraising, evaluating, and examining the validity and genuineness of each item of reality and each item of subjective experience that was mentioned. In so doing, the women were to feel under obligation to discredit and reject anything that seemed at all uncertain or questionable. For the one, emphasis was placed primarily upon subjective sensations and reactions with an interspersed commentary upon reality objects. For the other, attentiveness to reality objects as proof of wakefulness was emphasized with an interspersing of suggestions for subjective responses. In this manner, there was effected for each a progressive narrowing of the field of awareness and a corresponding increase in a dependence upon and a responsiveness to the writer. It became possible to induce in each a somnambulistic trance by employing a simple eye closure progressive relaxation technique slightly paraphrased to meet the special needs of each of the two patients.

The following sample of utterances, in which the emphasis is approximately evenly divided between subjective aspects and reality objects, is offered to illustrate the actual verbalization employed.

"As you sit comfortably in that chair, you can feel the weight of your arms resting on the arms of the chair. And your eyes are open and you can see the desk and there is only the ordinary blinking of the eyelids, which you may or may not notice, just as one may notice the feeling of the shoes on one's feet and then again forget about it. And you really know that you can see the bookcase and you can wonder if your unconscious has noted any particular book title. But now again you can note the feeling of the shoes on your feet as they rest on the floor, and at the same time you can become aware of the lowering of your eyelids as you direct your gaze upon the floor. And your arms are still resting their weight on the arms of the chair, and all these things are real and you can be attentive to them and sense them. And if you look at your wrist and then look at the corner of the room, perhaps you can feel or sense the change in your visual focus. Perhaps you can remember when, as a child, you may have played with the experience of looking at an object as if it were far off and then close by. And as associated memories of your childhood pass through your mind, they can range from simple memories to tired feelings because memories are real. They are things, even though abstract, as real as the chair and the desk, and the tired feeling that comes from sitting without moving, and for which one can compensate by relaxing the muscles and sensing the weight of the body, just as one can feel so vividly the weariness of the eyelids as fatigue and relaxation develop more and more. And all that has been said is real and your attention to it is real and you can feel and sense more and more as you give your attention to your hand or to your foot or the desk or your breathing or to the memory of the feeling of comfort some time when you closed your eyes to rest your gaze. And you know that dreams are real, that one sees chairs and trees and people and hears and feels various things in dreams and that visual and auditory images are as real as chairs and desks and bookcases that become visual images.'' In this way, with increasing frequency, the writer's utterances became simple, direct suggestions for subjective responses.

This technique of utilizing doubts and misunderstandings has been used with other patients and with experimental subjects. It is well suited to the use of hand levitation as a final development, since ideomotor activity within the visual range offers opportunity for excellent objective and subjective realities.

The above is an excellent illustration of the *interspersal approach* to introduce patients to their own subjective responses gradually and in a manner that *focuses attention inward* for trance. Associating their inner realities with outer objects, through which they could validate their experiences; enabled them to accept the former to a greater and greater degree. The senior author then uses a series of *open-ended suggestions* in a very general discussion of sensations, feelings, memories, dreams, and visual images as a means of *indirect associative and ideodynamic focusing* to deepen their involvement with whatever subjective realities were most available to them. The utilization of doubt and misunderstanding in the example serves as an introduction to a more general understanding of negative affects as indicators of personality change.

The experience of anxiety, confusion, doubt, uncertainty, and depression is characteristic of most patients involved in a process of growth and personality change (Rossi, 1967, 1968, 1971, 1972a, 1972b, 1973; Erickson, Rossi, and Rossi, 1976). Thus while the patient is uncomfortable with these manifestations, the therapist can recognize in them the hopeful indications of a much-needed process of personality transformation that is taking place within the patient. We could even conceptualize that the typical states of depression and uncertainty with which most people enter therapy are actually spontaneous manifestations of the second and third stages (depotentiating habitual conscious sets and unconscious search) of our general paradigm of trance induction and suggestion. They are entirely normal and necessary stages in the natural process of personality growth and transformation (Rossi, 1972a). Depression and uncertainty only take pathological forms when a problem is so overwhelming that one cannot work through these uncomfortable affects on one's own. In helping patients cope with these states we can again recognize how hypnotherapy can be understood as a facilitator of natural processes inherent in psychological growth.

6. Utilizing the Patient's Symptoms

Since the patient's symptom is usually a major focus of attention, we can sometimes utilize it to facilitate trance induction and rapidly resolve the problem. With this approach we are again utilizing each patient's inner realities—dominant frames of reference and fixed belief—to induce trance and facilitate therapy. Unusually elegant examples of this approach are the following, drawn from the senior author's work in teaching dentists:

A man in his thirties became interested in hypnosis and volunteered to act as a subject for some experimental studies at a university. In the first hypnotic session he discovered that he was an excellent hypnotic subject, but lost his interest in any further experimental studies.

Several years later he decided to have hypnosis employed by his dentist, since he needed extensive dental work and feared greatly the possibility of pain.

He entered a trance state for his dentist readily, developed an excellent anesthesia of the hand upon suggestion, but failed to be able to transfer this anesthesia or even an analgesia to his mouth in any degree. Instead, he seemed to become even more sensitive orally. Efforts to develop oral anesthesia or analgesia directly also failed.

Further but unsuccessful efforts were painstakingly made by the dentist and a colleague to teach this patient by various techniques how to develop anesthesia or analgesia. He could respond in this way only in parts of the body other than the mouth. He was then brought to this writer as a special problem.

A trance state was induced readily and the patient was casually reminded of his wish for comfort in the dental chair. Thereupon, he was instructed to be attentive to the instructions given him and to execute them fully.

Suggestions were then given him that his left hand would become exceedingly sensitive to all stimuli, in fact painfully so. This hyperesthetic state would continue until he received instructions to the contrary. Throughout its duration, however, adequate care would be exercised to protect his hand from painful contacts.

The patient made a full and adequate response to these suggestions. In additon to the hyperesthesia of the hand, and *entirely without any suggestion to that effect*, he spontaneously developed an anesthesia of his mouth, permitting full dental work with no other anesthetic agent.

Even in subsequent efforts anesthesia or analgesia could not be induced directly or purposely except as a part of the hyperesthesia-anesthesia pattern peculiar to that patient. However, this is not a single instance of this type of behavior. Other comparable cases have been encountered from time to time.

Apparently, psychologically, the patient's fixed understanding was that the dental work must absolutely be associated with hypersensitivity. When this rigid understanding was met, dental anesthesia could be achieved in a fashion analogous to the relaxation of one muscle permitting the contraction of another.

Hypnosis had been attempted repeatedly and unsuccessfully on a dentist's wife by her husband and several of his colleagues. Each time, she stated, she became "absolutely scared stiff, so I just couldn't move and then I'd start crying. I just couldn't do anything they asked. I couldn't relax, I couldn't do hand levitation. I couldn't shut my eyes; all I could do was be scared silly and cry."

A naturalistic approach employing "synergism" was utilized. A general summary of her situation was offered to her in the following words:

"You wish to have hypnosis utilized in connection with your dental work. Your husband and his colleagues wish the same, but each time hypnosis was attempted, you have failed to go into a trance. You got scared stiff and you cried. It would really be enough just to get stiff without crying. Now you want me to treat you psychiatrically, if necessary, but I don't believe it is. Instead, I will just put you in a trance so that you can have hypnosis for your dentistry."

She replied, "But I'll just get scared stiff and cry."

She was answered with, "No, you will first get stiff. That is the first thing to do and do it now. Just get more and more stiff, your arms, your legs, your body, your neck—completely stiff—even stiffer than you were with your husband."

"Now close your eyes and let the lids get stiff, so stiff that you can't open them."

Her responses were most adequate.

"Now the next thing you have to do is to get scared silly and then to cry. Of course, you don't want to do this, but you have to because you learned to, but don't do it just yet."

"It would be so much easier to take a deep breath and relax all over and to sleep deeply."

"Why don't you try this, instead of going on to getting scared silly and crying?"

Her response to this alternative suggestion was immediate and remarkably good.

The next suggestion was, "Of course you can continue to sleep deeper and deeper in the trance state and be relaxed and comfortable. But any time you wish, you can start to get scared stiff and silly and to cry. But maybe now that you know how to do so, you will just keep on being comfortable in the trance so that any dental or medical work you need can be done comfortably for you."

A simple posthypnotic suggestion to enable the induction of future trances was then given.

In both of these examples the therapist accepts the patient's dominant frame of reference (hypersensitivity in the first case and "scared stiff" in the second) and then utilizes it to introduce and facilitate therapeutic responses. He encourages the patients to do what they already know they can do and then displaces, transforms, or adds to it something they need to do. He uses questions, contingent suggestions, and associational networks to carry the patients from their well-rehearsed but maladaptive behaviors to the desired therapeutic responses. Other instructive examples that illustrate how this approach rapidly achieves therapeutic goals are as follows.

Another type of case in which this same general approach was utilized concerns a bride of a week, who desired a consummation of her marriage but developed a state of extreme panic with her legs in the scissors position at every attempt or offer of an attempt.

She entered the office with her husband, haltingly gave her story, and explained that something had to be done, since she was being threatened with an annulment. Her husband confirmed her story and added other descriptive details.

The technique used was essentially the same as that utilized in a half dozen similar instances.

She was asked if she were willing to have any reasonable procedure employed to correct her problem. Her answer was, "Yes, anything except that I mustn't be touched, because I just go crazy if I'm touched." This statement her husband corroborated.

She was instructed that hypnosis would be employed. She consented hesitantly, but again demanded that no effort be made to touch her.

She was told that her husband would sit continuously in the chair on the other side of the office and that the writer would also sit beside her husband. She, however, was personally to move her chair to the far side of the room, to sit down there and watch her husband continuously. Should either he or the writer at any time leave their chairs, she was to leave the room immediately, since she was sitting next to the office door.

Then she was to sprawl out in her chair, leaning far back with her legs extended, her feet crossed, and all the muscles fully tensed. She was to look at her husband fixedly until all she could see would be him, with just a view of the writer out of the corner of her eye. Her arms were to be crossed in front of her and her fists were to be tighty clenched.

Obediently she began this task. As she did so, she was told to sleep deeper and deeper, seeing nothing but her husband and the writer. As she slept more and more deeply, she would become scared and panicky, unable to move or to do anything except to watch both and to sleep more and more deeply in the trance, in direct proportion to her panic state.

This panic state, she was instructed, would deepen her trance, and at the same time hold her rigidly immobile in the chair.

Then gradually, she was told, she would begin to feel her husband touching her intimately, caressingly, even though she would continue to see him still on the other side of the room. She was asked if she were willing to experience such sensations and she was informed that her existing body rigidity would relax just sufficiently to permit her to nod or to shake her head in reply, and that an honest answer was to be given slowly and thoughtfully.

Slowly she nodded her head affirmatively.

She was asked to note that both her husband and the writer were turning their heads away from her, because she would now begin to feel a progressively more intimate caressing of her body by her husband, until finally she felt entirely pleased, happy and relaxed.

Approximately five minutes later she addressed the writer,

"Please don't look around. I'm so embarrassed. May we go home now, because I'm all right?"

She was dismissed from the office and her husband was instructed to take her home and passively await developments.

Two hours later a joint telephone call was received explaining simply, "Everything is all right."

A check-up telephone call a week later disclosed all to be well. Approximately 15 months later they brought their first-born in with greatest of pride.

Another example is that of an enuretic eight-year-old boy, half carried, half dragged into the office by his parents. They had previously solicited the aid of the neighbors on his behalf, and he had been prayed for publicly in church. Now he was being brought to a "crazy doctor" as the last resort with a promise of a "hotel dinner," to be provided following the interview.

His resentment and hostility toward all were fully apparent.

The approach was made by declaring "You're mad and you're going to keep right on being mad, and you think there isn't a thing you can do about it, but there is. You don't like to see a 'crazy doctor,' but you are here and you would like to do something, but you don't know what. Your parents brought you here, made you come. Well, you can make them get out of the office. In fact, we both can—come on, let's tell them to go on out." At this point the parents were unobtrusively given a dismissal signal, to which they readily responded, to the boy's immediate, almost startled, satisfaction.

The writer then continued, "But you're still mad and so am I, because they ordered me to cure your bedwetting. But they can't give me orders like they give you. But before we fix them for that"—*with a slow, elaborate, attention-compelling, pointing gesture*—"look at those puppies right there. I like the brown one best, but I suppose you like the black-and-white one, because its front paws are white. If you are very careful, you can pet mine, too. I like puppies, don't you?"

Here the child, taken completely by surprise, readily developed a somnambulistic trance, walked over, and went through the motions of petting two puppies, one more than the other. When finally he looked up at the writer, the statement was made to him, "I'm glad you're not mad at me any more and I don't think that you or I have to tell your parents anything. In fact, maybe it would serve them just right for the way they brought you here if you waited until the school year was almost over. But one thing is certain. You can just bet that after you've had a dry bed for a month, they will get you a puppy just about like little Spotty there, even if you never say a word to them about it. They've just got to. Now close your eyes, take a deep breath, sleep deeply, and wake up awful hungry.''

The child did as instructed and was dismissed in the care of his parents, who had been given instructions privately.

Two weeks later he was used as a demonstration subject for a group of physicians. No therapy was done.

During the last month of the school year, the boy each morning dramatically crossed off the current calendar day.

Toward the last few days of the month he remarked cryptically to his mother, ''You better get ready.''

On the 31st day, his mother told him there was a surprise for him. His reply was, ''It better be black-and-white.'' At that moment his father came in with a puppy. In the boy's excited pleasure he forgot to ask questions.

Eighteen months later the boy's bed was still continuously dry.

A careful study of these examples reveals the same pattern. In each case the senior author associates (1) what patients can do well with (2) trance behavior in which (3) they can now experience what they want in a hallucinated inner reality. This binds their real behavioral capacities to hallucinated wishes so that the wishes can become actualized. Therapeutic trance is the binding glue, the state of concentration or the medium in which fantasies and wishes are associated and bound to behavioral capacities so that what is desired can be actualized in real behavior. In hypnotherapeutic practice we are continually building bridges between what patients can do and what they want to do. This will become more and more evident in the next chapter on posthypnotic suggestion and in practically all the case studies that follow.

Exercises

1. Listen to tape recordings of your therapy sessions and determine to what degree you are utilizing the patients' own behaviors, interests, and personality characteristics to facilitate their therapeutic work.

2. As you study these recordings, consider where you might have introduced alternative remarks and suggestions that could utilize the patient's repository of life experiences and more highly developed functions to facilitate therapeutic progress. Explore those forms of indirect suggestions that fit easily within your own verbal repertory so that you can utilize them most effectively to facilitate the patient's inner searches and unconscious processes even without the formal induction of trance.

3. Study video recordings of your therapy sessions to discover

those moments of rapt response attentiveness when your patient was most focused on you. How well did you utilize these moments to introduce therapeutic remarks?

4. Plan how you could use these moments of response attentiveness to introduce indirect forms of suggestions that could facilitate free association related to therapeutic issues. Some simple examples are as follows.

Do your eyes feel like resting and closing for a moment while your unconscious mind explores that [*whatever*]?

I want you to be quiet for a moment, and as you think that over we will see what else your unconscious mind brings up about it. And you don't have to talk until you really feel comfortable about it.

Therapists must find the combination of words that is natural to them and their patients in order to facilitate the inner search and unconscious processes in a casual and comfortable manner.

5. The above approach easily lends itself to indirect forms of trance induction. During those moments of common everyday trance when the patients may be apparently absorbed within themselves, looking out a window, staring at their hands, the floor, the ceiling, or whatever, therapists can introduce options for trance via indirect forms, such as the following:

You are absorbed in something now, and if your unconscious agrees that this is a comfortable moment for you to enter trance, you will find that your eyes will seem to close all by themselves.

Does your unconscious want those eyes to close so you can just continue as you are even more comfortably?

Just let yourself continue as you are and your body won't even have to move until your unconscious has a surprising solution to that, even though your conscious mind may not yet know what it is, exactly.

During a moment of rapt response attentiveness, when the patient's attention is focused on the therapist, trance could be introduced as follows:

I know you are not entirely aware of it, but I'm noticing something about you that indicates you may be ready to enter trance. And if your unconscious really wants to, you'll find those eyelids closing [*handlifting, or whatever*].

6. Absolutely refuse to permit yourself to use any ritualized and mechanical form of hypnotic induction until you have noticed half a dozen or more of the patient's patterns of manifest behavior, interests, abilities, inner life experiences, frames of reference, "resistances," or symptoms that you can incorporate into the induction procedure. Then practice the process of integrating each patient's individuality into all the standard forms of trance induction such as eye fixation, hand levitation, and so on.

7. Study the patient's manifest behavior and symptoms to determine how they can be channeled into therapeutic responses. Practice building associative bridges between the known and possible to the unknown and desired.

8. Further study in the lore of hypnotic induction comes from many unexpected quarters. A volume on hypnotic poetry (Snyder, 1930), for example, presents the thesis that there are two basic types of poetry: hypnotic (spell-weaving) and intellectualistic. The former tends to induce trance, while the latter appeals more to the intellect. The author discusses many of the literary devices that may induce a hypnotic effect, such as (1) a perfect pattern of sound and stress, with heavy vocal stress falling at half-second intervals; (2) absence of abrupt changes or intellectual challenges; (3) vagueness of imagery, permitting each individual's personal unconscious to fill in the details; (4) fatigue for what we would call "depotentiating habitual mental frameworks"; (5) the use of repetition or refrain; and (6) giving an unusually clear and direct suggestion or posthypnotic suggestion only after lulling the listener into an agreeable state with the foregoing. He goes on to point out how poetic inspiration and perhaps artistic creation in general always involve an autohypnotic state. A careful study of the poems he presents gives the hypnotherapist a broader conception of the creative work involved in every hypnotic induction.

9. Classical studies like the above lend credence to the many current efforts to understand trance as a function of the specialized activities and interaction patterns of the left and right cerebral hemispheres (Ornstein, 1972, 1973; Hilgard and Hilgard, 1975; Bandler and Grinder, 1975; Erickson, Rossi, and Rossi, 1976; Rossi, 1977). Analyze the inductions in this and the remaining chapters of this volume for their relative appeal to the left and right hemisphere. We have introduced a number of speculations in this area in our commentaries on Case 12 in Chapter 9. volume.

CHAPTER 4

Posthypnotic Suggestion

Traditionally, posthypnotic suggestion has been used to assess the effectiveness of trance and to reinforce a therapeutic process. It was believed that a person who receives a suggestion during trance and then carries it out afterward proves by that very fact that an effective trance was experienced. Trance was conceptualized as a blank state during which an individual was easily programmed just as one might write upon a blank slate. We now recognize that this blank slate and programming model of hypnosis is misleading for psychotherapeutic work. Individuals retain their own personality dynamics during trance. Therapeutic trance is a means of focusing attention and utilizing personality dynamics in a manner that permits unconscious processes to mediate responses that are of clinical value. In the broadest sense we can speak of posthypnotic suggestion whenever we introduce an idea during a moment of receptivity that is later actualized in behavior. That moment of receptivity can occur during a formally induced trance or during the *common everyday trance* in which attention is fixed and absorbed in a matter of great interest.

1. Associating Posthypnotic Suggestions with Behavioral Inevitabilities

The traditional approach to direct posthypnotic suggestion usually takes the form, "After you awaken from trance, you will do [*or experience*] such and such." Indirect posthypnotic suggestion, by contrast, involves the use of the indirect forms of suggestion together with a number of other processes found in everyday life as well as clinical practice. The most useful of these are contingency suggestions and associational networks, whereby we tie the posthypnotic suggestion to inevitable patterns of behavior that the patient will experience in the future. These inevitable behavior patterns function as cues or vehicles for the execution of the posthypnotic suggestion. The patient's own associations, life experience, personality dynamics, and future prospects are all utilized to build the posthypnotic suggestion into the patient's natural life structure. An example from the senior author's own family life can introduce us to this concept of indirect posthypnotic suggestion in its broadest sense.

The first time an orthodontist worked on a daughter of mine I said to her, "You know, all of that baling wire in your mouth is miserably uncomfortable." Why shouldn't I tell her the truth? She knew it, she was certain of it. I then said to her, "That mouthful of hardware that you've got with all those rubber bands is wretchedly miserable, *and it's going to be a deuce of a job to get used to it.*" Well, what did I suggest? *You will get used to it. Getting used to it* was the indirect suggestion. She heard me agreeing with her misery, but her unconscious also heard the rest of the sentence. Always know how inclusive, how comprehensive your statement is. *It is a deuce of a job to get used to it.* When you put it that way, she accepts both parts of the sentence, though she doesn't know she has accepted the second part. Then I told her, "You are only a little girl now, but what kind of a smile do you think you will have in your wedding picture?" Mrs. Erickson and I kept that posthypnotic suggestion in mind for a long time until she was married. We never ever betrayed it by talking about it or telling anyone. When our daughter got married ten years later and saw her wedding pictures, she said, "Daddy, this is my favorite one. Look at the smile." That was an indirect posthypnotic suggestion that worked over a period of ten years even though she could not recognize it as such. When she first went to the orthodontist, marriage was the farthest thing from her mind. She wasn't thinking of marriage at all, but she did know that women get married and there was the remote possibility that she was making the beautiful smile she would have in her wedding picture. That's what goes into the most effective posthypnotic therapeutic suggestion. When you offer a posthypnotic suggestion in the form of a hopeful prognosis to a patient, tie it to a reasonable future contingency. Marriage was a reasonable expectation for us to entertain regarding our daughter.

This example illustrates a number of basic principles for offering posthypnotic suggestion. The process was initiated, as always, by first recognizing and fully acknowledging the individual's current ongoing experience. The daughter's attention was immediately fixated when her father gave expression to the current reality by acknowledging her misery over her new orthodontic treatment. He then utilized a compound statement to tie his indirect suggestion "getting used to it" to her ongoing and undeniable reality. He then reinforced the suggestion even further by associating it with a reasonable future contingency, when "getting used to it" would be rewarded with a beautiful smile on her wedding day. Four major factors facilitating this posthypnotic suggestion can be listed as follows:

1. *Fixing attention and opening a yes set* by recognizing and acknowledging current experience.
2. Associating a suggestion with this current experience by way of an *indirect hypnotic form* (compound suggestion).
3. *Utilizing* the person's own personality dynamics (need for a nice smile on her wedding day) as a vehicle for the suggestion.
4. *Associating the suggestion with a reasonable future contingency* (her future wedding).

A number of other illustrations of posthypnotic suggestions associated with behavioral inevitabilities are as follows. The suggestion proper is in italics:

Shortly after you awaken, *I'm going to say something to you.*

I'm going to arouse you and *put you back into trance.*

In spite of any thinking you do, *what I say will be true.*

2. Serial Posthypnotic Suggestions

It is most instructive to realize that it is more difficult to reject two or more suggestions given together in an associational network than it is to reject a single suggestion standing alone. Consider the following example by the senior author (Erickson and Erickson, 1941), which utilizes a five-year-old girl's interest in her favorite doll.

A five-year-old child who had never witnessed a hypnotic trance was seen alone by the hypnotist. She was placed in a chair and repeatedly told to *"go to sleep,"* and to *"sleep very soundly,"* while holding her favorite doll. No other suggestion of any sort was given her until after she had apparently slept soundly for some time. Then she was told, as a posthypnotic suggestion, that some other day the hypnotist would ask her about her doll, whereupon she was to (a) place it in a chair, (b) sit down near it, and (c) wait for it to go to sleep. After several repetitions of these instructions, she was told to awaken and to continue her play. This three-fold form of posthypnotic suggestion was employed, since obedience to it would lead progressively to an essentially static situation for the subject. Particularly did the last item of behavior require an indefinitely prolonged and passive form of response, which could be best achieved by a continuation of the spontaneous posthypnotic trance.

Several days later she was seen while at play, and a casual inquiry about her doll was made. Securing the doll from its cradle, she exhibited it proudly and then explained that the doll was tired and wanted to go to sleep, placing it as she spoke in the proper chair and sitting down quietly beside it to watch. She soon gave the appearance of being in a trance state, although her eyes were still open. When asked what she was doing, she replied, "Waiting," and nodded her head agreeably when told insistently, "Stay just like you are and keep on waiting." Systematic investigation, with an avoidance of any measure that might cause a purely responsive manifestation to a specific but unintentional hypnotic suggestion, led to the discovery of a wide variety of the phenomena typical of the ordinarily induced trance.

A series of subtle posthypnotic suggestions suitable for facilitating the trance training and the reinduction of trance for adults might run somewhat as follows.

1. **When you awaken, you will open your eyes. . .**
2. **Move and perhaps stretch a bit. . .**
3. **You can talk a bit about what interests you in your experience. . .**
4. **And forget all the rest. . .**
5. **Until I ask you to go back into trance. . .**
6. **So you can experience and remember something more.**

The first three lines of the above are a series of truisms that together form an associational network of behaviors that are inevitabilities. Since they are inevitable, they tend to initiate a yes set within the patient, who probably won't even recognize line 4 as a subtle suggestion for hypnotic amnesia. Line 5 is a fairly direct posthypnotic suggestion to reenter trance that contains an important contingency with the word "until." "Until" means that on reentering trance the patient will remember something forgotten due to a hypnotic amnesia when he was awake. Line 6 continues the associational network binding a future trance with the current experience, and it also contains a subtle ambiguity: Will the patient merely experience and recall what was lost in the amnesia, or will there be a new experience that will then be recalled? Will it be recalled only during trance or after trance as well? The therapist usually does not know the answers to these questions—they are a means of exploring the patient's unique system of responding. If it is found that significant amnesias are present that can be lifted by further suggestion, the therapist may decide to utilize this ability therapeutically. If new experience is forthcoming with each trance, this may become the ideal therapeutic modality for helping patients explore their inner worlds.

3. Unconscious Conditioning as Posthypnotic Suggestion

Most therapists automatically alter the tone and cadence of their voice during trance work. The patients, in turn, become automatically and usually unconsciously conditioned to experience trance in response to these vocal alterations. If the therapist adopts these vocal changes during an ordinary conversation, the patient will frequently begin to experience partial aspects of trance without quite knowing why. Since these minimal cues bypass the patient's conscious frames of reference, they are often surprisingly effective. When therapists notice these beginning manifestations of trance (e.g., eye blinking, minimal movements, blocking, some confusion, and so on), they can reinforce them with other nonverbal or verbal cues they typically use during the initial stages of trance induction. For example, when the patient is looking directly at the senior author during trance induction, he will frequently look directly at the patient's face but focus his eyes at a distance beyond. When he later does this during an ordinary conversation, the patient initially feels a bit disconcerted, then begins to experience a disorientation that can only be resolved by going into trance (Erickson, Rossi, and Rossi, 1976). At such moments the senior author may reinforce the process with a look of happy expectation and double bind questions such as the following:

I wonder just how awake you are now?

Just how much trance are you beginning to experience?

Is that a trance you're beginning to experience?

It's comfortable to just let that happen, isn't it?

You don't have to talk, do you? It's nice just to let yourself be.

When we begin to look into the matter, we realize that there are innumerable patterns of unconscious conditioning that are taking place between therapist and patient all the time. Many patients become conditioned unconsciously and automatically to begin the process of trance experience as soon as they enter the therapist's waiting room. The observant therapist need not engineer such patterns of unconscious conditioning or set them up intentionally. It is far more effective simply to observe them as they occur naturally and then to utilize them as important indicators of unconscious processes. Some patients, for example, position their bodies in certain characteristic ways during trance. Later, during an ordinary therapeutic session, the therapist may notice aspects of that trance position developing. Perhaps a head, arm, leg, hand, or finger falls into trance position. This may be a nonverbal and unconscious body signal that the patient is reexperiencing an association to trance on some level and now needs to do trance work. When therapists recognize these body cues, they can facilitate the process with an expectant look and questions somewhat like the following:

Are you aware of what's happening to you now?

Pause for a moment. Can you sense what's taking place within you?

Do you feel you are really completely awake?

How much trance are you beginning to experience?

When the patient's body language is, indeed, a signal that trance work needs to be done, the patient will frequently use the inner search initiated by these questions to enter more deeply into trance. If the body language meant something else (such as an important association to previous trance experience that now needs to be talked about), the therapist's question provides an opportunity for it to be expressed in the awake state or perhaps in a light trance state that is difficult to distinguish from the awake state.

4. Initiated Expectations Resolved Posthypnotically

A most effective approach to posthypnotic suggestion is to initiate expectations, tensions, or patterns of behavior that can only be completed or resolved after trance is formally terminated. This approach has experimental validation in numerous studies of the Zeigarnic effect (Woodworth and Schlosberg, 1954), which demonstrate how children will return to an uncompleted task after an interruption because of the tension or disequilibrium aroused by their set for closure. In the previous section we saw how unconscious conditioning could initiate partial aspects of trance that could only be resolved by the patient actually going into trance or that could only be resolved after trance by some therapeutic behavioral change. Our five-stage paradigm of the dynamics of trance induction and suggestion in Figure 1 is particularly evident in this approach (see page 4).

The senior author frequently uses this approach with patients experiencing trance for the first time. During their first trance he will casually remark how interesting and therapeutic it can be to experience a *"pleasant surprise."* He then obtains their willingness to experience a pleasant surprise after they awaken. A pleasant expectation is thus set up within the patients that can be resolved by a therapeutic shock or surprise after they awaken. This expectation is an unresolved tension that heightens their sensitivity to the therapeutic surprise that the therapist has planned. The expectation of a pleasant surprise tends to suspend patients' habitual sets and attitudes and to initiate unconscious searches and processes for the promised pleasant surprise.

After the patient has been awake for a while, the senior author guides the patient's hand and arm upward with a look of bemused expectation. The patient's arm usually remains suspended in midair because it has been given subtle but directive tactile cues to remain so (Erickson, Rossi, and Rossi, 1976). Patients usually do not recognize these tactile cues on a conscious level, however, so they are indeed surprised at the apparently peculiar behavior of their arms. The senior author will reinforce this surprise and imply that it means the patients are entering trance in fulfillment of the posthypnotic suggestion he gave previously with remarks such as the following:

Surprising, isn't it?

Does your hand always remain up when someone touches it?

And it can be a "pleasant surprise" to find yourself going back into trance without any effort.

Are your eyes beginning to close?

And that hand won't go down until the other hand goes up.

The patient's surprise and puzzlement about what is happening is essentially a confusion approach to depotentiating habitual conscious sets and frameworks so that an altered state is facilitated. In the following section we will further elaborate our conception of this use of surprise and expectation to facilitate the execution of therapeutic posthypnotic suggestions.

5. Surprise as a Posthypnotic Suggestion

Surprise in a posthypnotic suggestion heightens expectancy while providing a fail-safe channel for the expression of the patient's individuality after awakening. Consider the following posthypnotic suggestion, which is most appropriately offered at the end of a period of successful trance work during which the patient is in a positive mood and experiencing a yes set.

Would you like to experience a pleasant surprise after you awaken?

A patient who responds in the affirmative to this question (by head nodding, finger signaling, verbal response, smiling, and so on) is in the following situation:

1. The positive yes set of the trance work is carried over into the posthypnotic period.
2. Awakening is accompanied by a sense of heightened expectation and positive motivation to experience something new.
3. The patient's usual conscious sets do not know what the surprise, the new, will be. The patient's habitual conscious and limiting sets are therefore depotentiated in favor of something new that can only come from the patient's own unconscious. The suggestion for a "pleasant surprise" has been given in the form of a question which in itself initiates an unconscious search that may uncover and permit a new potential or another aspect of the patient's individuality to become manifest.
4. The suggestion tends to be fail-safe because whatever patients experience or report after a period of successful trance work can be accepted as a "pleasant surprise." If patients are happily excited, that can be a "pleasant surprise." If patients are more thoughtful and appear to lapse back into body immobility as they reflect on their trance experiences, the therapist can facilitate a surprise with a suggestion such as, "As you notice how quiet your body is, it may be surprising how easily your eyes can close as you go back into trance to reach a complete understanding of *that*." The therapist may not know what "that" is, but whatever it is can be facilitated.
5. When the patient experiences a surprise in some form after trance, a therapist's final comment such as "And that was a pleasant surprise, wasn't it?" tends to ratify the therapeutic work that has just taken place as well as the value of trance as a valid approach to solving problems.

A number of examples illustrating this surprise form of posthypnotic suggestion will be found in the cases of this book.

Exercises

1. Associating therapeutic suggestions with behavioral inevitabilities can be practical in everyday life as well as in the

consulting room. It is an approach particularly suitable for use with children provided the adult avoids sermonizing.

2. The serial posthypnotic suggestions require much thought and planning. Together with *contingency* suggestions, *associational networks*, and *double binds* they can constitute an almost impenetrable thicket for snagging practically any random association or behavioral potential the patient may have and holding it fast to the therapeutic endeavor. It becomes a fascinating exercise to interpenetrate each individual patient's *behavioral inevitabilities* with a serial pattern of suggestions so they mutually reinforce each other and, it is hoped, displace the patient's symptom.

3. Unconscious conditioning as posthypnotic suggestion requires a careful observation of patients' patterns of behavior and responsiveness whenever they come into the therapist's presence after having had a successful hypnotic experience. The therapist must then learn to follow up such careful observations with the type of questions that can facilitate inner search and deepening trance involvement. The beginner in this area may find it difficult to believe and to learn to see those spontaneous and conditioned patterns of trance behavior that develop in most patients when they meet the therapist again after a successful trance experience. Because of this it may be instructive to question every patient routinely on that "next meeting" in the manner suggested in this chapter. If ideomotor signaling has already been developed, it is very easy to ask within the first few minutes of that next meeting, "Now if you are already beginning to experience some trance, your right hand will lift" (or your eyes will close, and so on). It is important to assess the patient's state within the first few minutes of the next meeting, because after that, the initial conditioned response of trance may be rapidly extinguished, since it is displaced by the conventionalities of consciously relating to the therapeutic situation.

4. *Initiated expectations resolved posthypnotically* with *surprise* is a skill that develops along with the use of *contingent suggestions* and *associational networks*. They can be most easily learned by expressing the simple expectation of feeling rested and comfortable upon awakening. This is generally fail-safe, since such responses almost inevitable. To these inevitabilities one can gradually add suggestions particularly suited to the patient's needs and fitting the *patient's expectations* of what should be experienced.

CHAPTER 5

Altering Sensory-Perceptual Functioning: The Problem of Pain and Comfort

Recent clinical (Lassner, 1964; Melzack and Perry, 1975) and experimental research (Hilgard and Hilgard, 1975) has validated anew centuries of experience with the hypnotic alteration of sensory-perceptual functioning for coping with pain and facilitating comfort. Hypnotherapeutic approaches have been successful in reducing pain from obvious somatic sources (such as accidental physical trauma, surgery, dentistry, obstetrics, cancer, and so on) as well as psychosomatic problems. It has been established on an experimental basis that hypnotic pain relief is due to something more than the placebo effect (McGlashan, Evans, and Orne, 1969) or anxiety reduction (Hilgard and Hilgard, 1975). Since the usefulness of hypnosis in this area has been so well established, we will focus our attention on the practical approaches that have been developed by the senior author in clinical situations.

Introduction*

Hypnosis is essentially a communication to a patient of ideas and understandings in such a fashion that he will be most receptive to the presented ideas and thereby motivated to explore his own body potentials for the control of his psychological and physiological responses and behavior. The average person is unaware of his capacities for accomplishment which have been learned through the experimental conditionings of his body behavior throughout his life experiences. To the average person in his thinking, pain is an immediate subjective experience, all-encompassing of his attention, distressing, and to the best of his belief and understanding, an experience uncontrollable by the person himself. Yet as a result of experiential events of his past life,

---

*The following material was written by the senior author, and originally appeared in the *Proceedings of the International Congress for Hypnosis and Psychosomatic Medicine.* J. Lassner, (ed.) 1967.

there has been built up within his body, although all unrecognized, certain psychological, physiological, and neurological learnings, associations, and conditionings that render it possible for pain to be controlled and even abolished. One need only to think of extremely crucial situations of tension and anxiety to realize that the severest amount of pain vanishes when the focusing of the sufferer's awareness is compelled by other stimuli of a more immediate, intense, or life-threatening nature. From common experience, one can think of a mother suffering extremely severe pain and all-absorbed in her pain experience. Yet she forgets it without effort or intention when she sees her infant dangerously threatened or seriously hurt. One can think of men in combat who have been seriously wounded, but do not discover their injuries until later. Numerous such comparable examples are common to medical experience. Such abolition of pain occurs in daily life situations where pain is taken out of awareness by more compelling stimuli of another character. The simplest example of all is the toothache forgotten on the way to the dentist's office, or the headache lost in the suspenseful drama portrayed at the cinema. By such experiences as these in the course of a lifetime, be they major or minor, the body learns a wealth of unconscious psychological, emotional, neurological and physiological associations and conditionings. These unconscious learnings repeatedly reinforced by additional life experiences constitute the source of the potentials that can be employed through hypnosis to control pain intentionally without resorting to drugs.

Considerations Concerning Pain

While pain is a subjective experience with certain objective manifestations and accompaniments, it is not necessarily or solely a conscious experience. It occurs without conscious awareness in states of sleep, in narcosis, and even under certain types of chemoanesthesia as evidenced by objective accompaniments and as has been demonstrated by experimental hypnotic exploration of past experiences of patients. But because pain is primarily a conscious subjective phenomenon, with all manner of unpleasant, threatening, even vitally dangerous emotional and psychological significances and meanings, an approach to the problem can be made frequently through the use of hypnosis, sometimes easily, sometimes with great difficulty. Furthermore, the extent of the pain is not necessarily a factor.

In order to make use of hypnosis in dealing with pain, one needs to look upon pain in a most analytical fashion. Pain is not a simple uncomplicated noxious stimulus. It has certain temporal, emotional, psychological, and somatic significances. It is a compelling motivational force in life's experience. It is a basic reason for seeking medical aid.

Pain is a complex, a construct, composed of past remembered pain, of present pain experience, and of anticipated pain in the future. Thus, immediate pain is augmented by past pain and enhanced by the future possibilities of pain. The immediate stimuli are only a central third of the entire experience. Nothing so much intensifies pain as the fear that it will be present on the morrow. It is likewise increased by the realization that the same or similar pain was experienced in the past, and this and the immediate pain render the future even more threatening. Conversely the realization that the present pain is a single event which will definitely come to a pleasant ending serves greatly to diminish it. Because pain is a construct, it is more readily vulnerable to hypnosis as a successful treatment modality than it would be were it simply an experience of the present.

Pain as an experience is also rendered more susceptible to hypnosis because it varies in its nature and intensity and hence, through life experiences, it acquires secondary meanings resulting in varying interpretations of the pain. Thus the patient may regard his pain in temporal terms, such as transient, recurrent, persistent, acute, or chronic. These special qualities each offer varying possibilities of hypnotic approaches.

Pain also has certain emotional attributes. It may be irritating, all-compelling, troublesome, incapacitating, threatening, intractable, or vitally dangerous. Each of these aspects leads to certain psychological frames of mind with varying ideas and associations, each offering special opportunities for hypnotic intervention.

One must further bear in mind certain other very special considerations. Long continued pain in an area of the body may result in a habit of interpreting all sensations in that area as automatically painful. The original pain may be long since gone, but the recurrence of that pain experience has been conducive to a habit formation that may in turn lead to actual somatic disorders painful in character.

In a somewhat similar category are iatrogenic disorders and disease arising from a physician's poorly concealed concern and distress over his patient. Iatrogenic illness has a most tremendous significance because in emphasizing that there can be psychosomatic disease of iatrogenic origin, its converse cannot be overlooked: that iatrogenic health is fully as possible and of far greater importance to the patient. And since iatrogenic pain can be produced by fear, tensions, and anxiety, so can freedom from it be produced by the iatrogenic health that may be suggested hypnotically.

Pain as a protective somatic mechanism should not be disregarded as such. It motivates the patient to protect the painful areas, to avoid noxious stimuli and to seek aid. But because of the subjective character of the pain, there develop psychological and emotional reactions to it that eventually result in psychomatic disturbances from unduly prolonged protective mechanisms. These psychological and emotional reactions are amenable to modification and treatment through hypnosis in such psychosomatic disturbances.

To understand pain further, one must think of it as a neuro-psycho physiological complex characterized by various understandings of tremendous significance to the sufferer. One need only ask the patient to describe his pain to hear it variously described as dull, heavy, dragging, sharp, cutting, twisting, burning, nagging, stabbing, lancinating, biting, cold, hard, grinding, throbbing, gnawing, and a wealth of other such adjectival terms.

These various descriptive interpretations of the pain experience are of marked importance in the hypnotic approach to the patient. The patient who interprets his subjective pain experience in terms of various qualities of differing sensations is thereby offering a multitude of opportunities to the hypnotherapist to deal with the pain. To consider a total approach is possible. But more feasible is the utilization of hypnosis in relation first to minor aspects of the total pain complex and then to its increasingly severe and distressing qualities. Thus, minor successes will lay a foundation for major successes in relation to the more distressing attributes of the neuro-psycho-physiological complex of pain, and the understanding and cooperation of the patient for hypnotic intervention are more readily elicited. Additionally, any hypnotic alteration of any single interpretive quality of the pain sensation serves to effect an alteration of the total pain complex.

Another important consideration in the comprehension of the pain complex is the recognition of the experiential significances of various attributes or qualities of subjective sensation, and their differing relationships in such matters as remembered pain, past pain, immediate pain, enduring pain, transient pain, recurrent pain, enduring persistent pain, intractable pain, unbearable pain, threatening pain, etc. In applying these considerations to varying subjective elements of the pain complex, hypnotic intervention is greatly accelerated. Such analysis offers greater opportunity for hypnotic intervention at a more comprehensive level. It becomes easier to communicate ideas and understandings through hypnosis and to elicit the receptiveness and responsiveness so vital in securing good response to hypnotic intervention. It is also important to acknowledge adequately the unrecognized force of the human emotional need to demand the immediate abolition of pain, both by the patient himself and by those attending him.

Hypnotic Procedures in Pain Control

The hypnotic procedures for handling pain are numerous in character. The first of these most commonly practiced but frequently not genuinely applicable is the use of *direct hypnotic suggestion for total abolition of pain.* With a limited number of patients, this is a most effective procedure. But too often it fails, serving to discourage the patient and to prevent further use of hypnosis in the patient's treatment. Also, its effects, while they may be good, are sometimes too limited in duration which may limit the effectiveness of the *permissive indirect hypnotic abolition of pain.* This is often much more effective, and although essentially similar in character to direct suggestion, it is worded and offered in a fashion much more conducive to patient receptiveness and responsiveness.

A third procedure for hypnotic control of pain is the utilization of *amnesia.* In everyday life we see the forgetting of pain whenever more threatening or absorbing experiences secure the attention of the sufferer. An example is the instance already cited of the mother enduring extreme pain, seeing her infant seriously injured, forgetting her own pain in the anxious fears about her child. Then of quite opposite psychological character is the forgetting of painful arthritis, headache or toothache while watching an all-aborbing suspenseful drama on a cinema screen.

But amnesia in relationship to pain can be applied hypnotically in a great variety of ways. Thus one may employ partial, selective, or complete amnesias in relationship to selected subjective qualities and attributes of sensation in the pain complex as described by the patient, as well as to the total pain experience.

A fourth hypnotic procedure is the employment of *hypnotic analgesia,* which may be partial, complete, or selective. Thus, one may add to the patient's pain experience a certain feeling of numbness without a loss of tactile or pressure sensations. The entire pain experience then becomes modified and different and gives the patient a sense of relief and satisfaction, even if the analgesia is not complete. The sensory modifications introduced into the patient's subjective experience by such sensations as numbness, an increase of warmth and heaviness, relaxation, etc. serve to intensify the hypnotic analgesia to an increasingly complete degree.

Hypnotic anesthesia is a fifth method in treating pain. This is often difficult and may sometimes be accomplished directly, but is more often best accomplished indirectly by the building of psychological and emotional situations that are contradictory to the experience of the pain and which serve to establish an anesthetic reaction to be continued by post-hypnotic suggestion.

A sixth hypnotic procedure useful in handling pain concerns the matter of suggestion to effect the *hypnotic replacement or substitution of sensations.* For example, one cancer patient suffering intolerable pain responded most remarkably to the suggestion of an incredibly annoying itch on the sole of her foot. Her body weakness occasioned by the carcinomatosis and hence inability to scratch the itch rendered this psychogenic pruritis all-absorbing of her attention. Then hypnotically, feelings of warmth, of coolness, of heaviness and of numbness were systematically induced for various parts of her body where she suffered pain. And the final measure was the suggestion of an endurable but highly unpleasant and annoying minor burning-itching sensation at the site of her mastectomy. This procedure of replacement substitution sufficed for the patient's last six months of her life. The itch of the sole of her foot gradually disappeared but the annoying burning-itching sensation at the site of her mastectomy persisted.

Hypnotic displacement of pain is a seventh procedure. This is the employment of a suggested displacement of the pain from one area of the body to another. This can be well illustrated by the instance of a man dying from prostatic metastalic carcinomatosis and suffering with intractable pain in both states of drug narcosis and deep hypnosis, particularly abdominal pain. He was medically trained and understood the concept of referred and displaced pain. In the hypnotic trance he readily accepted the idea that, while the intractable pain in his abdomen was the pain that would actually destroy him, he could readily agree that equal pain in his left hand could be entirely endurable, since in that location it would not have its threatening significances. He accepted the idea of referral of his abdominal pain to his left hand, and thus remained free of body pain, becoming accustomed instead to the severe pain in his left hand which he protected carefully. This hand pain did not interfere in any way with his family life during the remaining three months of his life. It was disclosed that the displaced pain to the left hand often gradually diminished, but the pain would increase upon incautious inquiry.

This possibility of displacement of pain also permits a displacement of various attributes of the pain that cannot otherwise be controlled. By this measure these otherwise uncontrollable attributes become greatly diminished. Thus the total complex of pain becomes greatly modified and made more amenable to hypnotic intervention.

Hypnotic dissociation can be employed for pain control, and the usual most effective methods are those of *time and body disorientation*. The patient with pain intractable to both drugs and hypnosis can be hypnotically reoriented in time to the earlier stages of his illness when the pain was of minor consideration. And the disorientation of that time characteristic of the pain can be allowed to remain as a posthypnotic continuation through the waking state. Thus the patient still has his intractable pain, but it has been rendered into a minor consideration as it had been in its original stages.

One may sometimes successfully reorient the patient with intractable pain to a time predating his illness and, by posthypnotic suggestion, effect a restoration of the normal sensations existing before his illness. However, although intractable pain often prevents this as a total result, pleasant feelings predating the illness may be projected into the present to nullify some of the subjective qualities of his pain complex. Sometimes this effects a major reduction in pain.

In the matter of *body disorientation,* the patient is hypnotically dissociated and induced to experience himself as apart from his body. Thus one woman with the onset of unendurable pain, in response to posthypnotic suggestions, would develop a trance state and experience herself as being in another room while her suffering body remained in her sickbed. This patient explained to the author when he made a bedside call, "Just before you arrived, I developed another horrible attack of pain. So I went into a trance, got into my wheel chair, came out into the living room to watch a television program, and I left my suffering body in the bedroom." And she pleasantly and happily told about the fantasized television program she was watching. Another such patient remarked to her surgeon, "You know very well, Doctor, that I always faint when you start changing my dressings because I can't endure the pain, so if you don't mind I will go into a hypnotic trance and take my head and feet and go into the solarium and leave my body here for you to work on." The patient further explained, "I took a position in the solarium where I could see him (the surgeon) bending over my body but I could not see what he was doing. Then I looked out the window and when I looked back he was gone, so I took my head and feet and went back and joined my body and felt very comfortable." This particular patient had been trained in hypnosis by the author many years previously, had subsequently learned autohypnosis, and thereafter induced her own autohypnotic trance by the phrase, "You know very well, Doctor." This was a phrase that she could employ verbally or mentally at any time and immediately go into a trance for the psychological-emotional experience of being elsewhere, away from her painful body, there to enjoy herself and remain until it was safe to return to her body. In this trance state which she protected very well from the awareness of others, she would visit with her relatives, but experience them as with her in this new setting while not betraying that personal orientation.

A ninth hypnotic procedure in controlling body pain, which is very similar to replacement or substitution of sensations is *hypnotic reinterpretation of pain experience.* By this is meant the reinterpreting for the patient in hypnosis of a dragging, gnawing, heavy pain into a feeling of weakness, of profound inertia, and then as relaxation with the warmth and comfort that accompanies deep muscular relaxation. Stabbing, lancinating and biting pains may sometimes be reinterpreted as a sudden startle reaction, disturbing in character, but momentary in duration and not painful. Throbbing, nagging, grinding pain has been successfully reinterpreted as the unpleasant but not distressing experience of the rolling sensations of a boat during a storm, or even as the throbbing that one so often experiences from a minor cut on the fingertip with no greater distressing characteristics. Full awareness of how the patient experiences his pain is required for an adequate hypnotic reinterpretation of the pain sensation.

Hypnotic time distortion, first described by Cooper and then later developed by Cooper and Erickson (Cooper, L., and Erickson, M., *Time Distortion in Hypnosis,* Baltimore: Williams and Wilkins, 1959) is often a most useful hypnotic measure in pain control. An excellent example is that of the patient with intractable attacks of lancinating pain which occurred approximately every twenty to thirty minutes, night and day, and which lasted from five to ten minutes. Between the attacks the patient's frame of mind was essentially one of fearful dread of the next attack. By employing hypnosis and teaching him time distortion, it was possible to employ, as is usually the case in every pain patient, a combination of several of the measures described here. In the trance state, the patient was taught to develop an amnesia for all past attacks of pain. He was then taught time distortion so that he could experience the five to ten minute pain episodes in ten to twenty seconds. He was given posthypnotic suggestions to the effect that each attack would come as a complete surprise to him, that when the attack occurred he would develop a trance state of ten to twenty seconds duration, experience all of the pain attack, and then come out of the trance with no awareness that he had been in a trance or that he had experienced pain. Thus the patient, in talking to his family, would suddenly and obviously go into the trance state with a scream of pain, and perhaps ten seconds later come out of the trance state, look confused for a moment, and then continue his interrupted sentence.

An eleventh hypnotic procedure is that of offering *hypnotic suggestions effecting a diminution of pain,*—not a complete removal of the pain, since it had become apparent that the patient was not going to be fully responsive. This diminution is usually best brought about by suggesting to the hypnotized patient that his pain is going to diminish imperceptibly hour after hour without his awareness that it is diminishing until perhaps several days have passed. He will then become aware of all pain or of special pain qualities. By suggesting that the diminution occur imperceptibly, the patient cannot refuse the suggestion. His state of emotional hopefulness, despite his emotional despair, leads him to anticipate that in a few days there may be some diminution; particularly that there may be even a marked diminution of certain attributes of his pain experience. This, in itself, serves as an autosuggestion to the patient. In certain instances, however, the patient is told that the diminution will be to a very minor degree. One can emphasize this by utilizing the ploy that a one percent diminution of his pain would not be noticeable, nor would a 2 percent, nor a 3 percent, nor a 4 percent, nor a 5 percent diminution, but that such an amount would nevertheless be a diminution. One can continue the ploy by stating that a 5 percent diminution the first day and an additional 2 percent the next day still would not be perceptible. And if on the third day there occurred a 3 percent diminution, this, too, would be imperceptible. But it would total a 10 percent diminution of the original pain. This same series of suggestions can be continued to a reduction of pain to 80 percent of its original intensity, then to 70 percent, 50 percent, 40 percent, and sometimes even down to 10 percent. In this way the patient may be led progressively into an even greater control of his pain.

However, in all hypnotic procedures for the control of pain one bears in mind the greater feasibility and acceptability to the patient of indirect as compared with direct hypnotic suggestions, and the need to approach the problem by indirect and permissive measures as well as by employing a combination of the various methodological procedures described above.

Summary

Pain as a subjective experience is perhaps the most significant factor in causing people to seek medical aid. Treatment of pain as usually viewed by both physician and patient is primarily a matter of elimination or abolition of the sensation. Yet pain in itself may be serving certain useful purposes to the individual. It constitutes a warning, a persistent warning of the need for help. It brings about physical restriction of activity, thus frequently benefiting the sufferer. It instigates physiological changes of a healing nature in the body. Hence, pain is not just an undesirable sensation to be abolished, but rather an experience to be so handled that the sufferer benefits. This may be done in a variety of ways, but there is a tendency to overlook the wealth of psycho-neuro-physiological significances pain has for the patient. Pain is a complex, a construct composed of a great diversity of subjective interpretative and experiential values for the patient. Pain, during life's experience, serves to establish body learnings, associations, and conditionings that constitute a source of body potentials permitting the use of hypnosis for the study and control of pain. Hypnotic procedures, singly or in combination, for major or minor effects in the control of pain described for their application are: Direct Hypnotic Suggestion for Total Abolition of Pain; Permissive Indirect Hypnotic Abolition of Pain; Amnesia; Hypnotic Analgesia; Hypnotic Anesthesia; Hypnotic Replacement or Substitution of Sensations; Hypnotic Displacement of Pain; Hypnotic Dissociation; Reinterpretation of Pain Experience; Hypnotic Suggestions Effecting a Diminution of Pain.

Case 1   A Conversational Approach to Altering Sensory-Perceptual Functioning: Phantom Limb Pain and Tinnitus.

Our first case illustrates the simultaneous therapy of a married couple who presented two apparently different symptoms: The seventy-two-year-old husband (H) suffered from phantom limb pain; his seventy-five-year-old wife (W) was bothered by tinnitus, an unpleasant ringing in her ears that had bothered her constantly for years. The husband had seen Erickson (E) for the first time a week earlier and had experienced some relief. Erickson and Rossi (R) then asked him and his wife to join them for a hypnotherapeutic session that would be free of charge if they were willing to be tape-recorded for possible publication. This offer was gratefully received by them. The *rapport* that Erickson had already established with the husband was now enhanced since they both appreciated the therapy and special consideration they were receiving.

They entered the therapy room wide-eyed with hopeful *expectation* and immediately focused their entire attention on Erickson. Their *response attentiveness* was already at an ideal level. As can be seen from the transcript, they are both very respectful, cooperative, and eager for help. They have no evident misconceptions or resistances to hypnosis, so Erickson can introduce them immediately to the concept of learning to alter their own sensory-perceptual functioning for relief of their symptoms. He does this with a rather relaxed and seemingly casual conversation wherein he tells them interesting stories about his youth and the fascinating ways people can learn to regulate and alter many of their bodily processes. This enjoyable talk is actually a careful preparation during which Erickson is *structuring frames of reference* about their abilities to alter their own sensory-perceptual processes. He is preparing them for the relatively brief period of therapeutic trance that will follow, when he will offer suggestions to help evoke their repertory of sensory-perceptual skills that can be utilized for ameliorating their symptoms.

A Conversational Approach to Altering Sensory-Perceptual Functioning: Structuring a Therapeutic Frame of Reference

W: Well this phantom pain—if we could lick that, it would be wonderful.

E: All right. Now I am going to give you a story so that you can understand better. We learn things in a very unusual way, a way that we don't know about. In my first year of college I happened to come across that summer a boiler factory. The crews were working on twelve boilers at the same time, and it was three shifts of workmen. And those pneumatic hammers were pounding away, driving rivets into the boilers. I heard that noise and I wanted to find out what it was. On learning that it was a boiler factory, I went in and I couldn't hear anybody talking. I could see the various employees were conversing. I could see the foreman's lips moving, but I couldn't hear what he said to me. He heard what I said. I had him come outside so I could talk to him. And I asked him for permission to roll up in

my blanket and sleep on the floor for one night. He thought there was something wrong with me. I explained that I was a premedic student and that I was interested in learning processes. And he agreed that I could roll up in my blanket and sleep on the floor. He explained to all the men and left an explanation for the succeeding shift of men. The next morning I awakened. I could hear the workmen talking about that damn fool kid. What in hell was he sleeping on the floor there for? What did he think he could learn? *During my sleep that night I blotted out all that horrible noise of the twelve or more pneumatic hammers and I could hear voices. I knew that it was possible to learn to hear only certain sounds if you tune your ears properly. You have ringing in your ears, but you haven't thought of tuning them so that you don't hear the ringing.*

> Since *rapport* and *response attentiveness* were already established with this couple, the senior author was able to immediately *structure a therapeutic frame of reference* with this story about how the unconscious automatically learns to adjust our sensory-perceptual functioning in an adaptive manner even when we are asleep. He does not tell them in a direct and intellectual manner that they will have to learn to alter their sensory-perceptual functioning. If he did, they might find some issue to argue about or, as so commonly happens with patients who have experienced a great deal of failure, they might immediately plead that they could not alter their functioning; they would not know how to do it, or would not be able to believe that it could happen to them. His stories about himself and the illustrations he continues to present are all established facts that together structure the basic frame of reference which the couple will need for their therapeutic work. He continues now in a rather humorous vein.

Interspersing Therapeutic Suggestions

E: *Now this matter of tuning yourself.* I spent three months on the Mississippi River and I got invited into a home and I felt so cooped up after being out in the open. Getting into a room, everywhere you look, your looks come to an end. When you read the old-time sailing stories, where you look to the end of the earth with nothing interfering. And the old-time stories of sailors' claustrophobic reactions. Fear of closed spaces.

Also when I got back from that canoe trip . . . have you ever tried to sleep on a soft bed? You are miserable. I had learned to sleep on the ground, in brush piles, inside the canoe. My ribs fighting with canoe ribs.

104

When I got home and had a mattress, that was torture. The Indians did not like, in the early days, the white man's bed. They wanted the ground to sleep on. They *wanted comfort. Just nothing but sheer comfort.*

On the Tribal Eye program on KAET. Those nomads from Iran. How can they dress with all those petticoats? And be comfortable in the hot sun on those desert plains? *And you can get so used to the ringing in your ears that you don't hear it.*

I grew up on the farm. I had to be away from the farm for quite some years before I learned the barn smell on your hands when you live on the farm. I never smelled it when I was on the farm. I had to be away from it for a long time before I discovered the barn smell.

R: I guess that is why it is so hard to convince someone who doesn't wash often enough that he has to wash more often. He doesn't smell himself!

E: I can tell you a funny story about that. One year the boy in the next room at the rooming house had a fellow roomer who came from South Dakota. And Hebbie came from Milwaukee. And Hebbie told Lester, "You stink, go take a bath." It was the latter part of September and Lester said, "But I took a bath last July. I won't need one until at least Thanksgiving Day." But he really stunk, and Hebbie said, "You are going to take a bath if I have to put you in the tub myself." *What people don't know, that they can lose that pain and they don't know they can lose that ringing in the ears.* When I discovered that that barn smell had come back, I could really smell it. I wondered how long it would take me that day to lose it? Then by midafternoon I couldn't smell it. All of us grow up *believing that when you have pain, you must pay attention to it. And believing when you have ringing of the ears that you must keep on hearing it.*

> As the senior author continues with one illustration after another, he gradually begins to intersperse therapeutic suggestion (in *italics*) about how she can learn to *tune out* her ringing and he can *lose* his pain. Because these suggestions are interspersed within a network of stories they are interested in hearing, the patients tend to accept the suggestions (without even realizing that therapy is taking place) particularly since the senior author moves quickly on to another interesting anecdote before they can protest or reject or even think about the interspersed therapeutic suggestions.
>
> Although Erickson has not made any effort to induce a trance in a formal manner, it is evident that his stories are so absorbing the couple's attention that they are actually a bit entranced.

They simply sit quietly with their eyes fixed upon him. They are obviously relaxed and oblivious to anything else that might be going on around them. They are exhibiting a state of *response attentiveness* that is ideal, for the receptivity will enhance their experience of therapeutic trance.

Accepting the Therapeutic Frame of Reference

E: Now, the pain you feel, where? Where do you feel the pain?

H: Right at the present time, in my foot.

E: Yes.

W: Where there is no foot.

H: Where there is no foot.

E: All right, I had a friend named John. He was a psychiatrist, and we were visiting. He reached down and scratched his ankle. I said, "John, that really itches, doesn't it?" And he said, "Yes." We both knew it was a wooden leg.

H: My understanding is that when I was in the hospital there was a double amputee over there. I saw him twice. I had seen him at the hospital and I had seen him over at Good Sam's taking therapy. But the nurse taking care of him at St. Joseph, when he said his foot itched, she'd reach down and scratch his sheet and relieve it.

W: Where his foot would have been?

H: Where his foot would have been! She would scratch the sheet down there and said that it would relieve it.

After listening to the senior author recount his anecdotes and stories of the relativity of sensations and phantom limb pain, the husband now shows evidence of accepting and joining this therapeutic frame of reference by telling his own anecdote about it. He goes further as he now begins to make an emphatic effort to convince his own wife when she asks a doubting question.

Creating Expectancy by Introducing New Response Possibilities: Phantom Pleasure

E: Like I asked my friend John, "So you scratched it, how does your foot feel now?" He said, "Good." That nurse was very wise. *Because you can have good feelings in the foot.* Not just painful ones.

H: Oh, I hope so, Doctor.

E: That's what is overlooked in these amputees. They forget that they can also have good feelings.

H: I was at the leg man's yesterday. My leg wouldn't unlock. I went to him. He had three different rooms. No, two different besides mine. In each one they were talking about what can we do for this phantom pain that he got. He said, "It is driving me nuts." Of course, I never opened my mouth, because I was in another room. I didn't say I was out here or nothing. I knew I had had relief from what you done before.

E: All right. Now I want to have you two recorded so that Dr. Rossi could include it in the book. Now if you have phantom pain in a limb, *you may also have phantom good feelings. And they are delightful.*

H: That I haven't had yet.

E: That's right.

H: That I haven't had yet.

E: But you can learn them!

> Since the husband obviously accepted the therapeutic frame of reference, Erickson immediately pressed on with a further suggestion of how he can cope with phantom limb pain by converting it to phantom limb pleasure. Erickson introduces pleasure only tentatively as a possibility at this point. The patient certainly is not yet ready for a direct suggestion about experiencing pleasure. When the husband admits he has not experienced pleasure, Erickson utilizes the learning frame of reference he has so carefully developed earlier with his stories. With this background of illustrations he can now confidently say to the husband, "But you can learn them!" Since the husband enjoyed and accepted all those anecdotes about learning to change sensory-perceptual experiences, he cannot now reject Erickson's direct suggestion about his eventually learning also.
>
> Thus, even before trance experience is formally begun in this session, Erickson has structured the basic therapeutic frame of reference for the husband in such a way that he finds himself accepting it. It is now only a question of when he will begin to utilize that therapeutic frame. When the husband responds with, "Oh, I hope so, doctor," we can recognize that a high degree of *expectancy for a therepeutic response is being created.*

H: But I will say this, that in the afternoon I will lay down for an hour and I just go into a complete trance and I don't think of nothing.

W: After he [H] came to you [E].

H: After I come from you, I think of nothing. And it is not a sleep. I know I am not asleep. But I am in a trance. I have no pain whatsoever. And when I get up, I feel so much different.

E: All right. *And your next problem is learning to keep that good feeling a second longer.* And two seconds longer. Then four seconds longer. And six! And eight!

H: You know, doctor, you told me, the best that I can recall, when I was over here the other time, start in at twenty and count backward. That is what I do when I lay down. Now I don't recall all of what you said, but I remember something you said about nine, six, and three. I remember that before I went into this trance or whatever you might call it. And I try to think of those numbers each time that I lay down and try to count from twenty backward. I emphasize on that nine, six, and three. But as I say, I am not asleep. I can lay there. It seems to me as though I can lay there forever. Two or three hours, but I am not asleep, I am in a trance. My eyes are closed. I hear nothing. My wife can come in the room and I don't hear her. But after a certain length of time, I'm wide awake.

E: And we had it directly from his lips.

R: Yes. Isn't that beautiful. A good description of trance.

H: That's just the way it is. It has been with me, and I have only been out here since last Monday, wasn't it?

W: I think so.

> The husband now acknowledges the senior author's belief in the ability to learn to alter phantom pain sensations by describing his experiences of autohypnosis, which he learned just a week ago. Already he has learned to eliminate pain during the autohypnotic trance. Erickson seizes upon that and seeks to extend comfort for longer periods—second by second. This is one of his favorite therapeutic approaches—geometric progression. It is usually quite easy for patients to experience relief from their symptoms during autohypnosis. The problem is when

they come out of it. The senior author then asks them if they can extend their symptom-free condition for one second after trance today. Then double it to two seconds tomorrow. And double it again to four seconds the day after. If they continue doubling the amount of symptom-free time in this geometric progression every day, in eighteen days they will be extending it for more than twenty-four hours.

An interesting aspect of the husband's description of his autohypnotic trance experience is his emphasis on 9, 6, and 3 when he awakens. Erickson frequently trains people to go into trance by counting from 1 to 20 and to awaken by counting backward. He had no conscious awareness on this occasion of having said or done anything special with the numbers nine, six, and three. This appears to be a purely subjective, idiosyncratic response on the husband's part. It is accepted nonetheless as a valid and worthwhile part of his personal experience of trance. Precisely because it is a purely subjective experience, it is perhaps even more valuable in facilitating his trance experience, because in some way or other it utilizes his own internal associations in a constructive manner.

The husband and wife go on now to discuss their caring relationship for each other. Erickson utilizes this to talk about his daughter Roxanna who is studying to be a nurse. The point of his introducing Roxanna soon reveals itself as yet another example of someone who has done well in life because she was willing to learn.

Facilitating the Therapeutic Frame of Reference: Open-Ended Suggestions

H: Of course my wife is very concerned over me. She takes care of me just like she does a baby, you might say. I am concerned over her because she is concerned over me. So. But as she said as we crossed these steps out here a while ago, "We are going to make it, we are going to make it together."

E: Well. I tell my wife not to be concerned about me. I'm just in a wheelchair. That's all! I want to put her energy toward enjoying things.

H: She used to be very active. She used to swim. She didn't learn to swim till she was fifty years old.

W: Fifty-five.

H: Fifty-five. She swam five miles without stopping. Won a woman's trophy at the YWCA. She works with the retarded children. And stuff like that. That is what I want her to get back into, instead of thinkig that she has to stay at home to take care of me.

W: When he gets able, I will.

H: Well, I think I am able enough for you to start it. I really do.

W: When I worked with a little retarded child, it did me more good than it did him.

E: Where, in Sun Valley?

W: A little boy on the piano.

H: My wife would play a piece, and he would get down and look all round that piano and everything. She would put it on her cassette. When she would get through, she would say, "Now Kenny, you play it."

W: The piano would be in the auditorium. And I would say, "Now Kenny, just pretend like you are playing before a crowd of people. Close your eyes and smile." He would close his eyes and smile. Then sit there and play.

E: All right.

H: She enjoyed it and I enjoyed her doing that type of work. It done her more good than it done the child. It really did.

E: [Gives a detailed account of how his daughter put herself through many work and training experiences before she was certain she wanted to become a nurse.]
   Now my daughter was willing to learn.

W: Right!

E: Your husband knows how he can feel pain in that foot. He saw another patient learn how to get comfortable from a nurse scratching a sheet.

H: That he did.

E: That's correct. My friend John said, "It feels so good when I scratch my wooden leg." He had his Ph.D. and his M.D.

R: Scratching a wooden leg!

W: Sounds fantastic, doesn't it?

R: Yes, really! The power of the mind!

110

E: A true story. John was marvelous. And I discussed with him the importance of *having nice feelings in your wooden foot, your wooden knee.*

H: You discussed what, now?

E: I discussed with him *the importance of having good feelings in the wooden foot, the wooden knee, the wooden leg. Feeling it to be warm. Cool. Rested.* But most patients with phantom limb pain just think of only the pain. And if you can have phantom pain, *you can have phantom pleasure.*

H: Oh, boy!

W: It sounds good, dear, I never thought of it.

H: Yeah, I'll take the pleasure.

R: All right, sir!

E: And you saw someone else demonstrate scratching your sheet. It felt good. And that nurse was very successful.

> With these remarks the senior author reinforces the therapeutic frame of reference with further examples of altering phantom pain to warmth, coolness, rest, and the possibility of pleasure. He is introducing many therapeutic possibilities in an open-ended manner. At this point Erickson still does not know which of these response possibilities the husband's system will be able to utilize. He will allow the husband's own individuality to choose between them. This is a basic principle of therapeutic suggestion: *The therapist offers possibilities, and the patient's unconscious chooses and mediates the actual response modality of therapeutic change in keeping with his own capabilities.* Therapeutic suggestion cannot impose something foreign on patients; it can only help patients to evoke and to utilize what is already present within their own response repertory.
>
> The conversation now shifts to visiting nurses, their medical doctor, and the heart pacemaker that the husband has. The senior author utilizes this latter topic to give further illustration of our ability to alter physiological functions such as heart rate and blood pressure.

Further Structuring of the Therapeutic Frame of Reference: Altering Heart Rate and Blood Pressure

E: All right. Now a doctor from Michigan and one from Pennsylvania were visiting me, and my daughter Roxanna was then taking blood pressures all over the city. She asked them if she could take their blood pressure. And they both said, "Do you want it as it is normally, or would you like it ten points lower or ten points higher?" She said, "All three." So she got the normal reading and then they told her she would find out whether it is lower or higher. She found out.

W: How could they control it?

E: Blood pressure changes according to where the blood is. When you go to sleep at night, your blood drains out of your brain and into a plexus, a collection of blood vessels in the abdomen. You wake up and blood pressure is increased and shoves blood back into your brain.

H: That is what I have to do every morning, first thing I go in and she fixes me a cup of coffee. I take my pulse and it averages between seventy and seventy-one every morning. They told me if it got below sixty-nine to call them. My granddaughter lives up in Flagstaff, and I haven't been up there since they bought a business and are buying a home. I asked my doctor if I could go up there. He said, "Well go up there for an hour and a half or two hours, but be very careful with your heart condition and things." Well, I went over there an hour and half, and it was hard to breathe from there on down. I could only breathe from here on up, you might say. So they said let's get him to the emergency hospital, and I said no, I didn't want to go to an emergency hospital. I wanted to go home. So after we hit around 3,500-4,000-foot level, it began to come back. It was down to fifty-nine. It was down to fifty-nine. Then it came up a little bit when I came over Sunset Point. That is 5,000-foot altitude. I found I can't go any higher than that altitude.

W: I never feel it.

E: Now my friends have experimented, and they can raise the heartbeat for 5,000 feet or 10,000 feet voluntarily.

W: Really? Imagine that.

E: And I wanted your husband to realize that *there is a lot he can do for himself.* A friend of mine said, "I have never been able to blush in my whole life. Will you help me to learn to blush?" I told him I would. I often dropped by there in various hours of the day, and his wife was my secretary. One evening I dropped in when they were at the table. We exchanged news and all of a sudden I said, "Bill! What are you blushing about?" He turned bright red. Half an hour later he said, "Please turn it off. My face is still burning."

W: Sounds impossible, doesn't it?

E: But it isn't! Have you ever lived where it is cold weather?

W: Yes.

E: Well, you sit in a warm room and go into the cold, what happens? Your nose gets hard.

W: A complete change.

E: Your blood vessels in your face have been turning on and off. You learned that in the wintertime. Yes. You have got that learning. Ordinarily people don't use it. But this Michigan doctor and Pennsylvania doctor had worked with me, and then they started using the thing that they already knew but had never thought of using. You run, your blood pressure goes up. You rest, your blood pressure goes down. Your heart rate can go up, it can go down. *You can think about increasing your heart rate and you can speed it up. And you can do it comfortably and easily. So long as you know that you can do it.* And that is why I am having you here today. Just to give you more information about yourself.

> In these further examples, the senior author gives more suggestions about controlling physiological functioning. He deals with the important problem of H's coping with minor variations in the functioning of his pacemaker. Such variations, when they are not expected and understood, can panic patients and worsen their condition. Whenever he deals with symptom problems, Erickson always casually mentions how a momentary or temporary return of a symptom can be a normal signal about the body's functioning rather than the persistent return of the symptom or illness per se. This forestalls many lapses back into illness. In his example of blushing Erickson gives a humorous illustration of his surprise approach to altering physiological functioning (Erickson, 1964; Rossi, 1973; Erickson, Rossi, and Rossi, 1976).

Trance Induction: Modeling Trance Behavior

E: [To H] Now I would like to have you go into a trance. [To W] Watch him now.

Pause as the husband adjusts his body comfortably, closes his eyes, and goes into a trance. Just at this critical moment a youth from the street knocks loudly on the door of Erickson's office, opens it, and boldly invites us to attend his Baptist church. All of us are startled by his sudden intrusion except for H, who shows absolutely no reaction as he continues with his trance. In asking the wife who has never experienced trance to watch her husband enter trance, Erickson is using one of his favorite approaches to trance training. He simply has the new subject watch another more experienced subject go into trance.

Facilitating Normal Variations in Physiological Functioning

E: I've seen variations in blood pressure already. Now he wants to keep the heart rate about seventy. But it is all right when sleeping for his heart rate to be less than seventy. In the waking state, yes, seventy is all right, seventy-two is all right. If it drops below sixty-nine in his sleep, that's all right too. If it drops to sixty-eight, that is all right too. There is no occasion for alarm because the heart normally slows during sleep, and I don't want him to keep his heart at the waking level of beating. Now the heart can slow down in different ways. It can beat the same number of times per minute, but beat so it does not push as large a volume of fluid. It can beat the same number of times but beat less blood through the veins. He needs less blood circulating in his body when he is asleep, so the heart does not need to beat as hard as when he is awake. *And he can regulate that.* Now as you see, his entire body is at rest, and in the trance he can let one arm be awake while the rest of his body is in a trance. He can let his right leg go into a trance while the rest of his body is awake.

The senior author immediately notes a variation in H's blood pressure as he enters trance from the variations in his pulse that can be seen (usually some place on the temple, throat, arm, etc) by therapists who have trained themselves to look for it. His mentioning this variation tends to ratify trance as an altered state and lead into therapeutic suggestions about the normal variations to be expected in his heart rate. Note the easy manner with which the senior author is open-ended in his suggestion to permit the heart to vary in its functioning in any way that is necessary (number of beats, volume of fluid). In mentioning how one part of the body can be awake and move while the rest of the body is immobile in trance, he is indirectly suggesting how

114

patients can spontaneously shift for comfort now and then without feeling they are thereby waking up.

Dissociation Training

E: [To W] He said that he could be in a trance and you could come in and he would not know it. And Dr. Rossi knows that in a trance state I have a subject here, oh, she and I are here, but he isn't. She can't see him, she can't hear him, but she can see and hear me. In other words, human beings can isolate various parts of the body.

> With these remarks addressed to the wife Erickson is giving indirect suggestions to the husband for learning how to dissociate one's attention or a part of the body. Such dissociations are useful in facilitating trance depth as well as coping with symptomatic problems.

Indirect Open-Ended Suggestions

E: With enough experience he can go to Flagstaff and take with him his breathing habits of Phoenix. Because *you can take habits with you.* That's one of the problems that the airline pilots have. They all grow up with clock habits. And their sleep cycle is disturbed. They have to learn how to get a changing sleep cycle. I'm talking to you while he [H] is learning something. *He doesn't know what he is learning, but he is learning.* And it isn't right for me to tell him, "You learn this or you learn that!" *Let him learn whatever he wishes, in whatever order he wishes.*

> This is another illustration of the senior author's indirect and open-ended approach to offering therapeutic suggestions that permit the patient's unconscious to find its own individual mode of optimal functioning.

Facilitating Unconscious Search and Unconscious Processes: Suggestion by Surprise and Association

E: Now I mentioned the ringing in your ears. I mentioned blushing. I mentioned breathing. Elevating blood pressure, lowering it. You always have to be aware, and *we know a lot of things we don't know we know.* My friend Bill said he wanted to blush. He never had. I knew that he could get pale. He could get a red face in the heat. Blood would decrease in his face when he went to sleep. He had all those learnings. All I did was say something that took him by surprise. And he reacted that way. He did not know how to turn it off. But I so surprised him that the automatic working of his body wasn't in gear. All I said was "OK," and his body went back into automatic gear.

W: Yes

> In an indirect manner the senior author associates W's ringing-ear problem with the previous illustrations of successful coping with symptoms by learning to alter sensory-perceptual and physiological functioning. If he had directly told her at this point that she would have to learn to control the ringing in her ears, she would almost certainly have demurred and protested that she did not know how. She would be right. Certainly her conscious mind does not know how to alter the ringing. The control she will learn is still an unconscious potential at this point. By conversationally associating the ringing problem with the other anecdotes of successful perceptual alteration, however, the senior author is indirectly creating an associational network or belief system that will later enable W to accept further suggestions that will evoke and utilize whatever unconscious mechanisms she has available to effect a therapeutic transformation. Before she has any chance to discuss and possibly reject even this mild association, Erickson immediately shifts his remarks to the husband. Since she is intensely interested in learning trance by watching her husband, the wife's conscious attention is distracted to him, and the therapeutic association that Erickson just gave her remains lodged within her unconscious. This therapeutic association may now automatically begin a process of *unconscious search for the unconscious processes* that will eventuate in the therapeutic transformation to be experienced later as a *hypnotic response*.

Direct Suggestions in Trance

E: [To H] Now listen to me because you can listen to me. *You can have nice feelings in both feet, in both legs. You can enjoy having your heart beat strongly and gently. You can learn the feelings of breathing, the feelings of breathing that you have in Phoenix.* If your wife didn't learn swimming until she was fifty-five, I can tell her one thing she learned as soon as she got into the water. First time she went into the water up to her neck, she found it difficult to breathe.

W: I had to learn to relax.

E: And small children wading into the water find their breathing gets choked. And that scares them. After a while they learn to breathe with that water pressure against their chest. And when they learn to do that, then they don't use that learning outside the pool. As soon as they get back in the pool, they use that water pressure learning so they breathe normally. *Now he pays attention in the back of his mind to his Phoenix breathing patterns, habits, and when he goes to Flagstaff, he can keep on using those same muscle patterns, muscle habits.* **Now in med school when you got into an air chamber with decreased air pressure and you notice how your breathing changes, you pay close attention to it. When you come out, you notice the change. You can go back in the air chamber and breathe comfortably because you start using your new breathing patterns.**

> Erickson has carefully structured a therapeutic frame of reference about our ability to alter body functions before and during the initial stages of trance. H's response has been so positive that Erickson now judges that it is appropriate to drop a few direct suggestions into that therapeutic frame. Even now, however, he elaborates the direct suggestions with a further illustration about learning to alter body functioning while swimming. His choice of this particular example is very apt because it is very meaningful to both H and W; both have recently spoken of it. By choosing such illustrations close to the patients' personal life experiences, the therapist can make a sounder bond of contact with patients' inner lives and real potentialities.

Trance Induction and Facilitating Unconscious Processes

E: [To W] Now suppose you lean back and uncross your legs. Look at that spot there. Don't talk. Don't move. There is nothing really important to do, except go into a trance. You have seen your husband do it. And it is a nice feeling. Your blood pressure is already changing. You may close your eyes *now* **[pause as W closes her eyes and visibly relaxes her facial muscles] and go deeper and deeper into the trance. You do not have to try hard to do anything. You just let it happen. And you think back;** *there are a goodly number of times this afternoon when you stopped hearing the ringing. It is* *hard to remember things that don't occur. But the ringing did stop. But because there was nothing there, you don't remember it.*

Having prepared her for trance induction by using her husband as a model, the senior author now induces trance with a few instructions that have three objectives: to fixate attention ("look at that spot"), to depotentiate her habitual frames of references ("Don't talk. Don't move. There is nothing really important to do"), and to give free reign to her unconscious ("go into a trance").

He then states a common though little recognized fact about the experience of symptoms. Symptoms may seem constant and unchanging. Yet invariably there are moments when we are so distracted that they are outside the central focus of our awareness. This automatic mental mechanism that shifts our attention and thereby attenuates and usually completely obliterates the experience of the symptom is evoked as the senior author describes it. This little-recognized fact is usually received with a sense of surprise by patients—a surprise that further depotentiates their old symptom-laden frame of reference and initiates a *search on an unconscious level for those unconscious processes* that may now be utilized for symptom relief.

Relying upon Unconscious Learning: The Conditions for Direct Suggestion

E: Now the important thing is to forget about the ringing and to remember the times when there was no ringing. And that is a process you learn. **I learned in one night's time not to hear the pneumatic hammers in the boiler factory—and to hear a conversation I couldn't hear the previous day. The men had been told I had come in the previous evening, and I talked to them and they kept trying to tell me, "But you can't hear us, you haven't gotten used to it." And they couldn't understand. They knew I have only been there a short time—one night—and they knew how long it had taken them to learn to hear conversations. They put their emphasis upon learning gradually. I knew what the body can do automatically. [Pause]** *Now rely upon your body. Trust it. Believe in it. And know that it will serve you well.*

The senior author now strongly emphasizes that symptom changes will take place via an unconscious process. It is important for the conscious mind to "rely upon your body, trust it," and so on. He drops the direct suggestion "to forget about

118

the ringing" into the frame of reference he structured before trance induction in his story about learning not to hear the pneumatic hammers in his sleep at the boiler factory. Thus when direct suggestions are used, they are always placed like a key in the lock of a frame of reference that was previously structured by the therapist and accepted by the patient.

We can summarize the requisite conditions for the successful use of direct suggestion as follows:

—creating frames of reference as an internal environment or belief system that can accept the direct suggestion.

—patient's reliance on unconscious processes to automatically mediate the suggestion and new learning that is needed.

—therapist's partially evoking and thereby facilitating the utilization of such unconscious processes by illustrating them in ways that are personally meaningful in the patient's actual life experience.

Further Suggestions and Illustrations: Symptom Substitution; Synesthesia

E: Another patient of mine with ringing of the ears, a woman of thirty, said that she had worked at a war plant where there was music all day long, and *she wished she could have that music instead of the ringing.* I asked her how well she remembered that music. And she named a great number of tunes. So I told her, use that ringing to play those tunes softly and gently. Five years later she said, "I still have that soft gentle music in my ears." She worked at a war plant in Michigan. You described a little boy and piano playing and the cassette, and you demonstrated with your hands the way he moved his fingers. Part of the pleasure of seeing him, hearing him, became a part of your finger movements.

[Pause]

And you can put that part of pleasure with your finger movements into your ears. And you can do it so easily, so gently, without trying, without even noticing. *And you can really enjoy good feelings, good sounds, and good quiet.*

[Pause]

And you both can breathe for us, and neither of you need to be concerned about the other. You need to enjoy knowing each other. *And enjoying what you can do as meaningful to you.*

By now the reader can easily recognize how the senior author is offering further suggestions and illustrations of the sort of

119

sensory-perceptual transformations that may effect symptom relief. As we will see later, by the end of this session, W was actually able to utilize one of these illustrations successfully for symptom relief. Notice again how carefully the senior author intersperses his suggestions with the woman's own relevant life experiences in pretending to teach the retarded child to play the piano. In suggesting, "You can put that part of pleasure with your finger movements into your ears," he is actually trying to evoke and utilize unconscious processes of synesthesia whereby pleasure from one sense modality (kinesthetic or proprioceptive sensations from the fingers) could be shifted to another (her auditory perceptions).

Awakening from Trance: Facilitating Unconscious Processes by Learning and Utilizing Hypnotic Pain Control Without Awareness

E: **You go into a trance, I suggest, by counting to 20, and awaken by counting backward from twenty to one, but each person should go into a trance in the way he learns naturally by himself, and you have learned an excellent way and it's your way and be pleased with it and be pleased with extending usefulness of that trance in many different ways. You both can learn from each other without trying to learn. There are so many things we learn from others, and we don't know we are learning. And our main, very difficult learnings** *we achieve without knowing that we are achieving those learnings.* **And you both are very responsive people. Which in less technical language means** *you both can learn easily things about yourself and learn them without needing to know that you have learned them. That you can use those learnings without needing to know that you know those learnings.* **I am going to ask both of you to awaken gently and comfortably.**

In this awakening procedure the senior author incorporates many direct suggestions to emphasize learning without awareness. Ideally, learning to alter and transform the sensory-perceptual aspects of physical symptoms is an unconscious process that proceeds on an unconscious level. Consciousness usually does not know how to cope with these transformations and is best eliminated from the process. Erickson's last suggestion, "That you can use those learnings without needing to know that you know those learnings," contains some subtle implications. The patients can learn to use pain-transforming mechanisms on an unconscious level to such an automatic degree that they need not even know they are successfully dealing with pain. Since consciousness is not even aware of the automatic operation of these newly learned pain-control processes, consciousness need not know about the presence of current and future pain. The senior author has emphasized that pain has three components: (1) memories of past pain, (2) current pain, and (3) anticipation of future pain. His last suggestion can be understood as a means of coping with the latter two without giving consciousness an opportunity to dwell on the process and possibly interfere with it. This approach is to be used with appropriate clinical caution. With this couple the pain did not serve any useful function as a signal about body malfunction that their physician needed to know. Thus their pain could be eliminated completely for optimal relief. When pain is an important signal about a body process that the physician needs to know about, then the presence of pain should certainly not be eliminated from consciousness entirely. In such cases the pain can be transformed into a warmth, coolness, itch, numbness, and other symptoms. The aversive quality of pain is thereby eliminated, but its signal value is maintained.

Facilitating Amnesia by Structuring an Associative Gap and Distraction

[Pause as they both reorient to their bodies by blinking, stretching, yawning, and so on.]

E: My daughter spent three years in Africa. She is married to an Air Force officer. And he was assigned to Ethiopia. Shortly after her arrival in Ethiopia, she remarked to her husband, "You see that statue? That is just exactly what my Daddy likes." Yes, she knew I would like it. It was a statue of a woman, and how can you describe it?
[Shows statue to the group]

R: It's very unique.

E: It is a weird looking thing.

W: She knew you would like it?

E: She knew I would like it! I was delighted when I saw it. And my son picked out that little rug right there on the floor. He mailed it to me for a birthday present ten years ago. He knew I would like it. When I unrolled it, my two young daughters in grade school commented, "That is not North

American Indian? Is it South American Indian?" My wife said, "It isn't Indian!" I said, "It is Hindu. . . ."

The senior author demonstrates two means of facilitating hypnotic amnesia in these few remarks made immediately upon the awakening from trance. He first returns to a topic of conversation about his daughter that came just before trance induction. By picking up an associative thread from this period, the trance events are placed into an associative gap. Trance events and associations cohere together, but there are no associative bridges to the patient's mental framework (a conversation about Erickson's daughter in this case) which occur immediately before or after trance. Because of the relative lack of associative bridges, trance events tend to remain dissociated from the patient's habitual frameworks and may thus become amnesic. The following diagram may clarify the matter (Erickson, Haley, and Weakland, 1959), where the upper line is a conscious memory line with only a small gap that tends to cover the lower line of trance events.

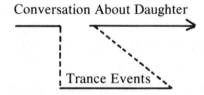

Conversation About Daughter

Trance Events

The senior author's second approach to facilitating amnesia is to distract the patient from trance associations by introducing topics of conversation that are far distant from the trance work that has just been completed (in this case gifts, rugs, Indians.) These distracting topics also tend to prevent the development of associative bridges between the contents of trance and the contents of the awake state, thereby facilitating an amnesia for trance events. This amnesia is often therapeutically valuable, since it prevents the patient's limited and maladaptive belief systems from later working and possibly undoing the suggestions accepted during trance. The amnesia also tends to vividly ratify trance as an altered state for the patient.

Spontaneous Acknowledgment of Therapeutic Change

H: Well, doctor, I'll say this. This has done as much good as that other one has done. This is going to be wonderful.

E: You'll be surprised at all the new learnings that both of you will develop.

W: Good, Good.

E: We will call it a day.
[The session is ended, but just before she leaves the woman comments as follows]

W: When I think of the ringing in my ears now, I'm beginning to think of a melody that I play. One of several that I like very much. Now the ringing is still there but the melody is there also.

This acknowledgment of an immediate experience of therapeutic change came spontaneously from both patients. This is the ideal situation, where the therapist does not have to ask about the change and by doing so possibly distort the change process itself. Some patients might take such a question as implying a doubt in the therapist's mind, while others would tend either to exaggerate or to underestimate the amount of change experienced.

The husband expresses an important and valuable expectation of present and future therapeutic gains ("this is going to be wonderful"), while the wife, more analytically, describes how a melody is being added to her ringing. It is hoped that future work may entirely replace the ringing with the melody. Since both spontaneously acknowledge a satisfactory therapeutic change, there was no need for the senior author to end this session with any further evaluation and ratification of therapeutic change. (This final stage of evaluation and ratification will be well illustrated in our next case.)

Case 2 Shock and Surprise for Altering Sensory-Perceptual Functioning: Intractable Back Pain

This is another case where Erickson worked simultaneously with husband and wife. This couple was in their early twenties, however, and they came to therapy in a very negativistic and doubting mood. Because of their extreme doubts Erickson used a very dramatic approach to establish rapport, response attentiveness, and trance induction.

Archie and Annie were high school sweethearts. They were idealists who went ahead with their plans to be married even after Archie's back was broken and his spine severed in the Viet Nam war. Archie had returned to civilian life permanently in a wheelchair with intractable back pain. His physicians said he would have to learn to live with it. They had warned him against any sort of black magic with hypnosis, which was certainly not worth his time. Archie and Annie nevertheless wanted to try, although by the time they came to their first interview they were in a hostile, negative, and doubting mood regarding their prospects.

The senior author's first task was to recognize and accept their hostility and doubt and, if possible, actually to utilize it in some manner. He had to accept their negative frame of reference and yet introduce his own belief in the potential value of hypnotherapy. Erickson watched a few of Archie's spasms of pain and recognized that they were of psychogenic origin, much like that of phantom limb pain. After listening to the outline of their story, he decided to demonstrate a dramatic form of trance induction with Annie in order to orient Archie to the genuine therapeutic potential of hypnosis.

Trance Induction: Displacing and Discharging Hostility and Doubt

Erickson first asked Annie to stand in the middle of a small Indian rug about a yard in diameter that was on his office floor. He then proceeded with an unusual trance induction.

E: Annie, you are not to move off that carpet. And you are not going to like what I am doing. It will be offensive to you. It will be offensive to Archie. Now here is a strong oak cane, Archie. You can hold it and you can clobber me at any moment that you think I am doing wrong. You won't like what I'm going to do, Archie, but watch me carefully and clobber me just as soon as you think it is necessary.

Now I'm going to take this other cane and you watch what I'm doing. You will feel what I'm doing Annie. Archie will see what I'm doing. I will stop as soon as you close your eyes and go into a deep trance.

> The senior author gently and tentatively touched about her upper chest area with the tip of his cane and then began to gingerly push the upper part of her dress apart, as if to expose her breasts. She closed her eyes, remained rigidly immobile, and apparently went into a deep trance. She had to escape the unpleasant reality of that cane. As soon as she closed her eyes and manifested a trance state, Archie was so surprised he almost dropped his cane.

124

What are the dynamics of such an induction? With his apparently shameless poking about Annie's dress, Erickson was channeling their very evident hostility and vague doubts about hypnosis in general into a very specific rejection of Erickson's initial behavior. Annie was so constituted psychologically that she had no alternative in the situation.

The poking cane certainly fixated her attention, and the shock of it all certainly depotentiated whatever conventional mental framework she had about how doctors behave and what hypnosis was about. As she stood there, desperately uncertain about what was happening, she was sent on an unconscious search for the trance-inducing processes within her own mind that would release her from her embarrassment. The senior author said he would stop only when she went into trance. She could only escape the unpleasant poking by going into trance. She need not reject the whole situation outright, because, after all, her husband was right there with a stout cane supposedly protecting her. By giving Archie the cane, the senior author was very carefully giving him a channel through which he could focus his hostility. He was also fixing Archie's attention so intently that the young man was in that state of intense response attentiveness characteristic of therapeutic trance as he watched the unorthodox proceedings with disbelief. Thus his general doubt and disbelief about hypnosis could now be channeled, displaced, and discharged onto the apparently ridiculous behavior he was witnessing. Without quite realizing it, he also became convinced that Erickson could perform the unspeakable, the unorthodox, and, by implication, an unusual cure.

A Two-Level Posthypnotic Suggestion to Utilize and Depotentiate a Doubting Conscious Framework

E: Annie, when you awaken, you can sit in your chair, and *no matter what you think, whatever I say is true.*
Do you agree to that?
[Annie nods her head "yes" repetitiously in the slight and slow manner characteristic of the perseverative behavior of trance.]
Whatever I say is true, no matter what you think.

This was a carefully formulated two-level suggestion: (1) "No matter what you think" is a phrase recognizing her conscious doubts that enables Erickson to focus her attention by utilizing her own mental framework of doubt and resistance. She could think whatever she liked within this doubtful frame. At the same time (2) on an unconscious level she was to make true or real whatever Erickson was to later suggest. We could also say that two realities or belief systems were permitted to coexist side by side in a more or less dissociated manner: (1) The conscious belief system of doubt and resistance to hypnosis that she brought to the therapy situation, and (2) the new reality of hypnosis Erickson was introducing in such a suddenly shocking manner that neither she nor her husband could properly evaluate and understand it. She was permitted to indulge in her previous belief system even while Erickson's reality was being introduced in a manner that she could not avoid or resist. Whatever the doubts or resistances of her previous beliefs, she was certainly not prepared to cope with a cane probing her dress while her husband stood poised with another heavy cane ready to clobber the crippled doctor. Since her conscious mental framework could not cope with the situation, her unconscious had to intervene with the appropriate responses of going into trance and accepting Erickson's suggestions.

The senior author assessed and deepened her trance by obtaining her positive response to his two-level posthypnotic suggestion. He then asked her to awaken and sit down. She sat down with a look of expectation, doubt, and hostility. He then addressed her as follows.

Truisms, Implication, and Not Knowing to Initiate an Unconscious Search

E: **Now you are awake, Annie. You don't know what has happened.** *You can think that you wish you knew, but you don't know.*

With this the senior author was stating the obvious. Certainly Annie did have questions on her mind about what, if anything, had happened. Thus the truth of the first part of the statement, "You can think that you wish you knew" opened a yes or acceptance set for the critical suggestion that follows, "but you don't know." This suggestion is critical because it implies that something important did happen, but she does not know what. The implication that *something happened* means she may no longer be what she has always experienced herself as being. The something that happened may be hypnosis; it may mean she now will be able to experience whatever reality Erickson is going to suggest. The *not knowing* thus opens a gap in her belief system that initiates an unconscious search for the internal resources (unconscious processes) that will be needed to carry out Erickson's further suggestions. Not knowing thus facilitates the utilization of inner resources that she had never been able to contact previously in a voluntary manner.

Surprise Question for Not Doing

E: Aren't you surprised you can't stand up?

With this suggestion in the form of a question, Annie did indeed experience amazement at not being able to stand up. The senior author said she would be "surprised," and she certainly was. His question quickly filled the gap and expectation that had been opened in her belief system by setting into operation mental processes that somehow prevented her from standing up. Annie probably did not know why she did not stand up. Neither was she aware that the senior author had also prescribed her reaction of "surprise" at not being able to stand up. Certainly it was true that she would be surprised at not being able to stand up. His question was thus another obvious truism that anyone would have to accept. Even without the previous gap having been opened in her belief system, this question of surprise could stand as beguilingly effective suggestion that anyone would have to accept as true. And most would also experience its implication of the involuntary behavior of not being able to stand.

Self-Test for Anesthesia

E: *No matter how hard I struck you with this cane, you would not feel it. And suppose you take your hand and hit yourself hard on the thigh. It's difficult for me to come over and do it myself, so go ahead. Hit yourself as hard as you can on your thigh. It won't hurt!*

With this Annie did indeed strike a numb thigh and was startled at the effect. She replied, "I felt it in my hand but I didn't feel anything in my leg." Having successfully experienced one fairly easy hypnotic phenomenon in not being able to stand, Erickson judged that she was now ready to experience the really important phenomenon of anesthesia. He made a veiled threat with the thought of striking her with his fearsome cane, so that she cannot help but feel some relief at being permitted to test the anesthesia by herself. Erickson then offers further relief with the fact that he really cannot come over to her (since he is crippled) and thus reinforces her further for a successful self-test of anesthesia. Erickson (Erickson, Rossi, and Rossi, 1976) has stated, "The unconscious always protects the conscious." Certainly Annie did feel a need for protection at this moment. The protection came from her unconscious, which effectively mediated the neuropsychological mechanisms that permitted her to say she had indeed experienced an anesthesia in her leg. Pressing on, the senior author now extends the anesthesia further.

Generalizing Anesthesia

E: *Now Annie, you can hit your thigh again but won't feel it in either your thigh or your hand.*

The senior author now generalizes her successful anesthesia of the thigh to her hand by associating them together in this strong direct suggestion. Annie then slapped her thigh again and exclaimed, "I heard that slap, but I didn't feel it in my hand or my thigh." Thus Annie spontaneously confirmed the reality of the anesthesia to her husband. He could doubt Erickson's explanations, but he could not doubt his wife's reactions. Hence the negative attitude induced by his physician was not disputed by his witnessing Annie's experience—it was depotentiated. That is, he was now experiencing a suspension of his previously doubtful and disbelieving frame of reference. Before he could reassert his doubt, Erickson quickly introduced him to a formally labeled trance.

Compound Suggestion Introducing Trance

E: *You heard that, Archie, you can go into trance now.*

Annie's experience was an effective use of modeling hypnotic behavior for her more resistant husband. The senior author then formally induced trance with a compound statement. "You heard that" was an undeniable truth that opened an acceptance set for the suggestion, "Archie, you can go into trance now." Archie could not deny the reality of his senses regarding his wife's experience, and thus had to accept Erickson's suggested reality of trance.

Utilizing Previous Sense Memories to Replace Pain: A Pun

E: Now, Archie, you've had many long years of happy feelings. Why not get those *happy feelings back*? You've had all the pain you need.

> With such suggestions the senior author began to evoke Archie's sense memories of previous years of good body feelings before his back injury. These memories of good body feelings will be *utilized* to replace his current pain. Notice the therapeutic pun contained in the phrase "happy feelings *back*." Without realizing it Archie was receiving associations of happy feelings with his injured *back*.

Realistic Expectations of Pain Relief and "Booster Shots"

E: I cannot guarantee you against all future pain, but I can tell you to use pain as a warning.

> With such suggestions Archie was able to experience considerable relief from pain. A few months later he caught the flu and telephoned Erickson for a "booster shot," since with the flu there was a recurrence of back pain.

R: Why was there a recurrence of back pain with the flu? Were his body and mind debilitated so he could no longer maintain the hypnotic suggestion of good feelings? Is it the same situation as with you, Dr. Erickson, that when you go to sleep you sometimes lose your own hypnotic control over your body pain? [E's pain is due to constantly atrophiating muscles associated with his second bout with anterior poliomyelitis.] Is hypnosis being mediated on the highest cortical levels which are sensitive to body illness as well as sleep?

E: Yes, just as I induce a trance on the highest cortical level.

R: People really are not asleep in trance; in fact, there is a high degree of mental activity. Perhaps those who say everyone cannot experience trance means you cannot put everyone in a sleeplike state of being an automaton responding indiscriminately to everything that is suggested.

E: Yes, you cannot put everyone into such a passive or submissive state.

R: By hypnosis and trance you mean focused concentration, focused attention. You certainly can facilitate that with anyone whose motivations and needs you understand.

E: Therapeutic trance is focused attention directed in the best manner possible to achieve the patient's goals.

Case 3 Shifting Frames of Reference for Anesthesia and Analgesia

E: When I want a patient to develop an analgesia, I'm very likely not to mention this question of analgesia. I'm very willing to let the patient tell me all about that pain until I can see from the expression on his face that he thinks I understand. I'm not averse to saying a few things, little things that makes the patient think I do understand. And then I'm very likely to ask him some simple question that takes him far away from this question of the pain: "Where did you spend last summer?" The patient can be rather surprised at that question about last summer. Last summer he didn't have that pain. We can go into the question of the pleasures and joys and satisfaction of last summer. Emphasize comfort, physical ease, joys, and satisfactions, and point out to the patient how nice it is to continue to remember the joys and satisfactions of last summer, the physical ease of last summer. When the patient seems to be getting just a little bit edgy, I remind him of when he was rowing the boat and got that blister on his hand. It hurt quite a bit but fortunately healed up.

I haven't been afraid to mention hurt or pain or distress, but it is far away from that backache the patient started telling me about. I've mentioned pain from a blister due to rowing a boat last summer and I haven't been shocked by that uneasy expression on his face. *Because you see in hypnosis your task is to guide the thinking and the association of ideas that the patient has along therapeutic channels.* You know very well that you can have a painful spot on your body and go to a suspenseful movie and lose yourself in the action on the screen and forget all about that pain in your leg or the pain in your arm, aching tooth or wherever. You know that, so why not do exactly the same sort of thing with your patient? If you are operating on a patient in your office and you are aware of the fact that it can cause pain, you can direct your patient's thinking to an area far removed from the pain situation.

I'm thinking of a patient of mine who said, "I'm afraid to go to the dentist, I agonize so much, I perspire so frightfully, I'm in absolute misery." I asked the patient immediately, "Did you do that as a child?"

I was listening to her complaint about pain, anxiety, distress, and I asked her what she did in her childhood. I made good contact with her by talking of the distress she was interested in, but I shifted to another frame of reference—childhood. She now talked about her childhood distress, but that was so far away that it was less disturbing and she felt a bit more comfortable. My next step was to ask her what her favorite pleasure was as a child. Now, how do you get from pain, anxiety, distress, to pleasure as a child? In this case it took only two associative steps. It was so delightful to switch and discuss with me a favorite activity of her childhood. Now she discussed this pleasure in immediate connection with my first question of her experience of distress in childhood. By that immediate succession of questions I tied the two together—distress and favorite activity.

After she told me all about her favorite pleasures as a child, one in particular, I suggested that when she went to the dentist's office, she should really settle in the dental chair. As she really squirmed around in the chair and really felt her seat on the chair seat, her back on the back of the chair, her arms on the arms of the chair, and her head on the headrest, she would have an overwhelming recollection of her favorite childhood activity that would absolutely dominate the entire situation. Now, what had I done? I had taken the painful realities of the dental chair, squirming around trying to get a nice comfortable seat (and I wiggled around in my seat to role-play the way I wanted her to find herself in that dental chair), and associated it with one of her favorite childhood activities. The thing that she remembered was playing in the leaves on the lawn. In the autumn you can build great big houses out of the leaves, nice pathways through piles of leaves, you could bury yourself in the leaves. You could squirm around and get nice and comfortable in those leaves and the rest of the real world would seem far away.

With that she simply went into a very nice anesthetic trance in the dentist's office without any direct suggestions for anesthesia. Now and then the dentist would ask her some stupid question when she really wanted to think about the leaves. The dentist thought that she was an awfully cooperative patient. Mentally she would notice that here was some stupid person trying to talk to her when she was burying herself in the leaves, probably some grownup yelling at her, but she was more interested in the leaves. She could have dental surgery done and not be bothered by it.

You can achieve anesthesia indirectly by shifting the person's frames of reference. In this case the critical shift was to, "What was your favorite activity as a child?" And then I could really elaborate on that. *In other words, you very carefully raise a question. You raise it in such a way that you can slide past the difficulty and start up another train of mental activity, of emotional activity, that precludes the possibility of feeling pain.* Some of my sophisticated subjects with training in clinical psychology and psychiatry, that I have used as subjects, will pick apart the technique that I have used on them. They then recognize the validity of it from their own experiences. They will have me employ precisely the same techniques on them again because they know that they are human and that you can do the same thing with pleasure, over and over again.

I think it is an error to always strive to get an anesthesia or an analgesia directly. I think you should be willing to accomplish them indirectly because every time you ask somebody "Forget that this is a watch," you're asking them to do a specific thing—to forget—to forget what? A watch. Now, remember, forget that watch. That's what you're saying when you say, "Forget the watch." But you can ask them to look at this, an interesting thing. It rather amuses me. It's rather fascinating how you can look at something and become tremendously fascinated with it, and then the topic of conversation changes, and you drift far away to that trip you had in Europe. Now what was it I came up here for? You drifted far, far away from your original preoccupation because you started following your different trains of thought.

Now the next thing that you should bear in mind is that when you take away the sense of feeling, anesthesia or analgesia, you've asked your patient to make a different kind of a reality orientation. In some of my earliest experimental work I asked students to discover what the mental processes were in picking up an imaginary apple and putting it on a concrete reality table in front of them (Erickson, 1964). What are the mental processes? A goodly number of the students complained of feeling funny all over and gave up the task; they left without completing the experimental situation. They were losing their contact with reality. Therefore, they felt funny. Now when you induce an analgesia, you are asking your patients to lose a certain amount of their reality contact. You are asking them to alter it. Then they begin to feel funny—they may recognize it or they may not. But they can react to that by getting out of the situation because it is strange and uncomfortable. Therefore, whenever you induce an analgesia or an anesthesia, you must see to it that your patients don't get frightened in one way or the other by the loss of their usual reality relationship. I let those students feel funny all over and let them run out on me because it was an important experimental finding that I wanted to study.

In working with patients in the office, when they get a funny feeling, whether they recognize it as a funny feeling or they just experience it as discomfort, they want to run out, too. But they can't afford it, and neither can you. Therefore, it is your obligation to tell them that one of the astonishing things is that as they begin to feel more comfortable or they get more and more interested in this or that, perhaps they will notice the light in the office is of a softer hue. Quite often I have told patients in my office, "I hope you don't mind here as we continue our work if the light automatically dims and becomes softer or lighter." Whenever their reality orientations are altered, I know patients are going to tell me the office is getting lighter or darker, or getting warmer or colder, or they feel afraid, or that they feel the office is getting bigger or smaller, that they are feeling taller or shorter. They get all manner of changes in their sense of reality whenever we explore anesthesia or analgesia. These spontaneous sensory-perceptual alterations are all indications that the patients' reality orientations are altered; trance is developing whether a formal hypnotic induction has been carried out or not. As patients learn to be more comfortable with these spontaneous alterations, they can allow themselves to go deeper into trance. They learn to give up more and more of their generalized reality orientation (Shor, 1959), and they become more capable of experiencing all the classical hypnotic phenomena as well as achieving their own therapeutic goals.

Case 4   Utilizing the Patient's Own Personality and Abilities for Pain Relief

E: I wanted to produce an anesthesia, a relief of terminal cancer pain for Cathy. She was suffering intolerable pain that could not be relieved by morphine, Demerol, or anything else. She was in a desperately debilitated state of mind in which she just repeated, "Don't hurt me, don't scare me, don't hurt me, don't scare me, don't hurt me, don't hurt me." A continuous, monotonous, urgent crying out of those two particular sentences. My opportunity of intruding upon her was rather small. What could I do in order to bring about a relief of the pain? I had to use Cathy's own learnings. I had to use my own thinking, and my thinking, of course, would not be in accord with the thinking of this high school graduate who knew she had only a couple of months left to live. She was thirty-six years old with three children; the oldest was eleven years old. Therefore, her thinking would be totally different, her desires would be so totally different, all of her understandings would be totally different from mine, and my task was, of course, to bring about a hypnotic state in which I could stimulate her to do something with her own past learnings. I didn't want to try to struggle in a futile way when the woman had already learned morphine had no effect on her, when Demerol, no matter how large the dose, seemed to have no effect on her. I didn't want to try to struggle with her and tell her she should go into a trance, because that would be a rather futile thing. Therefore, I asked her to do something that she could understand in her own reality orientations. I asked her to stay wide awake from the neck up. That was something she could understand. I told her to let her body go to sleep. In her past understandings as a child, as a youth, as a young woman she had had the experience of a leg going to sleep, of an arm going to sleep. She had had the feeling of her body being asleep in that hypnagogic state of arousing in the morning when you are half awake, half asleep. I was very very certain the woman had some understanding of her body being asleep. Thus the woman could use her own past learnings. Just what that meant to her, I don't know. *All I wanted to do was to start a train of thinking and understanding that would allow the woman to call upon the past experiential learnings of her body.*

I did not ask her to contend with me about going into a trance, because that, I thought, was futile. I did not ask her to try her level best to cooperate with me in going into a trance, because she didn't know what a trance was. But she did know what being wide awake was. She did know what a body being asleep was, because she had a lifelong experience of both states. The next thing I asked her to do after her body was asleep was to develop an itch on the soles of her feet. How many people have had itches on various parts of their bodies? Miserable itches, uncontrollable itches, distressing itches. We all have had that sort of experience, therefore I was again suggesting something to her that was well within her experience, within her physiological, psychological, neurological experience; within her total body of learnings. I was asking her to do something for which she had memories, understandings, and past experience. I was very, very urgent about this development of an itch. The woman shortly reported to me that she was awfully sorry she could not develop an itch. All that she could do was to develop a numb feeling on the dorsum of the foot. In other words the woman was unable in her state of pain to add to her state of pain. She did the exact opposite. She developed a feeling of numbness, not on the sole of the foot, but on the dorsum of the foot.

Now, what was my purpose in seeing her? That is the thing that all of you should keep in mind in dealing with patients. *You are seeking to alter their body experiences; their body awareness; their body understandings; their body responses.* Every change that develops should be grist for your mill, because it means that the patient is responding. When Cathy told me she had the numbness on the dorsum of the foot, I accepted that as a most desirable thing and I expressed regret, politely, that she had not been able to develop an itch. Why did I express a polite, courteous regret that she had not developed an itch? Why should I criticize or find fault with my patient's responses? I should be gracious about it, because Cathy had a lifelong history of experience with people who had been courteous, who had expressed regret, and who thereby put her at ease since earliest childhood in various situations. Cathy had a background of experience into which my courteous regret could fit.

Now the point I am trying to establish is this: When you talk to patients, talk to them to convey ideas and understandings in such a way that your remarks fit into the total situation with which you are dealing. You try to elicit an ever-widening response on the patients' part so that they respond more and more with their experiential learnings, with their past memories and understanding. Cathy could accept my apology and feel obligated. Since she failed me in one regard, she could feel obligated to put forth more and more effort on the thing that I accepted. While accepting Cathy's numbness on the dorsum of her foot, *I also utilized her own background and personality to intensify her efforts to please me*. Since I had been so gracious in accepting her failure to produce the itch, I intensified her motivation to cooperate with me in any further tasks.

The next thing I did was to suggest that the numbness extend not only over the dorsum of the foot but perhaps to the sole of the foot and the ankle. Well, of course, in suggesting the sole of the foot where Cathy had failed to put an itch, she would be all the more eager to produce the numbness. As surely as she did that, she would be obligated to develop a numbness of the ankle. Of course Cathy had had plenty of experience being unaware of the sole of her foot, unaware of her ankle. Cathy knew what numbness was, and she had body learnings of those things. Therefore, when I asked her to do those things, she could make a response. Now Cathy was not paying any attention to her bed, to the pictures on the wall, to the presence of the other physician with me, to the tape recorder that was in full view. Cathy was directing her mental attention to her body learnings. In the use of hypnosis you need to be aware of the total unimportance of external reality. Now as Cathy developed the numbness in the sole of her foot and the numbness in her ankle, she withdrew more and more completely from the reality of the room. She was giving her reality orientation to her body, not in terms of cancer pain but in terms of body learnings of numbness. Cathy became very greatly interested in letting the numbness progress from her ankles to the calf, to the knee, to the lower third of the thigh, the middle third, the upper third, having it cross over to the other side of her pelvis and go down the other leg so that she had a numbness from the umbilicus down. Now that interested Cathy. At that moment, of what interest was the ceiling, the bed, the doctor, the walls, or anything else? Cathy's interest was directed to that state of numbness just as dental patients should be so fascinated by the thought of the control of capillary circulation, by the thought of dental anesthesia, by the thought of learning how to chew their food with a different kind of bite so that they won't have temporal mandibular pain. The thing that interests the patients, the reason they are in your office, should be the point of orientation.

With Cathy oriented to the numbness of her leg and pelvis it was a simple matter to extend the numbness up to her neck. Cathy had metastases throughout her torso, she had lung metastases, metastases in the bones in the spine as well as the bones of the pelvis. When you consider that sort of thing, you make every effort to extend the numbness. Here is a patient who knows that she is going to die within a few months. She has been assured of that by physicians whom she trusts and believes, so death is an absolute reality, while the walls of the room, the bed itself might not be an important part of reality. This matter of impending death, this matter of her family, was an unforgettable reality, and so in dealing with her experience of pain it was necessary to include some of the ordinary reality of her daily existence. Cathy had had that cancer for about a year. If I want to help Cathy, I have to organize any hypnotic suggestions that I give her in such a fashion that they incorporate some of Cathy's own thinking, some of Cathy's own understanding. The first thing I did for Cathy in the matter of numbness of the chest was to mention that her cancer first started in her right breast and then to mention that there was still an area of ulceration at the site of the surgery and that that ulcerated area was painful. That is a bit of external reality but it is also a bit of body reality, because Cathy could look down at that ulcerated area, which made it external to her because it was something she was looking at. The pain was a personal experience within her body. The visual thing was external and unpleasant and disagreeable, and that external vision could threaten her life. The pain and distress was an internal experience so far as Cathy was concerned. Therefore, I made Cathy aware of some of the external environment. She was already aware of the internal environment, so I merely made certain to include external environment, but an important part of external environment. The walls in her bedroom, the pillows on her bed, weren't important parts of external reality, but her visual impression of that ulcerated area was a most important part of her external orientation, and so I directed her attention to that.

Cathy had expressed regret because she had not been able to develop an itch on the sole of her foot. What should I do? Now, too many operators, too many people who use hypnosis try to be perfectionists, they try to accomplish too much. That is one of the reasons for failure in many instances—the effect to try to accomplish too much. Any student in high school or college will tell you: certainly I can't make 100, I might make 95, or I might make 90, I can't do better than an 85, I am lucky to get an 80. We have that sort of an orientation. Even the expert marksman says: I hope to get 10 out of 10, but I am not at all certain of that. Expert bowlers would like to make a certain score, but they never really honestly expect in every game to have a perfect score; they expect a certain amount of failure. Those who use hypnosis had better bear in mind that the patients they are working on have a lifetime of experience in expecting a certain amount of failure. You, as the therapist, ought to utilize, you ought to go along with, the patients, and you ought to be the one that picks out the area of failure. It was tremendously important that Cathy be relieved of that pain, but she had an experience of going to high school Cathy knew by virtue of a lifetime of experience that she could not achieve perfection in her performances. Therefore, in suggesting relief I was very very careful to ensure a certain percentage of failure. What had failed Cathy in the first place? Her first failure was in that right breast, that is where the cancer started, that is where she had her first sense of personal failure. Her right breast had let her down. Her right breast had doomed her. There is no way of getting around that understanding on Cathy's part. That right breast had doomed her. So now I express my sorrow, my regret that I couldn't take away the pain at the site of that awful ulcerated area on her chest. I recognized aloud to Cathy that that was a minor pain, a minor distress, and I was awfully sorry that I failed. Now Cathy could agree with me, and she could agree with me when I wished that I could produce the same numbness there that I had produced elsewhere in her body. In other words I made use of the double bind: As long as she had distress at the breast area, she had to have numbness elsewhere in her body. Thus I had all of Cathy's general experience substantiating the numbness of most of her body.

Now, there is nothing magical about what I did—*it was a recognition of the thinking that Cathy would do* . . . the thinking and the understanding that would derive out of Cathy's ordinary life. A woman who grew up in this culture, in this age, would have certain learnings as a result of just being alive. Now, when I left that minor pain, that minor distress, it proved that I was not God. It just gave Cathy another goal to strive for, even though she had the feeling that she would fail as far as this minor pain was concerned. Cathy lived from February, when I saw her, until August. She lapsed into coma and died rather suddenly. But during that length of time, Cathy was free of pain except in this one particular area, but as Cathy said, she didn't hold my failure against me. Why should she? By letting her keep that minor pain, I ensured the success of the rest.

We need to understand the way we behave emotionally. We can take only so much, but there is always one last straw. In the use of hypnosis we make use of that particular learning: We get rid of everything but leave that last straw as a distraction because it is a minor thing. I removed the major part of her pain but just left that last straw which Cathy could consider unimportant. Now I have stressed this because I want to impress upon you the tremendous importance in *offering your suggestions not as the thing the patient is to do but as the stimulus to elicit patient behavior in accord with individual body learnings, individual psychological experiences.* I suggested an itch on the foot, which would be adding to her pain. My purpose was not really to produce an itch on the sole of her foot. My purpose in suggesting that was merely to start Cathy functioning within herself—to start Cathy using her own body learnings and to use them according to her own pattern of response. Then when Cathy developed the numbness on the dorsum of the foot and expressed her regret, I used that regret and numbness. I could use it intelligently to bring about the relief of pain that would meet Cathy's needs. When I first approached Cathy, I had no understanding at all about how I could produce a relief of pain for her, because I didn't know her. I knew nothing really about the uniqueness of her own individual learning. My initial task was to say something that would get Cathy's attention and allow her to make her own personal responses. I then utilized those responses. In the use of hypnosis in medicine, dentistry, and psychology there is a need to explore the kind of thinking and responding that is characteristic of the individual patient. We need to recognize the actual unimportance of what we say as being the goal to be achieved. *The importance of what we say lies in its being a stimulus for the elicitation of responses peculiar to the patient. We then help the patients utilize these responses in new ways to achieve their therapeutic goals.*

Selected Shorter Cases: Exercises for Analysis

In this section are summaries of cases by the senior author and others illustrating the basic principles we have explained. Some are reported here for the first time; others have been published elsewhere. The student would do well to analyze the dynamics of their effectiveness in terms of the concepts introduced in this and precedings chapters. Some guides for this analysis are placed in italics at the end of each case.

A Tiger Under the Bed

A woman dying of terminal cancer was brought to Erickson's office in an ambulance. She was in desperate pain, and drugs no longer diminished it. She was frankly skeptical of hypnosis and immediately told Erickson of her doubts upon entering his office. He proceeded impressively as follows: "Madam, I think I can convince you. And you know how much pain you are suffering, how uncontrollable it is. If you saw a hungry tiger walking through that doorway, licking its chops and looking at you, how much pain would you feel?" She was apparently stunned by this unexpected question and said, "Not a bit. In fact, I'm not feeling any pain now either." Erickson then replied, "Is it agreeable to you to keep that hungry tiger around?" She said, "It certainly is"! All the associations to hungry tiger had so focused her attention that she was in a "walking trance," from which she need not be awakened. She presented the entire appearance of being awake in all other respects. Yet she could see and experience the presence of that tiger at any time, day or night. The hypnotherapist simply evokes surprising sets of emotional, cognitive, or behavioral responses to interfere with the symptoms he needs to alter.

The senior author then told her that her doctors and nurses might not believe it, but she now experienced the truth of pain relief. And, indeed, her physicians and nurses did not understand. Whenever they came to offer her an injection for pain relief, the woman responded with a warm smile, "No, thank you, I don't need any. I have a hungry tiger under my bed." They suspected she was hallucinating and perhaps losing contact with reality, but in those last months of her life she lived in apparent comfort without the use of narcotics or tranquillizing medication. Her family thought she was just fine, however.

Shock; Surprise; Fixation of attention; Common everyday trance; Distracting associations; Altered frames of reference; Posthypnotic suggestion to protect the therapeutic work

Chin on a Chair

The senior author has had to deal with personal pain problems all his life because of poliomyelitis. He usually can control pain effectively during the daytime by simply going into autohypnotic trance. When he gets very tired or goes to sleep at night, however, the pain sometimes returns and wakes him up. He then has to rearrange his muscles and mental composure to get rid of the pain again. Sometimes in the middle of the night this is just not easy. On such occasions he confesses to having sometimes pulled a chair to the side of his bed, hooking his chin over the back of the chair, and pressing down until he could no longer stand the pain he produced voluntarily (Erickson and Rossi, 1977).

Hypnotic suggestion as a highly developed cognitive frame of reference that can sometimes fail during sleep; Distracting involuntary pain with voluntary control over pain

Shaggy Dog Stories

Then there was the patient with paralysis from the level of the twelfth thoracic vertebra who had severe recurring attacks of pain associated with an acute cystitis and pyelitis. He would endure his pain until he could no longer control his outcries. Since his general condition was chronic, narcotics were inadvisable. Because he was an earnest, sincere, considerate, socially-minded man, but totally lacking any sense of humor or capacity to understand wordplays and puns, his pain was handled by the simple procedure of instructing the nurses to tell him shaggy-dog stories, especially those employing word-plays and puns. He would listen earnestly, appreciative of the "sociability" of the nurse, and struggle absorbedly in trying to make sense of her narrative. As time went on the patient spontaneously would summon a nurse and state that his pain was starting up—could she spare a minute or two of her time to talk to him, and he would "try to understand" her story.

Fixation of attention; Distraction; Unconscious search and processes

Head and Shoulder to the Solarium

In a case of terminal-illness pain in a woman with a young daughter the senior author addressed the young daughter as follows: "Now your mother wants to be convinced that she can be free from pain. That is what you are going to do—convince your mother. Now just sit in this chair here, and while you're sitting in that chair, go into a trance and go over to the other side of the room. And I want you to lose all sense of feeling everywhere. You will be without feeling in a deep trance. You are sitting here, but you're over there on the other side of the room and you are watching yourself there. . . . Now you watch, mother. Your daughter is in a deep trance. She thinks she's on the other side of the room. Now keep your eye on me because I'm going to do something that no mother would ever want done." I rolled the girl's skirt up to expose her bare thighs. The mother looked on in horror as I did that. I raised my hand and I brought it down on her thigh with a terrific slap. The girl was watching herself on the other side of the room. Now I can't slap a girl on the other side of the room, can I? The mother was aghast that there was not a single wince out of the girl. Then I slapped the other thigh. The girl was still comfortable.

This mother was highly addicted to television so I eventually taught her that whenever she had a pain she could not tolerate, she was to leave her body there in bed and take her head and shoulders out into the living room and watch T.V.

This dissociative approach to pain relief was one of the senior author's favorites. In hospital practice he would frequently have patients take their head and shoulders out to the solarium while their surgeon did the necessary work on their bodies in the operating room.

Shock; Surprise; Modeling hypnotic behavior; Dissociation

Numb with Conversation

The conversational approach to fixating and holding the patient's attention can be very useful in traumatic stituations. There was an automobile accident in Portland, Oregon, and a man skidded on his face on a gravel road for about thirty feet. A gravel dirt road. He was brought into the hospital as an emergency case. One of the members of the American Society of Clinical Hypnosis—we will call him Dan—who does a great deal of plastic surgery and oral surgery was on emergency call that night. He went in and found that the man was conscious and suffering a great deal of pain. Those of you who know Dan know what a marvelous talker he is. He has a steady stream of words, of humor, of interest, of information, a tremendous wealth of knowledge and humor. Dan said, "You really filled your face full of gravel and you know what kind of a job that makes for me. I've got to take tweezers and pick out

140

every confounded little granule of sand and dirt and I am really going to have a job and I've really got to mop up that face and get half the hide off it and you have been suffering pain and you want some help out of it and you really ought to get some kind of pain relief and *the sooner you start feeling less pain the better* and I don't know what you ought to do while you're waiting for the nurse to bring something to inject in your arm but you really ought to listen to me while I am talking to you and explaining to you that I have to do certain things about your face. You know there is a gash here, that must have been a pretty sharp stone that cut that one, but here is a short one and here is a bad bruise and I really ought to mop it off with alcohol. *It will hurt at first a little, but after it is done a few times the sting will deaden the tip of the nerves that are exposed and you stop feeling the sting of the alcohol*, and did you ever try to make a violin? You know you can make violins out of myrtle wood, you can make them out of spruce wood. Did you ever try making one out of oak?" Dan had won a national award for the best tone violin that he himself built out of myrtle wood, and Dan kept up his steady stream. Now and then he discussed the tremendous difficulty of really mopping up that face and putting in the stitches and wondering when the nurse would get around to the hypodermic. All the while, behind him, the nurse was passing Dan the right sort of instrument, the right sort of suture, the right sort of swab, and so on. Dan just kept up that steady stream and the patient said, "You are awfully gabby, arent't you?" Dan said, 'You haven't heard me at my best I can talk with a still greater rate of speed just give me a chance and I'll really get into high." Then Dan started getting into high, "You know I think fast too and did you ever hear anybody sing the Bumble Bee? I'd better hum it to you." So Dan hummed the Bumble Bee and finally he said, "You know that is about all." The patient said, "What do you mean about all?" Dan said, "Here's a mirror, take a look." The patient looked and he said, "When did you put in those sutures? When did you clean my face? When did I get an injection? I thought you were just talking to me, just getting ready." Dan said, "I've been working hard for over a couple of hours, about two and a half hours." The patient said, "You didn't. You've been talking about five or ten minutes." Dan said, "No, take a look, count those stitches if you want to, and how does your face feel?" The patient said, "My face is numb."

Conversational approach; Fixation of attention; Distraction; Interspersal of suggestions; Time distortion

Calloused Nerves

Recently I had a patient sent to me with chronic hip pain. Very serious pain. I knew better than to try to induce a direct trance in the patient. What did I need to do? Everything I said to that patient, I think, was horribly unscientific, but the patient wanted certain understandings that she could accept, that could justify that chronic uncontrollable hip pain. I accepted the patient's absolute statements of uncontrollable pain. I accepted every one of her statements, so she knew that I believed and thought the way she did. Then I began an entirely specious explanation of how that pain came about, so that the patient could understand it in terms of her own frames of reference. I explained how that hypodermic shot of penicillin or whatever it was, probably had a needle with a ragged point and in being stuck in the hip, hit the sciatic nerve. I explained how the tip of the needle could tear nerve fibers, and I gave a long dissertation on the structure of a nerve. It is not just one single fiber; it is made up of many many fibers. I gave a dissertation on the different kinds of sensations that travel over the fibers. You get heat traveling on one fiber and cold on another, and a touch on another, and pressure on another, until that patient thought that I was rather erudite. Finally, when she was rather bored with this increasing hodgepodge of information, I threw in a suggestion here and there about pain wearing out, of the body becoming accommodated. A laborer with tender hands such as mine would have blisters very promptly using the pick and shovel. But with the pick and shovel wielded a half minute one day, a minute the next day, a minute and a half the third day, and a gradual progression in the length of time, there would be a callous formation until the pick and shovel could be handled all day long. I threw in all sorts of apparently sensible analogies. I pointed out that callous formations can be the skin of your hand and that one can also become used to emotional deprivation. In other words one can form emotional callouses, one can form intellectual callouses, dermal callouses, nerve callouses—all that sort of thing, until the patient listening to me began accepting all of those suggestions and began on her own to seek a way to use them to help herself lose pain. Every one of those things that I said about callous formation had the effect of the patient's thinking: "Yes, I know what callous is. I wish I could have a callous at the nerve in my hip where all that pain is. How nice it would be. How would my leg feel if I had a callous there? It would feel this comfortable, as comfortable as my other leg does." I presented ideas that the patient could find acceptable, but I wasn't asking her to accept those ideas. I was merely explaining possibilities, explaining them in such a way that the patient had to reach out and pull in whatever ideas she needed to facilitate her comfort. Now what is this suggestion? I think that this woman with hip pain was in the kind of trance that was effective for her. I did not dare attempt to induce a formal trance that she could recognize, because I knew she would then think the "calloused nerves" was just my idea that I was trying to force on her.

Yes set; Specious suggestion fitting the patient's frame of reference; Boredom depotentiating conscious sets; Interspersed suggestions initiating unconscious searches and processes; Indirect associative focusing; Indirect ideodynamic focusing; Open-ended suggestions

CHAPTER 6

Symptom Resolution

The basic view of modern psychosomatic medicine is that symptoms are forms of communication. As such, symptoms are frequently important signs or cues of developmental problems that are in the process of becoming conscious. What patients cannot yet clearly express in the form of a cognitive or emotional insight will find somatic expression as a body symptom. The conventional psychoanalytic approach to such problems is to facilitate "insight" so that the language of body symptoms is translated into patterns of cognition and emotional understanding. It is sometimes found that when patients can talk about their problems with emotional insight, they no longer need to experience their body symptoms.

Hypnosis has been an important tool in the evolution of this basic view of psychosomatic medicine (Zilboorg and Henry, 1941; Tinterow, 1970), and continues today as an important modality for the resolution of symptomatic behavior. The senior author's major contribution in this area is the discovery that while emotional insight is usually a very desirable approach in resolving psychosomatic problems, it is by no means the only route. He has developed ways of resolving symptomatic behavior "directly on an unconscious level." That is, symptoms may be resolved by working with a patient's psychodynamics in such a manner that consciousness does not know why the body symptom disappears. Moreover, the developmental problem that was expressed in the symptom is also resolved in an apparently spontaneous manner. Patients are usually pleasantly surprised by this. They say they did not even realize the therapist was working on their sexual problems, their educational problems, or whatever.

Two-level communication is our basic approach to working directly with the unconscious. We use words with many connotations and implications, so that while the patients' conscious frames of reference are receiving communication on one level, their unconscious is processing other patterns of meaning contained in the words. The senior author likes to point out that he uses "folk language" or "intimate language" to reach deep sources within the patient. He uses such mythopoetic processes (Rossi, 1972b) as analogy, metaphor, puns, riddles, jokes, and all sorts of verbal and imagistic play to communicate in ways that bypass or supplement the patient's usual frames of reference (Erickson, Rossi, and Rossi, 1976).

Why are such processes effective? We believe they work because they utilize the patient's own life experiences and previous patterns of learning in a therapeutic manner. A pun or a joke can bypass an erroneous and limiting conscious framework and effectively mobilize unconscious processes in ways that the patient's conscious intentionality could not.

Recent research in hemispheric functioning (Gazzaniga, 1967; Sperry, 1968; Galin, 1974; Rossi, 1977) suggests that the effectiveness of these approaches may be in their appeal to the right, or nondominant, hemispheric functioning. While the left, or dominant, hemisphere is proficient in processing verbal communications of an intellectual or abstract nature, the right hemisphere is more adept in processing data of a visuospatial, kinesthetic, imagistic, or mythopoetic nature. Since the right hemisphere is also more closely associated with emotional processes and the body image (Luria, 1973; Galin, 1974), the view has developed that it is also responsible for the formation of psychosomatic symptoms. These symptoms are expressions in the language of the right hemisphere. Our use of mythopoetic language may thus be a means of communicating directly with the right hemisphere in its own language. This is in contrast to the conventional psychoanalytic approach of first translating the right hemisphere's body language into the abstract patterns of cognition of the left hemisphere, which must then somehow operate back upon the right hemisphere to change the symptom. That approach sometimes works, but it is obviously cumbersome and time-consuming. All too often the patient develops marvelous patterns of intellectual insight, yet the body symptom remains. Even if the intellectual insight to the left hemisphere is correct, it may remain isolated from the right hemisphere's sources of symptom formation and maintenance. Thus, while the senior author developed the two-level communication approach long before our current understanding of left and right hemispheric patterns of specializations, we now believe that this "working directly with the unconscious" may be a means of communicating directly with the right, or nondominant, hemisphere, which is probably responsible for psychosomatic symptoms.

Case 5   A General Approach to Symptomatic Behavior

Miss X, who had plans to become a professional harpist, consulted the senior author for help with her problem of sweating palms and fingers. Her hands were usually damp, and when she tried to play in front of an audience, the perspiration was so great that her fingers would slip off the strings. The numerous medical doctors she consulted were both amazed and amused that she could hold one hand extended and soon form a puddle on the floor of the perspiration dripping steadily from her hand. They recommended a sympathectomy but could not be sure even that would solve the problem.

A salient feature of this initial session was the senior author's indirect exploration of the possible relation between the symptom of sweating and sexuality. His clinical experience has been that this symptom is usually associated with a problem in sexual adjustment. Since Miss X presented sweating as her only problem, however, his clinical judgment was to explore the possible relation between the excessive sweating and her sexuality indirectly by two-level communication. He did this by utilizing puns, certain words, and turns of phrase with double meaning, intonations, and pauses that may evoke sexual associations within Miss X if they are in fact associated with her problem. Rather than directly confront her with a clear statement about sexual problems in a manner that might arouse resistances, he simply provides contexts, implications, and association patterns that will enable her to bring up the sexual problem by herself. If he happens to be wrong in his clinical hypothesis about the sexual etiology of her symptom, nothing is lost; Miss X simply will not pick up and utilize the sexual associations.

There is a certain difficulty in presenting this material in a convincing manner in written form, because so many of the possible sexual associations are cued by intonation of voice, pauses, a certain smile or glance, etc. To facilitate the reader's understanding, words and phrases that could arouse latent sexual associations—if they are, in fact, present in the listener—will be italicized.

In the first part of the interview the senior author is involved in the process of preparation. A positive rapport and response attentiveness are established, and he begins to assess which of her abilities may be utilized. He facilitates therapeutic frames of reference and heightens her expectancy of receiving help. He initiates a process of two-level communication whereby he explores the possible sexual etiology of her problem and utilizes her special interest in music to enhance her first experience of therapeutic trance. We witness many of his approaches to depotentiating limitations in her conscious frames of reference and an interesting approach to symptom dynamics during what appears on the surface to be a simple process of hand levitation.

In the second part of this interview he leads her into a deeper experience of trance, during which she is very evidently engrossed in inner work. By the third and final part of this interview he is using ideomotor signaling to evaluate and ratify the process of therapeutic change that has already taken place. During this interview we witness with unusual clarity the logic of his general approach to symptomatic behavior:

1. He establishes rapport and focuses attention into a therapeutic frame of reference.
2. He demonstrates with the patients' own experience how their unconscious controls their behavior. This is a means of depotentiating their habitual framework and belief systems so he can then assign the locus of therapeutic change to the patients' unconscious.
3. He utilizes the indirect forms of suggestion (in this case particularly two-level communication) to evoke searches and processes on an unconscious level that may initiate a change in the dynamics of symptom formation.
4. He then demonstrates the resulting therapeutic change via ideomotor signals and/or the patient's obvious release from symptomatic behavior.
5. He then allows the patient to fully recognize and appreciate the significance of the psychodynamic insights about the source and meaning of the symptom that frequently come up spontaneously at this time. Ideas and attitudes facilitating a general enhancement of the patient's total life experience without the symptom are explored and integrated.

As will be seen, the first three steps may appear in varying order. They may appear almost simultaneously or in sequence, with varying degrees of repetition depending on the needs and responses of the individual patient. The successful demonstration of therapeutic change in Step 4, together with posthypnotic suggestions for the maintenance of this change, usually sets the stage for the broader patterns of new understanding and life reorganization that frequently take place in Step 5.

Together these five steps constitute a paradigm of our general approach to symptom resolution. Within this paradigm the therapist may explore one or more psychodynamic hypotheses about the source and maintenance of the symptom. The senior author's exploration within the two sessions of this case was so indirect, however, that we were not able to ascertain whether his hypothesis about the sexual etiology of Miss X's problem was correct. It wasn't until he received a letter three months after the termination of therapy, wherein Miss X confirmed that sweating was no longer a problem and that she had simulatenously resolved an important sexual difficulty, that we had confirmation that his two-level approach was correct and therapeutic.

This case thus arouses fascinating questions about the possibilities of a hypnotherapy based on the utilization of a patient's own creative

146

potentials rather than the older tradition of hypnosis as a form of direct suggestion. We observe that it is possible to release a patient's creative potentials in such a way that a problem can actually be resolved without patient or therapist really knowing the exact why or dynamics of cure. In the second session, however, the senior author does support the symptom-removal work of the first session by facilitating the growth of Miss X's insight regarding the etiology of her excessive sweating and related problems of claustrophobia, fears of flying, and her general life orientation. It will be seen in this second session that the idea of simple "symptom removal" is a gross oversimplification of what sound hypnotherapy can be. The hypnotherapist is more appropriately involved in the broader program of facilitating a creative reorganization of the patient's inner psychodynamics so that life experience is enhanced and symptom formation is no longer necessary.

SESSION ONE
Part One: Preparation and Initial Trance Work

Trance Induction with an Indirect Exploration of Sexual Associations by Two-Level Communication

E: Now the first step, of course, is to *untangle your legs*. And untangle your hands. Now *what do you think I should do*?

X: Well, to be perfectly honest with you, I guess I probably feel that *you ought to hypnotize me. In that if you don't, I might be aware of what you are doing*, and that would wreck it.

E: All right, now what is your education?

X: I have a master's degree in social work.

> E: "*Untangle your legs*," of course, has sexual associations. "Untangle your hands" means no more resistance.
>
> R: These simple changes of body position tend to lower resistance immediately.
>
> E: *What should I do*? Ever make love to a girl? Recognize the sexual connotation in that? It is pleasing to a girl to let her make the decisions. But these implications need not be consciously recognized. She feels I *ought* to, but she is not telling me I "have to." To hypnotize her would be the proper thing. *If you don't, I might be aware of what you are doing*, may be a two-level communication implying a recognition of sexual connotations right from her unconscious.

147

R: It can be a two-level communication even if she doesn't recognize it on a conscious level. This then is your first use of two-level communication to explore the possible sexual etiology of her problem.

Facilitating a Therapeutic Frame of Reference: Separating Conscious from Unconscious

E: **Then you know something about the conscious mind and the unconscious.**

X: **Yes.**

R: Here you begin the process of introducing a very important therapeutic frame of reference, distinguishing between the conscious and unconscious mind. Once patients come to realize and accept the reality of an autonomous and potentially creative unconscious system that is different from their conscious system (which is bogged down with a problem), they are immediately within a more therapeutic frame of reference, because they now have a rationale for giving up some of their older ways of doing things and are more open to new experience within themselves. Even for those readers who think of the "unconscious" as a mere metaphor, however, it is useful to make this separation between conscious and unconscious because of the therapeutic double binds you can later set up with this division.

The Pause as an Indirect Form of Hypnotic Suggestion

E: *And when you dream at night,** what part of your mind are you using?**

X: **The unconscious?**

E: **Yes, and that does not prevent you from knowing the next day *what you dreamed about, does it?***

X: **That's right, sometimes.**

E: **Yes. The conscious mind is usually pretty busy with itself, but it can be aware of the unconscious mind.**

---

*These breaks in the transcription approximate the natural pauses in the senior author's speech.

E: *When you dream at night,* your imagination is unfettered.

R: Therefore, the pause after the word "night" allows that first phase of the sentence to be momentarily associated with sexual connotations. The pause that isolates a phrase with its own implications and connotations is thus another indirect form of hypnotic suggestion.

E: The tone of my voice in saying *What you dreamed about, does it?* also carries sexual connotations.

Indirect Sexual Associations Interspersed in Trance Preparation

E: *All right, so that eliminates this question of preventing you from knowing what I'm doing.* You can know what I'm doing, but I can also do some things you don't know about. All right, what is *your favorite piece of music?*

X: My favorite piece of music? I think, uh, Y's Harp Concerto in F Minor.

E: Do you know what tone deafness is?

X: Yes.

E: I am tone deaf.

X: I know.   I noticed you are wearing purple.

E: The first sentence in a suggestive tone of voice reinforces the earlier sexual connotations. *Music* has sexual associations, as when you turn on soft music to make love. "Favorite piece" also has sexual connotations for some.

R: So this is actually an association on two levels: To the conscious mind it is an inquiry about her interest in music; to the unconscious, however, there are the sexual associations to music.

E: All this material is on two levels.

R: On the conscious level you are talking about preparation for trance and her interests. There are many implications and connotations to the particular phrases you use that can arouse sexual associations on an unconscious level, however.

Rationale of the Indirect Approach to Sexual Associations

E: I am also partly color blind. *I can enjoy purple.* And how well can you enjoy that piece of music?

X: Immensely.

E: You are sure of that?　　Lean back in your chair.　　I can daydream about things　*not really looking at anything.*　*Not really listening to anything.*　And I can listen to the *whispering*　of the wind in the woods.　*And you are in position to start*　listening　to some part　of that　*piece of music*.

> E: *Purple* love is a colloquial term for wife-swapping. I'm putting together my enjoyment (purple) with her enjoyment (music) and making them comparable.
>
> R: On the conscious level it is a conversation about things you enjoy. On the unconscious level, however, there are important sexual associations which *purple* and *music* have in common.
>
> E: *That's a good position* has obvious sexual associations. When you kiss a girl, she is *not really looking at anything*. When you look at many of these words and phrases from a sexual point of view, you can see they are really loaded.

Trance Induction Utilizing Internal Music

E: *Just listen slowly to it.*　*And you really don't need your eyes open.*　And really　thoroughly enjoy that piece of music.　And there was *a time*　*when you did not know that piece* of music.　A time when you were learning it　and *a time when you began enjoying it fully*　and more fully.

> R: Your trance induction is now well on its way with a comfortable body position, a fixation of her attention of her own inner music, and the casual suggestion that she does not need to keep her eyes open. Trance induction is thus a comfortable process that develops almost imperceptibly out of a conversation about her interest in music.

"Soon" to Introduce Suggestions

E: And soon you realize you are in a trance. It is a very comfortable way to be.

> E: "Soon" is the undefined future.

R: So you are always safe when you give a suggestion introduced with "soon."

Hallucination Training

E: And not only do you want to be in a trance,   but you want to hear that music   continue   *over and over again*   and then another piece of music comes to mind.

E: There is no music in this room.

R: But this suggestion reinforces the hallucinatory aspects of her inner music. She could become so preoccupied with it that she may hear it as filling the room like a tone hallucination. This is actually the first step in training her to experience an auditory hallucination.

E: *Over and over again* has sexual connotations.

Suggestions Bypassing Resistance: The Conscious-Unconscious Double Bind

E: And you don't really have to pay attention to me. You give your attention to the music,   but your unconscious mind will understand   what I say   and understand   things that you can't understand. First of all, I want your unconscious mind   to give to you   to give to you *a most comfortable feeling*   all over.   [Pause]

R: This is your typical approach to bypassing conscious sets and resistance to suggestions. While her conscious attention is focused on her inner music, another part of her mind is registering what you are saying without comment or resistance.

E: Yes.

R: Is this also an example of the conscious-unconscious double bind? Because she does not know what her unconscious mind can do or is doing (because it is unconscious), she can only agree with you. She has no basis for denying what you say.

E: Yes.

R: Her "unconscious understanding" what her conscious cannot is another double bind that depotentiates consciousness by greatly limiting the sphere in which it can understand and make judgments.

E: Relieving consciousness of the need for action.

Double Tasks and Confusion for Bypassing Conscious Attention

E: And the next thing I want   is for your unconscious mind   to know that there is a very significant purpose   for it to listen to me. And while your unconscious mind is listening to me,   your conscious mind will be very busy   listening to music of all kinds. Particularly phrases of music from here,   from there,   contrasting. But your unconscious mind   is going to be listening   to *anything*   that I say to it.   And it is very *meaningful* to your unconscious mind.   [Pause]
     Now your unconscious mind knows   that you can consciously lift your hands   and move them.

> R: You create a sharp division between the comfortable feeling her conscious mind can recognize and a strong request for attention from the unconscious. She is thus poised between comfort on one level and tension on another.
>
> E: Yes. It is an urgent solicitation for her unconscious through her conscious mind.
>
> R: Yet that urgent solicitation must reach her unconscious through her conscious mind?
>
> E: Her conscious mind will not pay attention; it won't even bother to remember, because I've assigned the music to her conscious mind. You can use a double task to depotentiate consciousness. *Confusion* as well as *assigning an absorbing task* are both ways of getting consciousness out of the way.
>
> R: You structure this even further with a compound sentence that begins with the suggestion "your unconscious mind is listening to me." The unconscious listening is then reinforced by the second half of the sentence, "your conscious mind will be very busy with listening to music of all kinds"—when she does, in fact, get engaged with her inner music. Recent research (Smith, Chu, and Edmonston, 1977) has established that it is possible to so occupy one cerebral hemisphere with music that the activity of the other is facilitated.
>   You seem to be so specific when you begin a sentence with the word "particularly," but then you end with the most general

"music from here, from there," so no matter what she hears, it will be within your suggestion. Then even while the conscious mind may be busy contrasting different phrases of music, you suggest her unconscious will be listening to you. You established within your own scientific research and clinical experience that the mind can be so occupied with two tasks at once. It is well illustrated in your 1941 paper on "The Nature and Character of Posthypnotic Behavior."

E: Yes.

Double Negative to Depotentiate Conscious Sets

E: But your unconscious mind knows that you don't know that   it can lift your hands.

R: This is a truism in double-negative form, the *not*-conscious (the unconscious) "knows that you *don't* know," which tends to confuse and further depotentiate her conscious sets.

Associating Symptoms with the Unconscious

E: Your unconscious mind knows   that it can produce sweating,   but I think your unconscious mind·should know more than that.   [Pause]   And I want your unconscious mind to be willing to learn *anything,* *just anything* **that I instruct your unconscious mind** *to learn.* **[Pause]** *That is very nice* **consciously to be busy with music   and various memories   from way back then   to the future of your dreams.**

R: In your first mention of her problem of sweating you immediately associate it with her unconscious. She, of course, knows it is related to her unconscious, since she cannot control it. What she does not realize is that you have been developing a relationship to her unconscious that she herself does not have. This implies that you will have therapeutic control over her symptom through your relation to her unconscious.

E: Yes. I mention the symptom and remove it [from the realm of her conscious mind's responsibility] to her unconscious mind and add *anything* to it.

R: You have assigned the symptom to her unconscious mind?

E: Very definitely, and I have assigned the symptom to *any-*

thing which has sexual connotations when expressed with certain undertones.

R: This is rather remarkable: You have associated her symptom with its unconscious etiology without her realizing what you were doing.

E: And if that association was inappropriate, her mind would simply not register it. I said "to learn" with a slight sexual connotation in my voice and then "that is very nice" with the same connotation.

Limiting Conscious Understanding

E: And your unconscious mind   is free   to limit itself   to things that I say.   [Pause]   I want to teach you something very much.   Your hands are resting on your *thighs*,   and your conscious mind is going to leave them *down there*.

R: In this compound statement your pauses are so spaced to first express a truism: "Your unconscious mind is free." This initiates an acceptance or yes set that opens the mind to accept the important suggestion that follows, "to limit itself to things that I say."

E: The phrase "to things that I say" also limited itself to conscious memories and conscious understandings.

R: Her unconscious is limited to the things you say, but why do you bring in the conscious?

E: I don't want her to know how freely I have been talking about sex.

R: By shutting off the conscious mind you obviate that possibility.

E: Yes, it can limit itself. The things I say are consciously heard but are understood on an unconscious level only. But the unconscious can keep those sexual connotations to itself. You don't allow the [conscious] self to become aware of it.

R: You then utilize the sexual connotations of *thighs*.

E: Yes. *Thigh* and *there; down there*.

Demonstrating Unconscious Control of Behavior

E: But your unconscious mind   is going to lift one   or the

other   or both.   I really don't know how your unconscious mind wants to learn.

> R: Here you name many possibilities of hand lifting to assure your suggestion will be acted on in some manner or other.

> E: Maybe it [the unconscious] is not going to lift up the hands because it wants to learn something *down there*.

> R: If there is a failure in hand levitation, can have psycho-dynamic significance; in this case sexual.

Threat and Enlisting Cooperation of the Unconscious

E: But I am going to find out   as rapidly as your unconscious mind wishes me to   learn. One or the other   or both of your   hands are going to lift up from your thigh   very slowly.

> E: "But I'm going to find out" is a threat. "As rapidly as your unconscious wishes me to" enlists the cooperation of her unconscious.

> R: You first raise a tension and then state that the condition for the resolution of the tension is the cooperation of her unconscious. Is this a way of activating her unconscious?

> E: Yes, when you offer a threat and then offer relief by cooperation, you have really enlisted the unconscious.

Separating Conscious and Unconscious: Not Knowing to Depotentiate Conscious Sets

E: Unconscious muscle movement is different from that of the conscious mind.   And you are not going to know   which hand is going to lift. You will have to wait and see,   but you'll be uncertain.   The mere tendency,   first one hand and then the other,   perhaps both,   then one,   then the other,   perhaps both.   Sooner or later   an elbow is going to bend a bit,   a wrist is going to lift up,   a hand is coming up.   [Pause]

> E: I'm again separating the conscious from the unconscious by pointing out how body movements are different with each. Not knowing which hand is going to lift depotentiates conscious sets because it removes hand levitation from her intentionality. This

155

ensures the involuntary lifting of the hand. It sets the conscious mind over in the other chair.

R: Where it can watch but not necessarily direct or control.

E: Yes.

Two-Level Communication

E: And it is going to be *very pleasant to wait*. And you've got a lot to learn about your hands. It is well worth the time, too.   And your unconscious mind is already beginning to *explore*. That's right. It's *lifting*.   A bit more. And sooner or later begin a minor *jerk*.   [X's hands begin minor jerking movement up off her thigh. Much facial frowning is evident.]

E: *It is very pleasant to wait* also has sexual connotations. You just keep in mind all these ploys from everyday experience.

R: You use verbal ploys from everyday life to facilitate hypnotic suggestion. You simply intersperse words and phrases having certain connotations. On one level you are talking about the process of hand levitation, and on another you are evoking sexual associations. This would be an example of two-level communication (Erickson and Rossi, 1976)

E: Yes. *Lifting* all by itself as well as *jerk* also have sexual connotations on another level.

Confusion and Mental Flux to Maintain Open Frames of Reference

E: That's right   [X's right hand begins momentarily to lift higher.]   It doesn't necessarily mean it is that hand.   It may be the other.   It is still too soon for you to know.   *Up it comes*.   That's right. That's a beautiful   unconscious movement.   [X's hands are lifting with the slow, very slight, and apparently spontaneous bobbing and upward jerking movement that enables an experienced observer to distinguish it from the smooth lifting that is more characteristic of conscious voluntary movements.]   That's another and another. You're really learning.   That's right.   And the wrist,   and the elbow.   That's beautiful.   And now the right hand, indicating that it wants to join the left hand.   I don't know if it will.   That's right.   Up toward your face.   Elbows bending.   And there is a bit of accommodation between the hands.

156

R: Your suggestions do not permit either hand to achieve a clear dominance in lifting. This tends to maintain her conscious mind in a state of confusion and creative flux. She is being maintained in a state of exploration and expectation rather than being prematurely fixated in the simple conviction that one hand is lifting. You are preventing her from forming a final and closed frame of reference around which hand is lifting. She does not realize it, but you are giving her an experience in maintaining a state of open, creative flux. This open state tends to facilitate the possibility of "creative moments" wherein she may break out of her old symptom-bound frame of reference to achieve a more adequate and therapeutic means of experiencing herself.

E: A common phrase in language is "not to let your right hand know what your left hand is doing."

R: So you are utilizing this form of dissociation to free her from conscious frames of reference that may be a source of her problem.

Utilizing Competition to Facilitate Hand Levitation

E: **Which one will reach your face first?** **Left hand began first.** **Is moving faster.**

E: Here I'm introducing competition between the hands. You work at a thing just so long, then you take a break. She has been working hard, so she can now take a break by doing something else.

R: She has been working hard at hand levitation, so now you give her a break by changing the task slightly to one of competition. The same goal of levitation is being achieved, but with a new attitude and source of motivation.

E: Yes, you are transforming one task into another. You alter the tension. [The senior author gives clinical examples illustrating how he utilizes patients' competitiveness to facilitate hypnotic experiences rather than have the patients' using their competitiveness to oppose the therapist. It is a basic principle of utilization theory to use a patient's personality characteristics to facilitate hypnotic experience.]

Two-Level Communication

E: **But will the right hand** **suddenly increase its speed** *and lift up?* **That's it.** **[Pause]** **And you can take pride in that. Your** unconscious is really taking over some control. And you are really beginning to learn   that the unconscious can control.   And it should be a pleasing thing   to note   how your hand moves,   and you are a harpist,   and *finger movements* are very important,   and your unconscious   is letting you know that.   And even if the left hand gets halfway to your face first, that doesn't mean that the right hand can't catch up to it.   [Pause]   It may be the right elbow needs to be reminded that it can bend.   Of course, the right hand can always have the *unconscious change its mind about the right hand movement.*

R: Here you are giving her unconscious a lot of apparent freedom by describing different possibilities of response; actually you are groping to find whatever response tendencies she has within her, and you then utilize them to facilitate the hypnotic experience of hand levitation.

E: And utilizing all the ploys of folk language: "*and lift up*" has a sexual connotation. Who will make the "first move" [in love play]? You want to make a girl blush? Talk about "*finger movements.*"

R: It has connotations of masturbation.

E: Right. Yet no one reading this would ever think of that. I have deliberately tested that out by asking patients, "Tell me about your finger movements." The flush in their faces indicates the question has a sexual connotation.

R: So this is another clear example of communication on two levels: On the surface you are apparently utilizing her finger movements as a harpist to facilitate hand levitation; on another level you are activating possible sexual associations that will enable her to discuss or do something about her sexual problems.

Implied Directive for Deep Trance

E: Now your left hand is approaching your face,   but the nice thing about it is   that your unconscious mind won't let your left hand touch your face   until you are really ready   to go very deeply in trance   and to do everything that needs to be done. Everything, even though you don't know what everything is.

R: This is an implied directive that facilitates deep trance: Her unconscious won't let her hand touch her face until she is ready to go into a deep trance. You are relying on the patient's own unconscious to determine the moment for entering deep trance; you are utilizing the patient's own internal, autonomous mental mechanisms to facilitate deep trance. You have also made the suggestion to enter deep trance contingent on an inevitability: Her hand is goint to touch her face from the way it is moving. The phrase "and do everything that needs to be done" is a very important all-inclusive suggestion that is hitchhiked onto the above in the form of a compound suggestion. "Even though you don't know what everything is" depotentiates consciousness further, so that the unconscious can work in its own way without the limiting preconceptions of her conscious sets.

The Negative to Displace and Discharge Resistance

E: And yet your left hand is moving up toward your face irresistibly,   but it won't touch your face until your unconscious mind is really ready. And irresistibly it moves closer and closer.   [Pause]   And even though your left hand is very close to your face,   that doesn't mean the right hand cannot beat it to your face.   [Pause]   A mere two inches to go,   and I still don't know if your unconscious is going to lift your right hand to touch your face first.   And that left hand less than two inches away.   And now your unconscious mind is showing   a *desire*   that you don't know you have.   That's right.

R: The use of the negative "but it *won't* touch your face until your unconscious mind is really ready" is very interesting. If she has any resistance your use of "won't" may pick up hers and redirect it in a constructive manner. Your use of the negative tends to displace and discharge the patient's resistance.

Inner Work as the Essence of Therapy

[Deep frowning and much grimacing by X.]
E: Your unconscious mind says there are some doubts,   but you don't know what the doubts are.   [Pause]   And isn't it surprising to know how *desperately urgent* it seems to be.

R: What is the meaning of such frowning and grimacing? Is inner work being done?

E: Inner work is being done without her knowledge just as a school boy goes to bed at night without having been able to work

159

out that arithmetic problem. He works it over and over in his mind. The next morning he notes the wrong digit and corrects the problem.

R: He did it in his sleep without being aware of it. So she is working on problems without being aware of them.

E: That is what she is doing: *All the therapy occurs within the patient, not between the therapist and patient.* "Desperately urgent" means she is going to be working on some important personal problem.

Implied Directive as an Ideomotor Signal

E: And now I know that your left hand is going to touch your face soon,   and that will signify   that you will be in a sufficiently deep trance.   That you will hear and understand every word   unconsciously   that I want you to.   [Pause]   That's delightful to see those doubts.   [Pause]   As in the *irresistible force that is moving your hand,*   and that's a relief.   [Her left hand touches her face.]

R: This is another use of the implied directive that allows her own unconscious internal-guidance system to work its ways into the therapeutic process. You're using her hand touching her face as an ideomotor signal that she is in "a sufficiently deep trance." Does your phrase "you will hear and understand every word unconsciously that I want you to," allow her to interpret your words on an unconscious level in the way you want her to with their sexual connotations?

E: Yes.

R: Her frowning suggests she is experiencing doubts, so you utilize that doubt by defining it as "delightful," which implies that it is somehow all right in the context of the inner psychological work she is undergoing. You then reinforce her for doing this inner work by mentioning that it is a "relief" when her hand finally touches her face.

Preparation for Therapeutic Results: Two-Level Communication and the Cerebral Hemispheres

E: And now you can begin to feel a sense of competence   And sureness   that you haven't had for a long time.   [Pause]   And

**your hand feels so comfortable there.   So comfortable you'll have to
take a couple of minutes to realize how comfortable it is there.   [Pause]**

E: Telling her she can have a sense of competence and sureness
prepares her for the therapeutic result.

R: Even before you deal with it?

E: I have dealt with it! She is frowning over it.

R: How have you dealt with achieving the therapeutic result?

E: By my two-level suggestions related to sexuality.

R: I see! By your use of two-level suggestion you have made
her work on the sexual problem to the point where she was
frowning even though she was not aware of it. That was the
essence of your therapeutic approach, and now you are telling
her that she will be well even though she may not know why.
This is really amazing! Under the guise of inducing trance by
hand levitation, you were actually giving two-level suggestions
to achieve a therapeutic goal. I notice you always seem to be
doing two things at once. Your two-level communication may
be selectively beaming suggestions to the left (conscious) and
right (unconscious) hemispheres at the same time.

Reward and Posthypnotic Suggestion

**E: And I am going to give you a special reward   after you awaken from
the trance,   and you can wonder what that is. But you can go   into a
trance   any time there is a good reason for it.   You can go in by
counting from one to twenty,   or if I count from one to twenty,   going one twentieth of the way each time.   You can come out of the
trance   at the count of twenty to one,   coming out one twentieth at a
time.   And you can   all ways go into a deep trance.   And you
don't need to know   any more than that   you can all ways go into a
trance   when it's purposeful and meaningful.**

R: Here you are facilitating a posthypnotic suggestion by
arousing expectancy and motivation by mentioning a reward.
"Wonder" is also a special word that tends to initiate an
unconscious search and unconscious processes that may be
useful. You then give your typical instructions for entering and
awakening from trance by counting from one to twenty. You

give an interlocking posthypnotic suggestion in a very casual manner that tends to depotentiate consciousness ["you don't need to know."] Your suggestions are made highly acceptable to her since they are so protective and respectful, permitting her to "go into trance when it is purposeful and meaningful."

E: "All ways go into a deep trance" is a two-level suggestion: On one level she hears "you can always go into a trance"; on a secondary level it means "you can go into a trance all ways",— that is, in many different ways. This is a posthypnotic suggestion that she will go into trance with whatever approach to induction you use. The secondary-level suggestion depends upon the literalism of the unconscious.

Indirect Suggestions for Amnesia, Hyperamnesia, and Posthypnotic Suggestion

E: And now, after you   awaken,   I want a bit of music   that you haven't thought about or remembered for a long time   to come suddenly in your mind   when you see me plainly.   And you can begin counting, mentally, silently   backward from twenty to one   beginning the count   now. [Long pause as X reorients to her body and awakens.]

R: This is a posthypnotic suggestion that utilizes her own well-developed internal programs about music. Since you are requesting music that has not been thought of or remembered for some time, you are also attempting to lift an amnesia. In this simple way you are testing her capacity for hyperamnesia as well as posthypnotic suggestion. You tie the posthypnotic suggestion to an inevitable behavior, "when you see me plainly," so she will have a clear cue to execute the posthypnotic behavior.

E: Yes, and I'm also tying in the first part of trance [where music is also mentioned].

R: With one sentence you are doing a number of things: You are probing for the possibility of a hyperamnesia in recalling a bit of music from childhood; at the same time you are structuring an amnesia for the actual content of her trance experience by tying the end to the beginning, so all in between tends to fall into a lacuna—an amnesic gap. When you administer posthypnotic suggestions, you typically use a buckshot approach, testing for many possibilities in order to assess what hypnotic talents a

162

patient may have. But you usually administer these suggestions in an indirect, fail-safe manner.

E: And it is all so disguised that even the intelligent onlooker does not realize what I am doing.

Evaluating Therapeutic Trance for Indications of Change: Questions Evoking Posthypnotic Responses; Shifting Tenses to Facilitate Age Regression

E: **Is it pretty?**   **Can you tell us about it?**

X: **The music?**

E: **Yes.**   **[Pause]**

X: **It changed.**

E: **Tell us what the change was.**

X: **From harp to an orchestra.**
[Pause]

E: **When was that?**
[Pause]

X: **When I was seven.**

E: **Where were you?**

X: **At home.**

E: **Who is in the room?**

X: **Who?**   **[Long pause]**   **My whole family, I think.**

E: **To your right or left?**

X: **To my right or left? To my left.**

> R: Your question uttered a moment after she focuses her gaze on you immediately reinforces the posthypnotic suggestion about music she has not heard for a long time.
>
> E: The word "pretty" is childhood language to evoke childhood associations. When she asks, "The music?" it implies there were other things in her mind.
>
> E: From harp, which is a solitary activity, to "an orchestra,"

which includes *others*. So she is saying [on another level] that the change includes *others*.

R: The music changing to something she knew at the age of seven indicates the success of your posthypnotic suggestion. You then carefully question her about the circumstances surrounding the music to further extend the hypermnesia?

E: Yes. But also to talk about safe things. We are not going to risk talking about the *others*. There are two meanings to "right" and two meanings to "left." They are loaded words. I'm using purposely double-barreled words.

R: Her conscious mind hears you questioning about the details of placement to the right or left. But on another level you are still on the track of "Is something right or wrong?"

E: Yes, and I'm directing it all to her. Notice how at a critical point I shift tense from the past (When *was* that? Where *were* you?) to the present (Who *is* in the room?). This shift in tense is an important approach to facilitating an actual age regression. Notice how her responses after that shift tend to imply she is reexperiencing the past.

Part Two: Therapeutic Trance as Intense Inner Work

In this first session the senior author has completed a basic unit of psychological work. He has established rapport and a good working relationship with the patient. He has made a preliminary survey of the problem and has introduced her to her first trance experience. Most surprisingly he has also made his first therapeutic approach via two-level communication without the patient's even realizing what he was doing.

This is an illustration of one of Erickson's basic approaches to hypnotherapy. He first sets up a therapeutic frame of reference by emphasizing and letting patients have an experience of the difference between the conscious and unconscious mind. With the process of hand levitation she is able to experience the difference between the voluntary lifting of the hand and the involuntary movements of the unconscious. While she is open to unconscious experience, he initiates a process of two-level communication: On one level he talks about hand levitation, while on another level he is using associations with sexual connotations. If her problem has a sexual etiology, these connotations will tend to activate her own sexual associations and lead her to the source of her problem.

At this point a number of alternatives are possible.

1. The Unconscious Resolution of a Problem.
The activated sexual associations may remain at an unconscious

level, where during trance they are turned over to effect an apparently autonomous resolution of the patient's problem. It is possible that hypnotherapy can take place entirely at an unconscious level without the patient (and sometimes even the therapist) knowing the "why" of the cure. The patient only knows a problem has been resolved. No insight in the conventional psychoanalytic sense is involved. This is probably the means by which the "miracles" of faith healing take place. Somehow or other something in the faith frame of reference touches off the relevant unconscious associations to effect an autonomous inner resolution of a problem. Of the many who apply themselves for such faith cures, however, relatively few experience these happy accidents. They are, indeed, so rare that they are called miracles.

With the two-level communication approach, however, the senior author is increasing the odds of a "happy accident" by making an educated guess about the sexual etiology of the problem. If he is right, then merely activating sexual associations during the relatively free and creative period of trance will increase the likelihood of a therapeutic interaction that can lead to an apparently spontaneous resolution of a problem on an unconscious level. The fact that the patient is in a therapeutic environment where cures are somehow effected by a not-too-well-understood process of trance tends to depotentiate her limited and erroneous conscious frame of reference and enables her unconscious to resolve the problem. This assumes that a therapeutic potential already present in the patient was blocked by the patient's erroneous frames of reference. Therapeutic trance is a relatively free period wherein patients can sometimes bypass these limitations so their own therapeutic potentials can operate without interference.

On its most basic level hypnotherapy can be effective simply by providing patients with a period of therapeutic trance so their own unconscious resources can resolve the problem. If the therapist has some understanding of the etiology and dynamics of the problem, then he may help focus the patient's unconscious resources by two-level communication. If the therapist is wrong in his assumptions, two-level communication is a subtle process that simply will not be "picked up" or acted upon by the patient's unconscious. It is thus something of a fail-safe procedure. The therapist is not likely to antagonize or bore the patient with erroneous and irrelevant ideas that may sound fine in a textbook but have little application to that patient.

2. *The Activation and Expression of Relevant Associations to the Problem: Insight Therapy*

A period of therapeutic trance with or without the help of two-level communication may stimulate associations to a problem that the patient wants to talk about. This route naturally leads to insight therapy. After an initial experience of trance the therapist may simply wait for the patient to bring up relevant associations. If none are forthcoming, the therapist may again review the nature and possible sources of the problem to ascertain if the patient now has more access to relevant associations. This was the course that the senior author began to explore by asking the harpist the details of her inner experience with music. Not much was forthcoming, and he felt the material was still too threatening for her to discuss it with the observers present; therefore, he again structures the conscious-unconscious therapeutic frame of reference and another experience of trance.

SESSION ONE

Part Two: Therapeutic Trance as Intense Inner Work

Structuring the Therapeutic Conscious-Unconscious Frame of Reference

E: By the way, are you right-handed?

X: Am I right-handed? Yes.

E: Are you right- or left-thumbed?

X: Right.

E: Put both hands above your head like this.   Up higher and interlace your fingers.   Lower hands. Lower them down.   Is your right thumb on top?

X: No, it's my left thumb.

E: Now you have known   that since you were a tiny tot.

X: That I was left-thumbed?

E: Yes. See, now that was your unconscious knowledge.

> R: Here you do your right- or left-thumbed routine to again assert the importance of her unconscious.
>
> E: Yes, I'm illustrating that there are things in her unconscious that she has known for a long time and did not know it. Further, I can prove it with her own behavior!

Spontaneous Ideomotor Responses Revealing Unconscious Knowledge

E: Are you a right or left kisser?

X: [X looks puzzled and then almost imperceptibly tips her head to the right with a slight quiver.] Left?

E: Oh, no! Did any of you see her?

R: I'm not sure I know what you are looking for.

E: Now again. Are you a right or left kisser?

X: [She now with more awareness tips her head slightly to the right.] Right!

E: What did you do the first time?

R: She tilted to the right very slightly and did not even know it.

E: So that proves she is a right kisser. It is startling how much we are learning about you. What time do you think it is? Don't look at your watch.

X: Twenty minutes of one.

E: Now look at your watch.

X: Not bad.

R: Only ten minutes off.

E: To explain that: A musician has a tremendous sense of time.

R: Yes. So she would not show so much time distortion.

E: How long did it take you to wake up?

X: Two minutes?

R: You use this approach with kissing to demonstrate the superior knowledge of the unconscious, but you are bringing it closer to the sexual area.

E: Yes, but harmlessly.

R: As you ask these questions, you watch her head and lip movements very carefully to detect the minor, unconsciously determined motor movements that will betray the answer. As I tried to answer that question about being a left or right kisser for myself, I noticed that I spontaneously made a slight tilt with my head. That tilt was an ideomotor movement that provided a kinesthetic cue I needed to answer the question. You ask questions that can only be answered by the kinesthetic knowledge of the body and point out how such knowledge belonged in

167

the "unconscious" before you brought it to conscious attention. This initiates a process of ideomotor signaling that is frequently unrecognized by the patient.

E: Now this is an awfully threatening situation.

R: That's why you immediately shift to the time question. You've made your point about the potency of unconscious knowledge, and you now reinforce it with the question about possible time distortion during her previous trance. When time distortion is present, it tends to ratify the reality of trance as an altered state.

Trance Reinduced by Catalepsy

[The senior author reaches over and gently touches the underside of her left hand. She takes this cue, and her left hand lifts slowly. It remains suspended cataleptically in midair.]

E: Do you always leave your hand suspended in mid air when a stranger touches your hand?

X: Do they always?

E: Yes.   Do they remain suspended in midair when a stranger touches them?

X: No, not usually.

E: "All ways of going into a trance."

R: Your earlier posthypnotic suggestion to enter trance in all ways is now effective in reinducing trance by evoking a catalepsy of her hand.

Ratifying Trance: Demonstrating Unconscious Control over Behavior

E: Were you in a trance?

X: I guess so.

E: What makes you think so?
[Pause]

X: I was aware of not having control over my hands.

E: Who had control over them?

168

X: I don't know. It wasn't me.   It seems like you did.

E: I don't know how to contract your muscles.

X: Maybe it didn't seem as if I have control.

E: Um hum. How can you develop another trance?

X: By recalling the same music?

E: All right. Now I'm not wasting your time, nor my own.   I am laying a background   for the development of your own conscious under-standing.   Now I am going to do something.

> R: You ask these questions only after she has had enough evidence of unusual behavior so she must acknowledge that something in her experience is different: She experienced an altered state that we now label as "trance." You are achieving an important aspect of your hypnotherapeutic paradigm. You are demonstrating to her conscious mind that the unconscious can control her behavior. This tends to depotentiate her habitual, everyday frames of reference. Your questions are directed to helping her realize that her ego is limited in its control, but her unconscious has potential for control and eventually cure.

> E: Her response, "I don't know. It wasn't me," is clear proof to her and the observers.

> R: By asking her how she can develop "another trance" you are by implication labeling her previous experience as trance. She acknowledges your ratification of her trance when she then suggests she can develop a trance by recalling music again. In a very subtle and indirect manner she comes to accept her experience as a genuine trance in a way that bypasses any critical doubts she may have had. With your final statement about the development of her unconscious understanding you again emphasize the importance of the unconscious and heighten her expectancy of what is to come.

> E: Yes.

Trance Reinduction by a Question: Initiating an Unconscious Search

E: **Do you know that you will be in a deep trance when I touch your face?** [The senior author touches his hand to her face. She closes her eyes and remains immobile.] **Now rest very quietly.   And enjoyably.**

R: You are again making use of your earlier posthypnotic suggestion that she could go into trance all ways. This time you reinduce trance by suggesting a cue [touching her face] in the form of a question. Such question inductions are particularly effective because questions are a marvelous means of fixing and focusing attention inward. In this case the question obviously initiated an unconscious search and the requisite unconscious process to lead to the desired hypnotic response of trance. One of your most effective forms of hypnotic suggestion is to ask questions that cannot be answered by the patient's ordinary conscious frames of reference. Questions that ask for an autonomous response [such as ideomotor signaling] on an unconscious level usually depotentiate consciousness and lead to trance experience.

Assigning the Locus of Therapeutic Change as Taking Place in the Unconscious

E: And you're beginning to understand   that your unconscious mind can develop control   and take charge of so many things.   Now in awakening I want you to do it easily and comfortably   in your own way.

R: You are again emphasizing and demonstrating unconscious control over behavior and making direct statements about it, so she will have a clear understanding of it as the means of your therapeutic approach.

E: I say "so many things" to emphasize the plural.

R: That implies the unconscious can also take control over her symptom, too.

Two-Level Communication

E: In a way that meets your *needs*.   But I want your unconscious mind   to continue   to listen to me   and to understand what I say   even though your conscious mind   may hear something different.   Now take it easily and awaken.   [Two-minute pause] Now.   [Long pause for at least five minutes during which X does not awaken. The fingers of her left hand move as if playing the harp, she grimaces and frowns and has the appearance of being in a state of intense inner concentration.]

E: The plural here again with "meets your needs." I'm actually talking about two-level communication without really explaining it.

R: That opens the way for two-level communication?

E: That tells her I am talking on two levels.

R: That the conscious mind can understand one thing while the unconscious can elaborate many other associations. The unconscious can elaborate whatever associations are necessary and pertinent to her particular problem. You are again using general words that can be interpreted in as many different specific and personal ways as possible relevant to particular problems. The success of this approach is suggested by the fact that her inner absorption was so deep at this point that it took her at least seven minutes to awaken. The activity of her face indicates that inner work was certainly being done. She was not asleep!

Unconscious Work During Trance: Unconscious Problem-Solving

E: Go right ahead [Pause] **and share that with your conscious mind.** [Another long pause as X remains in intense concentration] **Share it with your conscious mind.** [Another long pause] **This struggle is helping you. Even though you don't know consciously all of the struggle, that is all right.**

R: This was a relatively rare instance when a subject did not awaken immediately after you gave suggestions to awaken.

E: Her unconscious mind understood something different from the word "awaken." What does "awaken" mean? Wake up to your opportunities!

R: Wake up to your opportunity to do inner work?

E: "When the *hell* are you going to wake up?" is common folk language.

R: That is folk language for: When are you going to realize what is happening to you?

E: I told her to look for the double meaning, and her unconscious is doing that.

R: That is a double bind: You are forcing her to work on an unconscious level even though she cannot recognize it on a conscious level.

E: Yes. I set her up to place unconscious understandings on whatever I say. *They will be her unconscious understandings.*

R: This is beautiful! No matter what the problem is, no matter what the therapist's hypotheses are, you are encouraging the patient to do her own work, inner work that is valid for her unconscious.

E: She is not limited or biased by my ideas.

R: So this is a most general way of facilitating problem-solving.

E: *I don't need to know what your problem is for you to correct it.*

R: Valid hypnotherapy can be done without either the patient or therapist knowing what the problem was.

E: That's right. Note the strategy here of the pause after "Go right ahead," and then the longer pauses. That means there is no hurry, it can take place today, tomorrow, sometime. Do it at your leisure, in other words. Only you haven't said, "Do it at your leisure." But that is the understanding the patient gets.

E: It allows the patient to relax so inner work can be done.

E: I'm telling her it is a "struggle." Then I give reassurance with "that's all right" about something about which she knows nothing.

Therapeutic Trance as Intense Inner Work

E: [Another long pause as the intense inner concentration with wrinkled brow, frowning, and taut face continues.]
Now you can leave the struggle at this point.   But you can return to this point.   And there can be an interlude of conscious awareness. You can come right back to this point   any time.

R: Is more effective therapy done when a patient is obviously engaged in intense inner concentration, as is the case here, or when the patient appears more relaxed, passive, and asleep? What state do you prefer in doing therapeutic work?

E: I like to see this that we see in Miss X.

172

R: This is the more effective type of trance for doing inner work. Since she was frowning, did she have a conscious awareness of what was going on within her?

E: She knew she was doing some thinking, but she didn't know what it was. [The senior author gives analogous instances where certain wire puzzles can frequently be solved by taking them apart behind one's back or with eyes closed because visual interference with kinesthetic cues is eliminated. In a similar manner many emotional problems can be solved more easily without conscious thinking.] I tell her she "can leave the struggle" because she does not have to fight that battle every day, every night. She can always return and fight another day.

R: Here you carefully break into whatever inner work was being done and let her know she can return to it after an interlude of conscious awareness. This is another form of posthypnotic suggestion that assures that she will return to trance and continue her important inner work when you give the signal.

Two-Level Communication and Trance Depth

E: On my signal?   And I am going to ask you   *now*,   and I mean   to awaken.   Right *now!* [X finally opens her eyes]   You want to tell me anything?   [Pause as she continues awakening by reorienting to her body.]

X: Did you say things that I didn't hear?

E: That is an interesting question. Why do you ask that?   [Pause]

X: I don't know. I just have the feeling that you were talking to me, or somebody was, and I couldn't hear.

E: Who was talking to you? Take a guess. [Pause]

X: I don't know.

E: It was someone you knew, and everybody here is a stranger.

X: Was it somebody new or I knew? Did you say, or was it a stranger?

E: Everybody here is a stranger.   Somebody you knew?   Can you tell us?   [Pause]

X: It must be me.   I can't think of who else it would be.

Someone you know very well.   There is a bond between you.   Do you want to disclose that?

X: I'm shaking my head "no," but I don't know if I could disclose it.

E: Do you know who the person is?   [Pause]   Your unconscious doesn't want your conscious mind to know.

X: That is why I can't tell you?

E: Um hum.

> E: Who is the "someone else?" She has a sexual problem. Another person is involved.
>
> R: Her three-year followup proves you were correct in your assumption that there was "someone else" involved. How did you know, since she gave you no hints of it in your interview thus far?
>
> E: "Someone else" in that context could be a real person or another part of her personality. X came in. I got the least possible amount of information, knowledge, to understand something. Then I improvised thereafter. But I knew what I was doing. I laid each step carefully. I planned to say the word "music," and I planned to return to it.
>
> R: Yes, to produce a structured amnesia.
>
> E: I implied sex, and then I returned with there is "someone else."
>
> R: You continued with the sexual theme.
>
> E: But I said there is "someone else" to *you,* not to her!
>
> R: That made it a more potent indirect suggestion. That is how you use an audience, to give indirect suggestions to a patient. Under the pretense of giving a didactic lecture on hypnosis, you are actually administering indirect suggestions.
>
> E: That's right. If I don't have an audience present, I can elicit some memory of hers and make a few remarks about that harmless memory. And that is my audience. I can comment on her trip to Chicago, which has nothing to do with the problem at hand, but in commenting on that trip I can put in double meanings.
>
> R: The "audience" is actually another pattern of associations in her mind. This is another way of talking on two levels.

174

Conscious and Unconscious Head Signaling: The Unconscious Personality

[X shakes her head "no" in an absentminded manner.]

E: And there was an "I don't know" head movement   confirmed.

Now I am talking to someone else,   and she doesn't know to whom,   only I know.   [To the audience]   Wasn't that beautiful?

> E: Now when she shakes her head, that was an absentminded withdrawal to a trance state. If you recall, she was shaking it "no" very slowly.

> R: A very slow head movement is from the unconscious, while a fast head movement is from the conscious.

> E: Yes, and the unconscious response comes after a delay, while the conscious response comes immediately. I'm talking to her unconscious personality.

> R: In "talking to someone else," her unconscious personality, you are further depotentiating her everyday frames of reference about herself so that an unconscious search is initiated for this other aspect of her personality. This is, of course, an excellent approach for evoking multiple personalities or more repressed aspects of one's personality.

Facilitating Amnesia: Working with Associations

E: And now where were you born?

X: Arizona

E: How long have you been in Memphis?

X: Nine Years.

E: And doing social work, where?

X: St. Joseph's Home for Children.

E: There is a child guidance clinic somewhere in Memphis.

X: Yes.

E: My name ever been mentioned there?

X: Would your name ever be mentioned there?

E: Has it been?

E: "On my signal?" answers the patient's inner questions, "Should he alone signal me, or can I signal myself?"

R: Her questions about not hearing or who was speaking are very interesting. Would you say her remarks are an indication of deep trance in spite of all the other indications of tension and frowning, etc.?

E: Yes.

R: Does her remark about not hearing prove her consciousness was depotentiated since she has no conscious awareness of what you said?

E: That's right. I did effectively talk on two levels.

Hypnotic Amnesia

E: What do you suppose was said?   [Pause]

X: I don't know.

E: All right. Without looking, what time do you think it is?

X: Around 1:00.

R: About quarter to one. [Pause]

> R: Is she experiencing an amnesia, or was she so deep in trance that she just was not receiving, simply did not hear or record what you said even on an unconscious level?
>
> E: She is saying, "I, the conscious me, does not know."
>
> R: How would you prove that? You could ask for ideomotor signals from the unconscious to determine if it was receiving things the conscious mind could not recall.
>
> E: Yes.

Variation in Trance Depth: Therapeutic Suggestions Bridging Conscious and Unconscious

E: How deeply in a trance were you?

X: How can you tell?

E: What do you think is all I want to know. [Pause]

X: Like how well done is the steak—medium to deep or medium to well done?

176

E: [To R] She illustrates very nicely how a second trance very greatly deepened. And she further illustrates the wealth of activity that is really cut off from her conscious knowledge.

R: I have had the difficulty of putting people so deeply into a passive sort of trance that I am not sure they are receiving what I say even on an unconscious level because they do not respond to posthypnotic suggestions. How can I be sure patients are actually receiving what I say?

E: You can put people very deep, but you talk so there are islands which they can use as a highway. They are on the bottom of the deep ocean. They need to come up and jump from this island to the next.

R: There are variations in trance depth from deep ocean to conscious island that you utilize to give suggestions.

E: You say something they can hear in deep trance that they can relate to consciously. For example, a bit earlier I said, "And there can be an interlude of conscious awareness."

R: That suggestion brought up an island of conscious awareness?

E: Yes, something that can be seized upon.

R: How does that help them follow a posthypnotic suggestion? It raises them momentarily to consciousness where they can receive the suggestion?

E: It leads into consciousness.

R: Are you building an associative bridge from the unconscious to the conscious?

E: Yes, it builds a bridge between the struggle taking place on both conscious and unconscious levels.

R: In deep trance it is possible to place suggestions so deeply that there is no bridge to consciousness where they can be expressed. Those suggestions cannot be therapeutically effective.

E: That is why I build bridges.

Two-Level Communication Utilizing an Audience or Memories

E: [To R] And there were thoughts of someone else,   and very sensitive thoughts. Now shall I continue   describing   what I saw: [To X]

X: I don't know. I am only familiar with it by name. I have never been there. I have been inside, but I am not really familiar with it.

E: I lectured there a number of years ago. Now I am engaged in social chitchat for the passage of time.

X: I was just thinking that.

E: With that first question she is back at an infancy level. [The senior author gives personal examples illustrating how such questions invariably evoke important early memories and associations.] When you ask, "Where were you born?" you are really massively changing the train of conversation. You are massively augmenting any amnesias. I'm taking her far back to Memphis, far from this room, thus augmenting amnesias for what has happened here. Then, by having her search her Memphis memories about whether my name was mentioned there, I'm keeping her in Memphis.

R: This clearly illustrates how you are always working with the patient's associative process—putting it here and there. You appear to be making casual conversation, but you are actually doing something with the patient all the time.

E: Then I identify what I'm doing as social chitchat. I was just thinking that she was an intelligent girl.

R: So you acknowledge her intelligence by telling her what you are doing.

Training for Deeper Trance

E: [To R] Now you are witnessing that training for a deeper and deeper trance.

R: What do you mean by your remark about deep trance training?

E: You've just seen me waltz her from Phoenix to Memphis. Now I've waltzed her back with this remark to you! When she says, "I was just thinking that," she is really talking on two levels. She is the observer. I've waltzed her from being on the subjective [immersed in her subjective memories of Memphis] to being the observer.

R: Why is that training for deeper trance?

E: When you can waltz a person about like that from Phoenix to Memphis, from subjective to objective, you have changed her whereabouts and status very simply.

R: That is training her for deeper trance in the sense that you are training her to follow you? Anything that causes the patient to follow the therapist, or any approach that enables the therapist to change the patient's mental status, is training for deeper trance?

E: Yes.

R: This has nothing to do with the trance state per se; it is the skill with which the therapist changes the patient's associative processes. This is a basic skill any therapist should have quite apart from any use of hypnosis.

E: That's right.

Ratifying Trance and Two-Level Communication

E: And you are witnessing the training for   a two-level communication.   [Pause]

E: As I say this to you, she is also being the observer, since she is being talked about. It reinforces what happened before.

R: By talking about "training for a deeper and deeper trance," you are ratifying the fact that she has experienced some trance. With this remark about two-level communication you are ratifying that two-level communication has taken place. But why?

E: Because I don't want her unconscious mind to ever think, "He didn't mean those sexual allusions."

R: You are ratifying the two-level communication.

E: And it can be related to this waltzing from Phoenix to Memphis and back to Phoenix. And from patient to observer.

R: Her three-year follow-up does indicate that the changes from Phoenix to Memphis are related to the "someone else" and the sexual problem alluded to in your two-level communication. It is hard to believe that you were not using some form of ESP.

E: I had no way of knowing that, but I can suspect it with my knowledge of human beings.

Questioning for Unconscious Ideomotor Head Signaling

E: Now do you mind thinking,   just thinking about something highly emotional?

X: Thinking about?

E: Um hum.   Now,   my question was, Do you mind thinking about a highly emotional matter?

X: A highly emotional what?

E: Matter.
[X's head bobs about uncertainly and apparently absentmindedly.]

E: And your head movements were not really understandable.   In response to my question, "Do you mind thinking about a highly emotional matter?" your head moves yes,   no,   I don't know, maybe.

X: That's right.

E: May I ask you   to think of a highly emotional matter?

X: Anything in particular?

E: [To R] We will just discuss that. I ask a specific question,   and she said,   "anything in particular?"   Now what does that mean? There are some things that she chooses not to talk about, not to think about, and some she can. [To X] You see, I don't need to know them. But you need to know them.

X: I'd rather you knew them.
E: You'd rather I knew them?
[To R] Well, I didn't ask her to confide in me,   but the effect is what?

R: She would rather you know.

E: She told me she was willing to confide in me. That is much better than pressing a patient to give you information. I'm explaining a technique of dealing with patients.   And let them have every right that they ought to have.   The main purpose is to help the patient.   Not to satisfy one's *curiosity*. And I was just showing, illustrating, the way one puts questions that gives the patient the right   to choose whether or not to confide.

180

[To X] How do you feel about my using you for a demonstration?
[Long pause]

> E: These are soldering questions. In the previous trance there were sexual allusions. Now I'm getting in the words "highly emotional."
>
> R: You are now binding sexual allusions to "highly emotional."
>
> E: Then I reassure her that I don't know.
>
> R: That is characteristic of your approach. You build up high tension with some provocative remarks that send the patient on some frantic unconscious search, and then you reassure and lower tension so that the unconscious process thus initiated can proceed in peace on its own.
>
> E: When "I ask a *specific* question" and she responds with "anything in particular?" she is indicating that there is a *particular* thing.
>
> R: But evidently she does not want to reveal it.
>
> E: Then I reassure her again with, "I don't need to know them."
>
> R: And you put the responsibility on her by saying, "But you need to know them."

Dissociation and Rapport

X: I guess I feel kind of, sort of separate, even though it doesn't bother me that I am aware of.

E: No, you and I are together, and those people are outside. It is a very nice way of illustrating that we are here and [To R] you fellows are over there.

R: Yes.

E: And you did that so nicely, [To R] and I didn't tell her to do that.

R: Her sense of separation is a form of dissociation which indicates she has a separate and different relation with you than the observers? She has a special rapport with you that tends to exclude others.

E: Yes.

Facilitating Hypnotic Phenomena: Double Bind and Questions to Evoke Immobility and Caudal Anesthesia

E: Now I am going to say something to you. You are not going to understand it consciously. Doesn't it surprise you that you can't stand up? [Pause as X looks surprised]

X: Can I try?

E: Oh, you could *try*.
[Pause as X makes a slight forward movement in her chair with the upper part of her body only and then stops]   It does surprise you, doesn't it?   Some day when you get *married and are having a baby*, you can use the same measure.

X: Oh, really?

E: Um hum. I just gave you a caudal anesthesia or a spinal anesthesia.

X: [Nervous laughter]

E: *I don't lay on hands, I lay on ideas.* That is kind of a surprise to know that you can't stand up.

X: Let me know when I can.

E: I will always let you know   when you can't. I'll always let you know when you can.''[To audience] Now   when a caudal anesthesia like that can be induced,   you know you've got a perfectly good subject.

R: It is a beautiful double bind when you say you are going to say something to her that she is not going to understand consciously: She is bound to listen, but since she cannot understand consciously, she must respond on an unconscious level.

E: Yes.

R: You initiate a hypnotic phenomenon with a question. It is usually better to evoke a hypnotic phenomenon with a question than a direct suggestion? It is a fail-safe approach.

E: Yes.

R: What cues do you use to know when to attempt such a question to initiate a hypnotic phenomenon?

E: You always give praise to the unconscious.

R: Just previous to this question you did give her unconscious praise when you remarked, "And you did that so nicely, and I didn't tell her to do that." The way you say the word "try" with a subtle, dubious tone in your voice implies she can try but will fail.

E: Yes.

R: Were there any other cues you used to know when to evoke this immobility? Did you notice that she was already manifesting signs of being in a trance, slow eyelid movements, etc.?

E: I praised her unconscious, and if she has picked up some sexual allusions, I can be pretty sure the sexual allusions here [getting married, having a baby] will be involved.

R: So you suggest a hypnotic phenomenon where she can be involved. That is why you used this hypnotic phenomenon rather than something else?

E: Yes, it was a specific application for her.

R: Because you were building up sexual associations.

E: I needed to see if I could confirm it.

R: Since she succeeded in experiencing this hypnotic phenomenon, would you take it as a confirmation that your sexual associations were picked up?

E: Yes, with a minimum of words I induced a spinal anesthesia. If I was right in all my double-talk, she is going to develop caudal anesthesia. Since she has studied [a medical specialty], she knows what a caudal anesthesia is. I'm literally asking her, "Does my talk on two levels about sex have meaning?" She says, "It did." No direct words have been said. Nobody listening can know it. But her unconscious and I can know it.

R: So you have been preparing her for some time to experience this hypnotic phenomenon of caudal anesthesia. It is not just a casual intrusion. This reminds me of your preparation for having a patient experience visual hallucinations: You usually activate many trains of association regarding the subject of the hallucination before you try to evoke it.

E: Yes. *Hypnotic technique is giving the stimuli that can be resolved by the subject into the hypnotic experience you wish her to have.*

Depotentiating the Clinical Problem

E: And the next question is   she's got a definite and limited problem. And that has interfered with her as a personality very much. Now is that personal problem a serious emotional problem,   or is it a superficial emotional problem?   I can think of a serious case of claustrophobia. The solution was somebody walking   rapidly across the floor and down the steps, clicking her shoes at each step. When she was a little girl, her mother punished her by putting her in the closet   and then walking   noisily out of the house and down the steps.

R: Um. So really a very superficial thing.

E: A very superficial.

R: Not a deep emotional disturbance.

E: Not a deep emotional experience.   Now your sweating may be   caused by some superficial thing,   or it may be   a   very dramatic thing. By the way,   how many doctors have you seen about your sweating? [Pause]

X: All- told about ten. Ever since I was little, I asked every doctor I happened to run into.

E: And   your sweating has been sufficient so you could hold your hands out allowing a *puddle to form on the floor.* Have you been able to let a puddle drip on the floor? Have you seen other doctors and did you puddle?   How have you done here?

X: What?

E: How much sweating have you had here?

X: Oh,   not a puddle.

E: Your hands were moist when you came in. But you haven't puddled.

R: In this section you limit and depotentiate the sweating symptom with direct remarks as well as clinical cases from your experience.

E: This was an actual case of claustrophobia.

R: You tell such actual cases to develop a positive expectancy in the patient.

E: When I tell her the sweating can have a superficial origin, I'm telling her that her sweating is not the scary thing she thinks it is.

R: This is a way you depotentiate her previous rigid sets and fears about her problem.

E: What does a baby do?

R: Puddle on the floor. It has sexual associations when you talk about puddling on the floor?

E: Yes, I'm still keeping the sexual associations in there.

R: You continue to depotentiate her symptom frame of reference by downgrading it with your casual but concrete comments about how little sweating she's had here.

Puns to Initiate Unconscious Search and Creative Moments

E: To the last puddler I saw   I said, "You really are ambitious,   you don't like the puddle you are in.   It pays well.   You hate to give up all that pay. As long as you can lead a band in Las Vegas,   you will have puddles.   You can give up Las Vegas. Go to New York.   Live by yourself in an apartment.   Write music and arrangements.   You'll be free."   A year later he was turning out a lot of music and arrangements   and free of his puddling. Now you weren't embarrassed by my talking about you, were you?

R: "You don't like the puddle you are in" is actually a pun relating symptom (sweating) to personality problem (ambition). Such puns may seem funny and even superficial to some readers, yet in one stroke they can fixate a patient's attention, depotentiate erroneous frameworks, initiate an unconscious search, and facilitate *a creative moment* (Rossi, 1972b) wherein startling insight may be achieved.

Assigning the Unconscious as Locus of Therapeutic Change

X: I didn't know you were talking about me.

E: Have I talked about you?   [Pause]

X: I think so.

E: You don't have to be concerned.

[Erickson now engages Miss X in a five-minute period of chitchat about her family and her general interests. He is apparently "taking a break," allowing her to relax from the very intense period of trance work. Such alternations in the rhythm and intensity of conscious and unconscious work are important. There is a natural ninety-minute biorhythm of rest and activity, fantasy, intensity, and appetite that we all experience continuously (Kripke, 1974). It sometimes seems as if Erickson recognizes that natural variation in the patient's "biological clock" and adjusts his rhythm of alternating trance and conscious work to coincide with it.]

E: She ought to think I've been talking about her. She really has got a lot of amnesias when she makes remarks like, "I didn't know you were talking about me."

R: In other words, her conscious mind is confused here, and as a result she is open to therapeutic work on an unconscious level since her conscious limitations are in disarray.

E: She doesn't "have to be concerned" since her unconscious does all the listening.

R: That is right, you are giving potency to her unconscious because that is where the important work is going to be done.

SESSION ONE

Part Three: Evaluation and Ratification of Therapeutic Change

In the previous section the senior author continued structuring the conscious-unconscious double bind and his two-level communication approach. He assigned the locus of therapeutic change to the unconscious and let the patient have a very intense trance experience during which therapeutic change could take place. He depotentiates her symptom and then notes that she has not, in fact, been manifesting her symptom during this session. The entire procedure has been so casual that she does not yet realize consciously just how much therapy has been taking place. The stage is therefore set for an evaluation and ratification of the therapeutic change.

Demonstrating a Therapeutic Change: The Double Bind in "Try" Related to Hemispheric Specialization

E: Do you think you could make a puddle with your hands now?   Try it.

X: Try? I did make a puddle for some doctors once. This doctor told me it was the worst he had ever seen and he went and got a bowl. Four other doctors came around to watch me make a puddle.
[X places her hand in position to create a puddle, but no significant moisture appears.]

E: I said *try* it!   You are beginning to have some doubts?

X: About a puddle, yeah. I could give you a little stream.

E: Try it.   Just a little puddling stream.
[Pause]
Looks like your poorest performance on the record.

X: I can't understand it.

> R: Right after a short period of chitchat you ask a very challenging question to demonstrate a therapeutic change: Her sweating has decreased.
>
> E: I said, "try it," implying she is to make an effort and at the same time to negate it.
>
> R: You had her in a double bind, didn't you?
>
> E: Yes.
>
> R: The word "try" evokes a double bind situation when it is said with the appropriate inflection and dubious tone of voice. The word "try" means make an effort. The dubious tone of voice says, "Do not succeed in that effort." She is thus placed in a bind where nothing happens. Even the symptom is turned off. I sometimes wonder if such double binds that function in two modalities are related to the differences in cerebral hemispheric functioning (Diamond and Beaumont, 1974; Rossi, 1977). The cognitive meaning of "try" would be processed by the left hemisphere, while the emotionally laden tone in which it is said would certainly be processed by the right hemisphere. Since psychosomatic symptoms are now thought to be mediated primarily by the right hemisphere (Galin, 1974), your negative tone of voice would be able to block the symptom at its right hemispheric source. Much research certainly needs to be done in this area (e.g., Smith, Chu, and Edmonston, 1977).
> When you next say "try it" with emphasis, you immediately double bind it with the negation, "You are beginning to have some doubts." When you say "try it" the third time, you immediately double bind it with the joking tone with which you

say "just a little puddling stream" and your "poorest performance on the record." Her final response of not understanding why she does not experience the symptom indicates that her conscious mind is puzzled and rather depotentiated. It has been caught in the double bind that made her symptomatic behavior impossible, but she does not know why. It is important that consciousness be depotentiated when you challenge the symptom, since that allows it to drop into the unconscious which you have prepared as the locus of therapeutic change.

A Pun Associating Symptom Cure with Appropriate Psychodynamics

E: Do you suppose your hands are unfolding for you to become a *dried-up old maid?*

[Pause as X continues to try but with no success]

E: Who is a dried-up old maid? Someone without a sex life.

R: It is another pun to facilitate a creative moment: "dried-up" means symptom cure, and on another level it relates to sexual activity. Again you are tying symptom cure to a sexual association. You are not dealing with a simple symptom removal by direct suggestion. You are associating symptom cure with the appropriate psychodynamics that are related to it.

E: "Old maid" is the question.

R: Your question with a pun catches her attention on many levels; it associates symptom change with the appropriate sexual psychodynamics underlying the symptom and directs her unconscious to work on that association. Her follow-up letter does, in fact, indicate that she was well on her way to becoming a dried-up old maid if she did not deal decisively with her romantic life at this time. As her followup letter indicates, however, she was later able to deal effectively with her love life.

Depotentiating Conscious Doubts About Symptom Change: Depotentiating the Symptom

E: Discouraging, isn't it?
[Pause]

X: Yes it is.
[Pause with more futile trying]
Too bad we didn't have a harp here, so I could play.

188

E: Do you type?

X: A little bit.

E: Do your hands drip on the typewriter? [To R] Do you have a typewriter with you?

R: No, I don't, unfortunately.

E: Do you suppose if I got a typewriter for you, you could feel your fingers getting wetter? Do you really suppose you could?

X: I don't, I don't think they are going to get any wetter than this.
[Pause with more futile trying]
I don't know.

> E: By saying, "Discouraging, isn't it?" I'm making light of it and depotentiating the symptom. When she says it's too bad we don't have a harp, it indicates that she is on my side now and wants to demonstrate symptom cure by actually playing the harp.
>
> R: You then by implication generalize the symptom cure from harp to typewriter. It is important to demonstrate symptom cure concretely in the here and now.
>
> E: Yes, and without reassurance. Reassurance only implies "You can fail." If you say, "You *can* get over this," that implies you have it.

Ideomotor Signaling to Ratify Symptom Cure: The First Round

E: Lifting your right hand means "yes," lifting your left hand means "no." Does your unconscious mind think that you can make a puddle with your hands?   Which one will lift?   Wait and see.
[Pause]
You can even watch to see which one is going to lift.

X: I can watch?

E: Yes.
[Pause as her right hand lifts a bit, then her left hand lifts a bit too. She has been looking at her right hand.]

E: [To R] The fixation of her gaze shows her conscious action. She only shows one slight look at the other hand. We know what her conscious

answer is. She doesn't know what her unconscious answer is. [To X] But your unconscious will suddenly give you a correct answer.
[Her right hand lifts more strongly.]

> R: You are now using ideomotor signaling as a further demonstration of symptom cure? You are trying to eliminate any further doubts about her symptom cure?
>
> E: Yes, and I create a state of uncertainty by asking, "Which one will lift?"
>
> R: That uncertainty tends to depotentiate her conscious (and problematic) frames of reference so her unconscious has an opportunity to respond.
>
> E: Where a person looks in finger or hand signaling indicates their conscious expectation.
>
> R: If you have no concrete way of demonstrating symptom cure in the therapy situation itself, then this sort of ideomotor signaling is a good substitute (Cheek and LeCron, 1968). She finally lifts her right hand more strongly, indicating that her unconscious believes she can puddle her hands. Yet she cannot actually do it. How do you explain this discrepancy?
>
> E: She knows from long experience that she can puddle. I haven't taken anything away from her.
>
> R: By lifting both hands she is saying that you haven't taken anything (her symptom) away from her; the capacity for the sympton is still there.
>
> E: Yes, the capacity is there, but there is no longer fear.

Depotentiating Conscious Doubts About Symptom Cure: The Double Bind

E: And now you are seeing a demonstration of what it means when people say it is hard to believe. All past experiences made only one answer possible. But the unconscious is going to give a forcible answer.
[Pause]
It is difficult to change one's set frame of reference.
[Pause]
And you are afraid to know the answer.
[Pause]

It is perfectly all right to think one thing consciously and to know exactly the opposite unconsciously.

[Pause]

And does it put a strain upon you?   And yet there is no sweating in spite of the strain. So now you will have more courage.

[Pause]

That really takes a great deal of courage.

E: I'm using folk language to express what people feel.

R: It is hard for a patient to really believe a long-term symptom can disappear so quickly. By giving voice to this inner doubt you are depotentiating it.

E: Yes. It is difficult to believe these changes have been made.

R: She is afraid to know the change has really been made, lest she be disappointed.

E: That's right.

R: Here you are allowing room for conscious doubts, but reinforcing the fact that the unconscious recognizes there has been symptom change. This is another use of the conscious-unconscious double bind.

Then, even though the ideomotor signal of the right hand lifting means she still has the capacity for sweating, you point out that at present "there is no sweating in spite of the strain." You then give strong ego support for the courage to believe, but you don't actually say "believe," since that would imply doubt.

Posthypnotic Suggestion

E: I am going to ask you to awaken,   and I'm going to tell you an apparently meaningless story.   But your unconscious mind will understand. Now awaken now.   one, two, etc. to twenty,   nineteen, eighteen,   seventeen,   sixteen,   fifteen,   thirteen, nine,   eight, seven, six, five, four, three, two, one.   Awaken.

R: This is an interesting form of posthypnotic suggestion whereby you are able to later give her unconscious a message that will not be meaningful to her conscious mind. In this way you may be able to bypass the limitations or doubts the conscious mind may have.

"Until": Posthypnotic Suggestion for a Continuation of Psychotherapeutic Work on Symptom Cure

E: You know the comic strip of Mutt and Jeff? Do you   know them?

X: Yes.

E: One day Jeff was searching his pockets desperately, and Mutt was watching.   Over and over again   Jeff searched his pockets. And Mutt asked him why.   And he said, "I lost my wallet and I looked in all my pockets except one. I can't find it." And Mutt asked him, "Why don't you look in that one?" Jeff answered, "Because if it ain't there, I'll drop dead."
[Pause]
When did you decide I would be the last hope?

X: I know my unconscious knows what that story means.

> R: This is one of your favorite anecdotes to deal with the patients' conscious doubts about symptom cure. You depotentiate their conscious doubts with bits of humor and simple acknowledgment of the doubt.

> E: Yes, that is a perfect example. I've also said to patients, "And you are going to doubt it all the way home until."

> R: Why do you end the sentence with "until?"

> E: Now you want to know the end of the sentence, don't you? The patients who doubt symptom removal will doubt all the way home, and then they start looking for the "until." "Until" something happens, you see. They start looking for "what it is that will tell me that it is gone." They are expecting.

> R: You have them looking for and expecting a confirmation of symptom cure.

> E: Yes, I'm setting them up for that.

> R: So when the patient walks out of the office he is still doing psychotherapeutic work. This is a form of posthypnotic suggestion to search for convincing proof of symptom removal.

> E: All the way home "until" they know.

Ratifying Symptom Change

E: And when did you decide I was your last hope?
[Pause]

192

X: When I was reading this book [Haley's *Uncommon Therapy*.]

E: As soon as I get shut of you, the better.

X: As soon as what?

E: I get shut of you, get rid of you, the better, which isn't complimentary, is it?   Or is it?
[Pause]

X: You mean complimentary to you?

E: To you.

X: To me. Oh! Yeah, I guess I do have a feeling that, yeah.

E: The sooner I can get rid of you, the happier I'll be and the happier you'll be. Which raises the question in my mind, when do you leave?

X: Saturday afternoon, late.

E: How are you traveling to California?

X: Flying.

E: Did you do any puddling on the plane?

X: I don't think actual puddles, but some streams.

E: And you came in here with only a faint mist.

X: Yes.

> E: This question reinforces her hope and makes it real in another way. I was her last hope. I was her *reality* hope; I was a hope made into a reality. I'm ratifying her hope and making it real.
>
> R: Your question then was another way of ratifying that we have done our therapeutic hope. Such remarks made in a humorous vein tend to speed up the therapeutic process and further ratify that therapy is being done.
>
> E: I'm derogating the symptom as a way of depotentiating it with my comment about "only a faint mist."

Indirect Posthypnotic Suggestion via a Momentary Common Everyday Trance

E: Holding onto me, aren't you?
How soon will you forget me?

X: To be perfectly honest, I don't think I will.

E: To hold onto me means keeping me in some way; it means keeping what I did for her, not literally keeping me. "Holding onto me, aren't you?" and "How soon will you forget me?" are both posthypnotic suggestions. "Forget me" and "holding onto me" are two opposite things. "Holding onto me" is holding onto therapy. "Forgetting me" is forgetting me personally.

R: The careful apposition of opposites is one of your ways of focusing behavior, but what makes them posthypnotic suggestions?

E: They are questions; they fixate attention and call upon thoughts and associations that are inevitable in her future.

R: Fixating attention and initiating an unconscious search within define those questions as hypnotic. Even without inducing trance in a lengthy and formal way, you can so fixate attention with a question that you initiate a momentary form of the "common everyday trance." Since she will inevitably have thoughts about her therapy with you in the future, these questions will tend to bind her future associations to this moment in therapy when you are actively depotentiating her symptom.

Distraction to Protect Suggestions

E: [To R] And how do you like that for a posthypnotic suggestion? [Pause]
[To X] How do you like this kind of therapy?

X: I don't like any kind of therapy. You mean to do it or be on the other end?

E: How do you like my way of doing therapy?

X: I like your way.

E: And you promise not to forget it.

X: Um hum.

E: [To R] Reinforcing the posthypnotic but it certainly doesn't look like it or sound like it.
[To X] Now why do you insist on referring to past streams?

X: The past?

E: Streaming in the past.

X: You mean streams instead of puddles?

E: Un hum.

X: Two things I think. I guess I object to the word. The other thing is that mist, stream, or puddles, they are all just as bad for me.

> E: Here I am defining it as posthypnotic to have more effect on her at the conscious level. With an altered tone of voice this question "about this kind of therapy" now makes the situation a personal kind of thing and a friendly relationship.
>
> R: You are also immediately distracting her from the posthypnotic suggestions you have just given, lest her conscious mind starts to argue or interfere with them. This is highly characteristic of your approach—you make a suggestion and then immediately distract before consciousness can take issue with it.
>
> E: My remark, "And promise not to forget it" refers back to my earlier question, "How soon will you forget me?"
>
> R: That tends to reinforce the earlier suggestion while structuring an amnesia for all that took place between the two statements.

Depotentiating Conscious Doubts About Symptom Cure with Dramatic Hypnotic Experience

X: I am aware of wanting to get rid of it, but on the other hand   I guess I feel hopeless about it,   about being able to change.

E: I know that.   You also hope you will always be able to stand up, don't you?

X: Yes.

E: And before you met me, you believed that you could always stand up, and you found out   that there are times when you can't stand up.   Just try it.
[Pause as X again tries unsuccessfully to stand up]
You can do anything I tell you to do, can't you?

X: It seems like it.

E: Then you can stand up.

X: Can I?

195

E: Yes.
[She does stand up]

X: Yep.

E: Stand up again.
[While she is standing, the senior author continues as follows]
Try to sit down.
[She stands with knees slightly bent but immobilized, and she cannot sit down]
[Pause]

X: I think my legs are made out of steel.

E: Now you can sit down.
[She sits down.]
Now do you know that you can do anything that I tell you to do?
Do you suppose that comes to having dry hands?

X: Could you make me have dry hands?

E: Um hum.

X: Maybe you can.

E: *Maybe?* What is your relationship with this fellow that came in with you?

X: I'm not sure.

> E: I'm allowing her to express her hopelessness, then I proceed to demolish it with this demonstration.
>
> R: You use a dramatic hypnotic experience (not being able to stand up) to depotentiate her negative, doubting, conscious framework of hopelessness about being able to give up her long-standing symptom. That is a major purpose in evoking hypnotic experience: to effectively demonstrate that something can change, to depotentiate the erroneous rigidities of a patient's conscious framework.
>
> E: I demonstrate that there is something else besides her negative thoughts. It is further demolishment when she cannot sit down because she has known for a long time that she can stand up and she can sit down. I am not preventing her, it is a hypnotic experience: She is using something she didn't know

196

she had. When she asks if I can make her hands dry, my "um hum" is not forceful but casual.

R: It is all the more convincing by being soft.

E: But I don't let her get away with "maybe." I depotentiate it by repeating "maybe?" with a doubting tone and then immediately distract her from any remaining doubts by reference to her boyfriend.

Developing the Objective Observer

E: **A longtime friend?**

X: **We were colleagues, not really. I guess you would say he is my boyfriend.**

E: **Do you mind if I ask him now?**
[**Erickson asks him a series of general information questions for a few moments, and then returns to Miss X as follows**]

Tell me, any special thing that causes you stage fright or embarrassment?

X: **My hands.**

E: *Now?*

X: **Now? No, because we are talking about them.**

E: I'm also still exploring the sex theme. I first let her define him. Then I let him define himself. This also allows her to sit back and see him objectively.

R: That develops the objective observer in the patient. Your incredulous response "*Now?*" again depotentiates the mental framework that makes her symptom possible.

Depotentiating the Symptom's Habitual Framework: Jokes and Unconscious Values

E: **Let's remain silent. Then will they cause embarrassment?**

X: **No. Everybody in the room knows what my problem is, so I don't.**

E: **Is or was?**
[**Pause**]

X: **Is.**

E: Let's see those streams then.

X: They are just misty.

E: You couldn't irrigate anything with a mist. The only useful purpose for a mist is on the house plants.

X: But you can't play the harp with house plants either.

E: Therefore you reserve the mist for the house plants.

[Pause]

Struggling to believe is very difficult, isn't it?

R: Yes.

X: I have always had the feeling that if they could really dry up, it would never happen again.

E: Well, let's correct that.

> E: Now we are transforming the symptom to the situation of talking about her hands. I am shifting the cause of the symptom: before, harp playing caused the symptom; now, talking causes it.
>
> R: This is another way of gaining control over the symptom and depotentiating it: You take the symptom out of its usual context and shift it to a new framework where you can deal with it more easily—in this case simply by using silence. You then success-fully challenge the symptom, and she finds she can only produce a mist.
>
> E: I'm not abolishing the mist, I'm giving that mist a value removed from the harp.
>
> R: You are displacing the symptom from a disturbing place to a useful one. The conscious mind may take your remark about the usefulness of mist to plants as a kind of absurd joke in this context, but you are accomplishing something very important on the unconscious level. For the unconscious, symptoms have an important value. You are letting the unconscious retain the value of the symptom (now diminished to a mist) by displacing that value to another concrete function: A mist is good for house plants. This kind of displacement works in the literal and concrete unconscious, even though it is absurd from a con-scious rational frame of reference.

Reversals, Implications, and the Positive Values Inherent in Symptoms

E: Your hands can dry up, but do you want them to have the freedom to get wet again? Isn't that right?

X: Um hum.

E: Wet not only from putting them in water but by perspiration.
So don't try to rob your hands of rightful perspiration.
[Pause]
Your hands have been overperspiring for a long time.
Let's give them at least two hours to learn the right amount. And you can already see that they have been doing a lot of learning.
[Long pause]

> R: Is it a double bind when you ask if she wants the freedom to let her hands get wet again? It is a peculiar reversal when you tell her she can get wet hands.

> E: I'm giving her freedom—even to get wet hands!

> R: But if she is free to get wet hands, that must imply she has dry hands. So you've used implication to give her a suggestion for dry hands.

> E: Since there is no restriction on wet hands, it also means there is no restriction on dry hands. She is not put into any rigid situation—there are situations where wet hands are acceptable. Until she met me, all wet hands were horrifying.

> R: You are giving a positive value to something that was all negative before. You are helping her recognize the positive value of the physiological function that was formerly only a negative symptom.

Depotentiating Future Resistance: Being in a Trance Without Knowing It

E: By the way, how many times have you been in a trance today?

X: I was just trying to figure that out.
[Pause]
I don't know. I'm not sure.

E: More than once?

X: Yes.

E: More than twice:

X: Yes. I think so.

E: More than three times?

X: I'm not so sure.

E: More than four?

X: No, I don't think so.

E: More than five?

X: No.

E: Can you stand up?
[She stands.]

R: Why do you ask how many times she has been in trance today?

E: She cannot know for a certainty whether this idea came while she was awake or in a trance state. If you are going to hunt a deer, you had better know which field it is in, because you can't kill it in a field it is not in. She can't direct any resistance to any idea until she knows whether it was in trance or waking state.

R: So you are again depotentiating any possible expression of resistance here.

E: Future resistance! To resist any idea she first has to define it as trance or unconscious.

R: So you are making it difficult to determine whether the important suggestions were placed in the conscious or trance state. You are essentially using a confusion technique to protect your suggestions from her conscious resistance. Asking her this question about the number of times she has been in trance can put her in a doubtful position about her unconsciousness. Thus it is very valuable therapeutically if patients do not know whether or not they were in trance. That confusion stops them from holding onto therapeutic suggestions in a way that allows them to repudiate them.

E: Yes, it is very valuable.

Hypnotic Immobility Conditioned to "Try"

E: *Try* to sit down.

X: I can't.

E: Are you in a trance?

X: I don't know.

E: You don't know.
That's right. You don't know.
That's why you don't know how many times you have been in a trance.
Now you can sit down.
[She sits down]

X: Oh, I see.

R: Being in a trance without knowing it?

E: Yes.   If it were a boyfriend who told you you could not sit down, you would wonder if he was in his right mind, wouldn't you?

X: Yes.

R: Is this inability to sit down due to a momentary trance?

E: If I can put a trance in her hips, she has to recognize I can put a trance in her hands.

R: But why were you able to put it in her hips? She was in the normal awake state when you asked her the question.

E: "*Try* to sit down."

R: The word "*try*" uttered in that soft and doubting way you have is a cue that she could not. You had conditioned her to immobility when you use the word "*try*" in that way.

E: Yes, the hypnotic response hits her hips or her hands, and she knows that. I have also gotten across the idea that she does not know whether she is in a trance or not.

R: What is your actual belief about being in or out of a trance without knowing it? If we had a machine that could detect trance, do you believe she would be going in and out of trance throughout the session?

E: Yes.

Dynamics of Indirect Suggestion: Demonstrating Unconscious Control of Behavior

E: **And you are really becoming aware of how effectively your unconscious mind can control you.**

> R: All these demonstrations of the effectiveness of the unconscious to control behavior are to convince her conscious mind that her unconscious can also control her symptom? This is your basic approach to dealing with symptoms by hypnotherapy. You don't directly suggest symptoms out of existence. You arrange a series of experiences that demonstrate the potency of the patients' unconscious. You give them an opportunity to witness the therapeutic control their unconscious minds have over their symptom and then leave it to their unconscious to continue its therapeutic regulation. Therapy thus comes from an adjusted interplay of psychodynamics within patients rather than the patients trying to accommodate themselves to a therapist's direct suggestion from the outside. These are the actual dynamics of indirect suggestion.

> E: Yes.

Open-Ended Suggestion to Cope with Problems

E: **Now think of a few more of the things that you would like to have your unconscious take charge of.**

X: **Short of my hands?**

E: **Other than your hands.**
[A comfortable chat now takes place about family matters and apparently unrelated topics for about ten minutes. He is giving her another rest.]

> E: Here I'm getting at any other problems she may have.

> R: This is an open-ended suggestion to let her unconscious resolve other problems the therapist may not even know about.

Ideomotor Signaling to Evaluate and Ratify Symptom Cure: The Second Round

E: **Now, before I asked you what your unconscious   answer was about sweating,   I told you about your hands.**
Your right means "yes," your left means "no."

"Yes" you would have sweating, "no" that you would not have sweating.
Watch your hands and see if they will signal yes or no.
Rest them on your thighs.
Which is going to lift?
[After a minute or two of waiting, X's left hand begins to lift ever so slightly and very, very slowly with minor jerks.]
Your confidence is growing.
Growing more powerful.
[The right hand also begins to lift, but the left hand remains higher.]
You can close your eyes now.
Your unconscious can know the answer, but you don't have to know the answer.   All right.   Now drop your hands in your lap. The question has been answered.   Now you can feel very rested and very comfortable.   Now what is that smile for?
[Pause]

R: This is the second time you have utilized ideomotor signaling to ratify symptom cure. The first time she lifted her right hand, indicating she felt the symptom was still present. You therefore back up and do further work, (1) depotentiating her conscious doubts about symptom cure, and (2) depotentiating the habitual mental framework in which her symptom occurred. (3) You ratify your therapeutic work with various forms of indirect suggestion and protect these suggestions by distraction, etc. (4) You let her experience other dramatic hypnotic phenomena, such as being unable to stand up or sit down, to open other channels for therapeutic change that could bypass the erroneous symptom-producing structures of her ego. (5) You give her a breathing spell, and now you feel ready for another ideomotor test of the degree to which she is willing to give up her sweating. A change toward cure is evident, though the situation is still unclear: She does lift her left hand slightly, indicating the symptom is going, but then her right hand lifts, indicating it is still present to some degree.

E: The right hand lifting was a token answer for any remaining conscious doubts that she had.

R: This time the left hand lifts higher, indicating the answer has shifted more toward an acknowledgment of a significant symptom change. You then tell her to close her eyes and her conscious mind need not know the answer. Why?

E: [The senior author illustrates with a story indicating that the conscious mind interferes with therapeutic work.]

Ratification of Symptom Change

E: Those doubts come into your mind, don't they?

X: Yes, they do.

E: It is nice to watch growth.

R: Yes, absolutely.

E: Now I am going to tell you another story.
[**The senior author now tells a clinical case history of how he helped an eleven-year-old control her bed-wetting. A major point of the case was that symptom control comes about gradually. He then continues.**]

> R: You now acknowledge her conscious doubts and bring them out into the open. You openly acknowledge the truth about her inner situation. She responds with an affirmative "yes." You have thus also opened up a yes set. She is in an affirmative mood. You then immediately follow up with, "It is nice to watch growth," which is a direct reinforcement of the fact that her left hand did go up, that she is changing and in the process of giving up the symptom.

> E: With what part of the body does she wet?

> R: Your story of the bed-wetter was particularly appropriate because the symptom of wetness and a number of details were similar. You are again bringing in sexual connotations.

> E: Yes, wet genitals and wet hands.

Utilizing Time and Failure for Cure

E: Give yourself plenty of time.   Now your hands have fizzled out for today.   They can have some wetness tomorrow,   the next day. And you will be surprised at the increase in length of dry times.
[**Pause**]
After a while you will have a drought on your hands. Now and then it rains even in the desert.

> R: You are utilizing time for symptom cure.

E: Yes, and giving her permission for failures. *All the failures will prove an improvement.*

R: The failures will prove the improvement because they come after increasing lengths of dry times.

Ideomotor Questioning to Ratify Symptom Cure: The Third Round

E: Drop your hands.   Now let's see,   which hand is going to move up.   [The left hand lifts only. She frowns while it lifts.]   The wrist, too. And the elbow will bend.   Come toward your face. Higher, higher,   up,   well, that is really hard to believe, isn't it? That your unconscious says: Sweating is not for your future. And your unconscious knows that.   Your unconscious knows that you will have a gradual growing conscious realization of that,   that only at the speed that your conscious mind can tolerate. Close your eyes.

R: You test a third time, and finally only the left hand lifts, indicating that the sweating has been effectively dealt with. This is a clear case illustrating how you return again and again to deal with her doubts and internal resistance until you get a clear ideomotor response of symptom cure.

E: Yes.

R: You now extend the ideomotor response and, by implication, the cure by having her whole hand levitate higher and higher.

E: "A gradual growing conscious realization" means that she can learn as rapidly or as slowly as he wants to.

Trance Rest to Reinforce Therapeutic Change

E: Go deeply in trance.   And now awaken at your convenience.   (X closes her eyes, visibly relaxes for a few moments, and then awakens.)

R: After the successful ideomotor indication of symptom change you give her a period of trance rest. She had been under an evident strain (frowning) during the ideomotor signaling, so you now let her have a few moments of therapeutic trance as a way of rewarding her inner work with relaxation and inner freedom.

Humor to Facilitate Unconscious Psychodynamics

E: Now for a bit of flippancy.

X: Yes.

E: I embarrassed Dr. Bertha Rodger in New York. I was lecturing there at a banquet in my honor.   Someone asked me where I was going to sleep that night. I said with Bertha.   And I think you are very much surprised to find out how often you sleep with me.   You are constantly going to sleep with me, aren't you?   Rather shameless, aren't you?

X: No, I don't think I'm shameless.

E: It only seems as if I'm relating a personal narrative.

R: But in fact you are indirectly bringing sex in again. But what is the purpose of this direct sexual confrontation here?

E: I tell her she is going to sleep with me. Consciously she knows she is not.

R: She knows the absurdity of that.

E: But I have said it so convincingly. I have been very convincing to her unconscious so her unconscious says, "He's not really talking about sleeping with him, he's talking about sleeping with someone else!" I'm nakedly hammering on the sexual aspects.

R: You are using flippancy and humor to facilitate the inner resolution of the sexual psychodynamics of her problem. Humor depends for its effect on engaging unconscious processes. You use humor here to initiate an unconscious search and facilitate the unconscious processes intimately related to the psychodynamic source of her symptom reaction.

Ratifying Therapeutic Work

E: We *have* done a lot together, haven't we?

X: Yes.

E: We have done a lot together. You have been here two and a quarter hours. Do   you believe me?

X: Yes.

E: Why, just because I said it?

X: No. I know that too.

E: Now can you come back tomorrow? You have a lot of resting to do.

X: Here or at home?

E: Preferably in Phoenix.

X: Do you want me to rest overnight so I can sleep with you again tomorrow?

E: Tomorrow because I want you to get some good phsysiological rest.   You have done a lot of work. Far more than you know.   You have altered a lot of your brain pathways.   You have set up new ones.   You need to sleep.   You are going to think about your hands in a different way.

> R: You now directly help her acknowledge that a lot of therapeutic work has been done. You end this session with these marvelous waking suggestions that will facilitate conscious rest and further therapeutic work on an unconscious level throughout her sleep. Her attempt at extending your joke by asking, "Do you want me to rest overnight so I can sleep with you again tomorrow?" actually places sex where it belongs in the context of doing further therapeutic work with you; she is beginning to associate sexuality with therapy without quite realizing it.

SESSION TWO:

Insight and Working Through Related Problems

The next day X returned for another two-hour session with Erickson. Her friend L is present as an observer. The session begins with the spontaneous admission of her enduring feelings of confusion about yesterday's therapy. Such confusion is characteristic of the patient's mental state during the initial and middle stages of therapy with Erickson. Confusion is an indication that the patient's habitual frames of reference and generalized reality orientation have been loosened so that their psychodynamics are now in an unstable equilibrium. A process of deautomatization is taking place wherein many of the patient's erroneous sets that have been responsible for symptoms and maladaptive behavior are loosened to the point where new associations and mental frameworks can be formulated to achieve therapeutic goals.

Recognizing that a great deal of insight therapy needs to be done in this session, Erickson begins by giving her some "mental warm-up exercises": He requests that she recall in exact detail the furniture of the place she slept the night before and then all the things she saw on a shopping tour yesterday. All of this may seem irrelevant to the patient, but Erickson is thereby "warming up" search operations in her mind with nonthreatening material. These search operations will be used later in the session, when she will need to seek and express insights.

The senior author then induces trance with an ideosensory approach ("How soon will you warm up your hands?") that is uniquely suited to X because the sensation of "warmth" is tied to the theme of sexuality that touches one of her basic unconscious complexes. He then embarks on the work of undoing repressions in a variety of ways. His object, as always, is to help the patient loosen the rigid mental frameworks that are responsible for symptom formation, so that the unconscious can restructure a better reality. He utilizes ideomotor signaling, analogies, stories, and other devices to move her associative processes continually toward introspection in critical areas. Here we witness Erickson at his best as a therapist facilitating the process of insight. He continually offers one approach after another, like a locksmith trying different keys until the patient finally unlocks her own repressions. After a great deal of initial resistance, X experiences a flood of insights about her family dynamics and the reasons for her symptoms.

The senior author then closes the interview and effectively terminates therapy by working through many of her conscious doubts about symptom removal (her claustrophobia and fear of planes as well as sweating). In a respectful way he then finally discloses to X many of the therapeutic approaches he has used with her. The "mysteries of hypnosis" are dispelled with a simple statement of the Utilization Theory of Hypnotic Suggestion: He has only helped her utilize her own associations and mental processes to achieve her own therapeutic goals.

Confusion as a Prelude to Mental Reorganization

E: What have you done since yesterday?

X: Not very much. I went to bed relatively early. My mind seemed confused. I was recalling snatches of things that had been said, words mostly. Some of your stories. I didn't want to go to the bathroom in the middle of the night. I don't know if that had anything to do with what you were telling us yesterday, but I didn't want to go swimming last night either. I didn't want to go in the water. I just generally felt confused. I haven't been able to stop thinking about yesterday.

E: What particular thinking have you done?

X: Well, I'm kind of amazed at the feeling that there is sort of another entity inside that could listen and could understand things that I don't, and is maybe more hopeful than I am consciously.

E: Where are you staying?

X: With a social worker friend of mine in Tempee.

> R: When she says, "My mind seemed confused," you recognize it as a typical effect of the initial stage of your therapy. It is a good sign, since it means that her conscious frames of reference have been depotentiated and her unconscious has had an opportunity to reorganize itself along therapeutic pathways.
>
> E: Yes.
>
> R: Her conscious mind is confused, but since she has not been able to stop thinking about yesterday, it must mean that her unconscious has been very actively at work.
>
> E: She feels "there is sort of another entity inside," and then gives her prognosis.
>
> R: Clearly indicating you have been on the right track in guiding her to make contact with this inner source that could understand more and be more optimistic than her conscious mind.

Training in Thorough Mental Examination
E: Name the items of furniture in the house.

X: Well, in the living room there are giant pillows instead of furniture, but there is a rocking chair there, too.   There is a couch in the kitchen.   There are tall bar stools in the kitchen.   There are three bedrooms, so there are three beds. Two regular and one water bed. There are three dressers. I think that's all.

E: No other objects?   You haven't named a table yet.

X: OK, there is a table and four chairs in the kitchen, etcetera.

E: Now, any special thing you did yesterday?

X: I went shopping by myself for about an hour and was sort of wandering around in a daze, just taking my time. Other than that, no.

E: Where did you shop?

X: A little place, well not little. It is a giant conglomerate department store.

E: What objects did you look at?

X: Food, cheese, meats, flour tortillas, wine, tomatoes, beans, *pants*.

E: Any other things?

X: No.

X: The pants that I bought were men's pants, but I looked at a pants suit that would be for a woman.

> R: What's the purpose of this seemingly irrelevant question about house furniture?
>
> E: When you think about a thing you think inclusively; don't exclude anything.
>
> R: Oh, that's the implication! By having her think in extreme detail about her friend's house furniture, you are training her unconscious to go into something very thoroughly without telling her conscious mind what you are doing. You don't directly say, "I want you to thoroughly explore your problems." Instead you put her through another task in a thorough manner. You then expect that process of thorough examination to automatically generalize to her own self-examination of her personal problems.
>
> E: She came to me with a problem, and I tell her she is going to have to do some thinking. And then I demonstrate to her exactly the kind of thinking.
>
> R: You then do the same thing by requesting she make a detailed examination of her shopping.
>
> E: She makes a remarkable listing: she ends up with "pants."
>
> R: Oh, the sexual implication of pants?!
>
> E: Yes! It is put in so beautifully. Why would she buy men's pants? It is like choosing a man.

Developing Insight

X: Once you asked me about how soon I would forget you. I didn't quite understand what you meant by that, but I think my response was that

I didn't think I would, and L was giving his explanation of what he thought it meant.

E: And what was his explanation?

X: Two parts of it, I think. One that I should not let you get in the way of me using myself or something.   You are using yourself as sort of a metaphor to sort of assist me to do what I need to do for myself.   Is that right?

E: He is sharper than a razor.

X: Yes, he is.

E: Anything else?   [Pause]   Only those things that you can say to the group.

X: Well, again I was surprised that it seemed as if my own conscious mind was a separate kind of thing, and I kept asking L if he thought that my unconscious could understand what my conscious mind couldn't. Then he sort of laughed and explained, of course, that would be true.   Your use of the word "courage" sort of fit for me,   partly because I think I found myself just recently overcoming a very difficult situation in my work by some sort of supreme exercise of my will and courage, too. I think.   Oh, I know something else too. About the little girl with blond hair [X has blond hair and is here referring to a childhood memory] who was laying down on the stairs, and I think L said something about her having claustrophobia, and my response was, "How does he know I have claustrophobia?"

E: Do you really have claustrophobia?

X: Um hum.

E: How sure are you of that?

X: Well, I'm assuming that it is a matter of degree. Once when I was up in the arm of the Statue of Liberty, which is a very narrow passage, I blacked out because it was a very small area, and I don't like planes for the same reason.   I always thought if somebody really wanted to torture me, all they had to do was to lock me in the closet.

E: Whereabouts in the plane do you have the strongest feelings?

X: When I am sitting by the window and look out. I guess that that is the worst.

E: How much plane traveling do you do?

X: I fly to the west coast about twice a year.

E: Now what kind of stores did you pass yesterday?

X: A department store, a Broadway, a supermarket, bakeries, liquor stores, sporting goods, hub caps, dune buggies, drug stores, water bed store   um   tropical fish.

E: Did you pass any places of business that you didn't like?"

X: The only thing that comes to mind, and I'm not sure I didn't like it, but what came to mind was a purple nude dancing place on a corner that we passed.

E: What in particular did you see in that place?

X: What did I see?   It looked like a building made of cement bricks that had just been washed in purple. And there were nude women painted all over the outside of the building, and I think it said topless.

> E: She is starting to pick up my double meanings when she begins to wonder about my question of how soon she would forget me. She is right about the fact that she should not let me get in the way of her using herself.
>
> R: She is gaining insight into her claustrophobia, her fear of heights, and the operation of her own conscious-unconscious system. Her final comment about noticing the "purple nude dancing place" is not elaborated, but it is hard to believe that she does not realize its possible connection with the fact that you always wear purple clothing [The senior author is partially color blind, but he can distinguish shades of purple] and the sexual connotations in your remarks. In any case it strongly suggests her unconscious is picking up the sexual associations present in your two-level communication. You are evidently still concerned about her readiness to deal with the sexual issues, so you do not use this possible opening to talk about sexual matters.

Ideosensory Induction Utilizing a Psychodynamic Complex

E: How are your hands?

X: Misty.

E: **Must be you have a warm heart.**   **How soon will you warm up your hands?**   **[Pause]**

X: **They are getting warmer.**   **[Pause]**

E: **Close your eyes.**   **[Pause]**   **Lean back in your chair.**   **[Pause] And just keep sleeping deeper and deeper.**

> R: Here you deliberately associate her sweating with warm heart and, by implication, sex. Then, before she can respond or interfere in any way with this association, you immediately begin an ideosensory induction to trance by asking how soon will her hands warm up. That question is trance-inducing because to feel an adequate response of warmth, she must first go into trance. Since you have already associated warmth with heart, sex, and sweating, this choice of induction reinforces and extends these associations. Your initial association of misty and warm heart put her on an inner search for your meaning. That inner search is characteristic of the everyday trance when people pause for a moment's reflection over a puzzling question or task. You then immediately make use of this momentary inner focus to initiate a trance induction that also utilizes the inner associations (warmth) that are occupying her at that precise second. We could summarize the whole process as follows. You gave her two trance-inducing tasks simultaneously: (1) The association between symptom (misty) and warmth (sex) puts her on an inner search, and (2) the question about warming up her hands requires trance for an adequate response. These two approaches are interlocking and mutually reinforcing because they have the common theme of warmth. This common theme is itself trance-inducing because you tied it to a central psychodynamic complex (warmth, sex, sweating) that is present in her unconscious. Whenever we touch upon a person's complexes, of course, there is a spontaneous *abaissement du niveau mentale* (a lowering of consciousness) that also facilitates trance. No wonder, then, that she immediately responds with the ideosensory response of warmth and enters trance.

Autonomous Trance Training

E: **While you are sleeping   more and more deeply,   I am going to make some calls. [E dials and makes some telephone calls of a professional nature, discusses setting up future appointments with R, etc. After about five minutes he returns to X].**

213

R: In the initial stages of trance training you sometimes give the patient a free period to learn to go deeper into trance in an autonomous manner, by whatever means they have at their disposal (Erickson, Rossi, and Rossi, 1976).

Exploratory Ideomotor Questioning

E: Breathe very deeply, X.   And either nod or shake your head   gently   in answer to my question.   Do you mind being with me?   [She nods her head "yes."]   You do mind. Is there somebody else you want with us?   [Pause, no response]   All right, I will repeat my question.   Are you willing to be alone with me?   [Shakes head "no."]   Do you know why?   [Pause, no response]   All right, another question.   Do you know why you have what you call claustrophobia?   [Shakes head "no"]   Do you know when your sweating first began?   [Shakes head "no"]   Do you know when you'll approach the harp to play?   [Nods "yes"]

> R: After five minutes of autonomous trance-deepening you judge her ready to respond to some exploratory ideomotor signaling. You usually like to use head nodding or shaking because that utilizes well-learned and automatic movements that people frequently carry out without realizing it in everyday life. Patients, therefore, may tend to be more amnesic for head signaling that they cannot watch versus finger or hand signaling, which they can witness when their eyes are open.

> E: When I begin by asking about being alone with me, I'm trying to affirm the sexual associations of the first session. I'm letting her go into her sexual dynamics.

Posthypnotic Suggestions: Consciousness Need Not Control; Undoing Repressions in Central Psychodynamics

E: Later, after you are awake, you will suddenly   but not immediately   give me the date   and place, doing so out of context of the general conversation.   Do you understand me?   [Nods "yes"]   That is, we could be talking about gourmet foods,   Minnesota as a gopher   state, and you will suddenly   intrude upon   that conversation   the date and place,   and after having

**uttered those things,   you will realize that is the time and place when
you will approach a harp.   Now do you understand? [Nods "yes"]**

R: Why do you use this approach to breaking through her amnesia about when her sweating began? Are you giving the unconscious the opportunity to intrude itself with the help of any chance association that may be related to the significant material?

E: In training a rifle team for the international shoot, I told them to let the sight wander back and forth, up and down, all over the target. You don't know just when you'll squeeze the trigger.

R: The conscious mind will not know just when, so the unconscious will have an opportunity to intrude and squeeze the trigger at just the right moment. You are taking pressure off the conscious mind and giving responsibility to the unconscious. Did you explain that to the riflemen?

E: I did not explain it to them. I said to them they might not even know when their finger squeezed the trigger. It takes all the pressure off because it is not necessary for them to know. The only necessary thing is for the bullet to hit the target.

R: The conscious mind need not know the precise moment. You are allowing the unconscious to play a bigger part in the response.

E: And the conscious mind can be more comfortable because it isn't pressured to do it at an exact moment. A small child always asks, "Can I do it when I want to?" The feeling of comfort and freedom is very important. You don't have to know the exact time.

R: You allow this freedom for the unconscious to make its own response in its own way in its own time. You depotentiate the erroneous sets of the patient's conscious mind that presumes to control everything and thereby open freedom for the individual's creative unconscious.

Structured Amnesia

**E: Another question: Are you willing to be alone with me
briefly?   [Nods "yes"]   That is nice.   Now would you   within
your own mind think about the happiest   event in your life.   Just
think about it.   You don't need to tell me.   Also think about   the**

most wretched   moment of your life.   And you don't need to tell me.   [Long pause]

> R: After giving her an important posthypnotic suggestion, you return again to the question of her willingness to be with you. It continues the sexual connotation, but placed here it tends to structure an amnesia for the posthypnotic suggestion that came between the two forms of the same question.

> E: Yes, all this through here has sexual connotations [happiest and most wretched moments].

> R: An immediate absorption into sexual preoccupations would serve as a distraction that might also facilitate an amnesia for the preceding posthypnotic suggestion.

Serial Posthypnotic Suggestion for a Negative Hallucination Training

E: Shortly you will awaken,   wondering where the others have gone.   [Pause]   It will rather surprise you.   Why did they leave?   Was there any purpose?   Now slowly awaken.   [Pause as she opens her eyes and reorients to her body a bit.]

> R: You feel it is usually more effective to give a posthypnotic suggestion in a serial form where the posthypnotic behavior is integrated with ongoing waking behavior or typical patterns of waking behavior (Erickson and Erickson, 1941). In this case you don't directly suggest she won't see the others when she awakens. Only the very best hypnotic subjects would be capable of such a strong negative hallucination this early in their training. You give a more subtle form of suggestion that can utilize many already existing mental patterns like surprise, and questions about why they left, etc.

Trance Awakening with Amnesia by Distraction

E: What do you think is my favorite gourmet food?

X: Chicken?

E: Take a slice of bread, butter it generously with peanut butter, then cover it with a thick layer of cheese. Put it under the broiler until the cheese is melted. Butter it with peanut butter, cover it with a thick layer of cheese, put it back under the broiler until the cheese is melted.

216

X: Trying to remember if I ever had cheese and peanut butter.

    E: Here I begin with a breathing spell about my favorite food.

    R: This also serves as another distraction which tends to render the preceding trance material amnesic.

Confusion and Unconscious Search: Depotentiating Conscious Control

X: I don't know what you are about?

E: What do you think I am about?
[Long pause]

X: I don't know right now.

E: What don't you know?

X: Well,   like yesterday, I thought I knew what you were about, oh, in some ways.

E: How do you feel about containing another entity?

X: Mixed. I feel relieved in some ways and frightened in others.

E: What should you be frightened about?

X: I guess it is a lack of control. If there is another entity, then there are things over which I don't have control.

E: Why must you have control?   [Pause]

X: Well, it is very frightening for me to be out of control.

E: How much is it frightened less?

X: For me to be out of control?   Quite a bit, I think.

E: Now let me clarify that for you.   In this room you have relinquished control to me.   Out of this room you will have all your own control, and you have relinquished it in this room to enable me to help you, that's all.

My first daughter-in-law was a marvelous hypnotic subject. I took her to a study group in Phoenix   to demonstrate and discuss hypnosis.   I intended to use her and I couldn't get a single response from her.   After we got back home,   she said, "Will you forgive me, Dad, I had to find out if I had control."   I have had that happen on several occasions. They had to find out if they had full control.

R: She tries but cannot figure out the relevance of this conversation for her therapy when she says she doesn't "know what you are about." Your effort to give her a breathing spell actually confuses her and sends her on an unconscious search. That sort of inner exploration is actually the kind of mental set you try to enhance for trance work. You therefore immediately return to therapy work with your question about "containing another entity." She then confirms the basic problem of many patients: They are usually afraid to give up conscious control, they do not trust their own unconscious to find solutions and new ways of coping.

E: With the example of my daughter-in-law I give her another breathing spell. I'm also assuring her that she does have control, that's all right. But you really do have it. I want her to be absolutely confident about herself.

Paradoxical Suggestion and Distraction

E: Now what you want is more control of yourself. If you relinquish control in relationship to your hands, you have relinquished control in your relationship to what you call claustrophobia.   But you can now have full control.   You didn't even tell me to go to hell.

E: You give a seemingly paradoxical set of suggestions when you tell her she can have control, and yet if she relinquishes control of her hands, she relinquishes control of her claustrophobia. You mean that if she allows her unconscious to deal with her hand problem, it will also deal with the claustrophobia. But you don't state it in a clear, rational way for left hemispheric understanding, as I have here. You present it as a seeming paradox of having control yet relinquishing control. Such a paradoxical presentation will momentarily jam her critical faculties so her unconscious again will have an opportunity to interfere. Then, before she can recover her critical faculties, you are off with another provocative statement about telling you to go to hell. This now distracts her further, so your suggestion about the connection between sweating and claustrophobia cannot be dealt with consciously and must remain within, where only her unconscious can receive and work with it.

Trance Induction by Depotentiating Conscious Sets: Evaluating Posthypnotic Capacity
[X is immobile with a trancelike stare.]

218

E: Is there anybody else here?

X: In this room?   [Long pause]   I can't give you a simple answer.

E: Then give me a complex one.

X: Well there are three or four other people here,   but they are not.

E: They are not what?

X: Not impinging or something.

E: Not impinging.   [To R] Would you like to ask a question on that point?

R: How are your hands feeling right now?

X: Wet and warm.

E: They are warmer.   Let's let them keep on being warmer and warmer.

> R: The effect of your double depotentiation of her unconscious sets with paradox and immediate distraction is that she is sent on such an intense inner search that she is, for all practical purposes, in a trance. You recognize this and ask a question about the presence of others to evaluate her capacity to follow your subtle posthypnotic suggestion about wondering where the others have gone.

> E: She is saying, "I'm in a trance but I don't know it." Reality isn't reality. She is defining: I do not know my conscious state, I do know my trance state, my unconscious state.

> R: Her answer about people "not impinging or something" is a bit like the trance logic when a subject sees a hallucinated person seated in a chair but also sees the chair as if the hallucination were transparent [Orne, 1962]. She is aware yet not aware; she is following your negative hallucination suggestion to a mild degree. You therefore deepen her trance involvement by requesting ideosensory behavior that can only be accomplished by the unconscious: she is to allow her hands to get warmer.

Hypnotic Enhancement of Psychodynamic Complexes

E: Where are you going to put your hot little hands? Answer.   [Pause]

X: On my face?

E: That wasn't your first thought.   Do you know now?   You don't have to bury your thoughts, do you?   Even though some are unfamiliar. How soon would you have those hot little hands?

X: How soon would I have them?

E: Um hum.

X: Where I was thinking of putting them?

E: No, how soon when you can have hot little hands to put somewhere.

X: They are hot now.

> E: It is perfectly socially acceptable to tell her to let her hands get warmer and to speak of "hot little hands," but now we all know!
>
> R: You are actually getting her sexual psychodynamics involved in this apparently innocent ideosensory exercise. This is again two-level communication to deal with issues you are not sure her conscious mind is ready to cope with.
>
> E: When I ask how soon she would have those hot little hands, I'm asking, "How soon will she get down to the sex?"
>
> R: When she responds with, "Where I was thinking of putting them!" she appears to be getting closer to the naked sexual question.

Undoing Repressions: Facilitating Inner Dialogue by Double Bind Questions

E: Quickly, without thinking,   quickly without thinking, give me a date.

X: March 17.

E: Year?

X: 1958

E: Now what happened then?

X: That would be St. Patrick's Day.   [Long pause]   My boyfriend dyed his hair green.

E: All right.   Now there are a lot of things that you are willing for me to know.

E: How many things are there about you that you don't want me to know?   [Pause]

X: Quite a few.

E: Do you know the reason why?   [Pause]

X: I would be embarrassed.

E: Now the important thing.   What do you know about you that you don't want to know?   Don't tell it. You don't want to know it. How many things are there about you that you don't want to know?   [Long pause]

X: How many?   [Long pause]   Two.
E: All right.   Do those two include something about a harp?   Do those two include something about your hands?   And you don't want to know, do you?

X: I don't want to know.

E: Why?

X: It would force me to look at something I don't want to look at.

E: Do you think it is awful bad?

X: Pretty bad.

E: And don't you want to know all the good and all the bad about you?   It is only your knowledge of it.

X: It is too much.

E: What are you most afraid of?   Don't tell me, tell yourself what you are afraid of.   Have you done that?
Can you share it with me?   [Long pause]   Don't answer that question.   Can you share it with others here?

X: Um hum.

E: Do you want to?   [Pause]   Is it as bad as it first started out to be?

X: No.

E: [To R] You see what I did.   I protected her all along the line, and it reduced the seriousness of it.

R: Yes.

E: Have your remembered something bad?

R: This question, of course, is designed to bring up in her mind all the most intimate associations she is not yet ready to talk about. But by simply bringing them up in her own associative process, it is an increment toward eventual expression. This is another form of paradoxical or double bind approach (Erickson and Rossi, 1975). By asking a person about what they are not willing to talk about, you bring them closer to talking about it. After she has had an opportunity to turn it over in her own mind, you again ask if it is possible to talk about it. Her inner associations are by now primed for expression since they have been brought to the fore of her awareness. Since there is a long pause, however, you realize she is not yet ready to speak, so you finally tell her not to answer the question. You are always carefully watching patients and accepting where they are. You try one approach after another to facilitate their inner work, but you always accept whatever responses they make.

Desensitization by Indirect Suggestion

E: [Turning to L, who has had some training in psychology] What do you think about desensitization?   [Pause]

L: Is that a question?   I just heard the word.

E: Have you seen it?

L: Yes, it is a good way to do it.

R: You give her a rest here as you ask her boyfriend, L, about the process of desensitization you have just been involved with. You have been desensitizing X to her fears about revealing herself. This is also an indirect suggestion to X that lets her know she is desensitized and may be ready for more self-revelation.

Control and Fear of Self-Revelation

E: [To X] Is there anything unspoken?   That you can do safely? [Pause]

X: I'm afraid that my hands are going to be this way for the rest of my life.

E: And what way is that?

222

X: Misty.

E: What is bad about that?   [Long pause]

X: Well, it is revealing of me.   And very uncomfortable.   It is revealing because in other ways I seem to have so much control, and then there is this way in which I have absolutely none.   It is as if at any moment   this sort of sign emerges   that I am not what I seem or something like that.

E: That you are not what you seem.   And what exactly is that big lie? Do you know it?   Have you admitted it fully to yourself?

X: I guess not.

E: Do you want to?

X: No.

> R: In this section X clearly reveals her need for control and her fear of revealing herself. There is sometimes a tendency for the hypnotherapist to err in the direction of uncovering unconscious material too quickly. You carefully avoid this danger by emphasizing that patients need not tell until they are ready to do so with a feeling of comfort and safety.

Giving up Conscious Control

E: So you want to have a lack of control in that regard.   And earlier today you said you wanted full control.   What are you going to do about that?   [Pause]

X: I want to say give it up, but it doesn't make too much sense.

> R: You always have this apparently peculiar tendency to point out how patients do not want control even when they thought they did. You are again trying to release the rigid grip of their conscious mind over their unconscious.
>
> E: I point out that contradiction. Now when does a girl want to have a lack of control?
>
> R: During orgasm.

Automatic Writing

E: I can only remember the girl's last name when I was teaching in

Michigan State University in a class of psychologists working for their Ph.D.'s.   In one class a girl named Erickson, no relation to me at all, said, "I have some hideous secret and I don't want to know it   but I ought to know it.   Can you do anything about it?"

I said, yes, easily.   I said take a pencil and while you are looking at me, let your hand write automatically that big troublesome secret.

Her hand wrote it and I saw her take the piece of paper and she folded it and refolded it and refolded it and she slipped it into her purse.   Some months later she said, "Why am I telling you this secret? I broke my engagement."   I said, "Well, you have broken your engagement. Why are you telling me? I bet anything there is something in your purse that will tell you." She said, "You are ridiculous."   I said, "It is fun to be ridiculous."   She very carefully emptied out her purse.   She said, "Where did this piece of paper come from?"   She unfolded it and it read, "You are not going to marry Mel, you are going to marry Joe."   And she did. But she was engaged to Mel.

I think it was important for her to know her secret.   All kinds of secrets.

> E: I tell this seemingly irrelevant story about automatic writing, but it illustrates an identical psychic situation of having a "hideous secret" I don't want to know.
>
> R: The incredible aspect of your telling this story as an illustration is that in her followup letter written three months after this session, she reports almost the identical situation: She gave up one boyfriend to marry another. I almost feel ESP is operating in you, but you deny that.
>
> E: I believed she was in a sex conflict, and you can't have a conflict without two opposing objects. When I said, 'All kinds of secrets,' I made it apply to X as well.

Working Through Conscious Resistance

E: A recent patient of mine told me she was afraid to fly on a plane. And do you really know   your fear?   This great big lie you are telling yourself.   Don't you think you ought to know all of it?   When do you think you will have enough courage to know it?   [Pause]

X: Later.

E: How much later?   [Pause]

X: Tomorrow.

E: All right, now tell me. Jeff searching through his pockets all except for the last one.   He didn't dare look in the last pocket for fear he would drop dead.   Do you understand how Jeff felt?   Do you really think you will drop dead if you know it?   [Pause]   It just seems that way.   How much time do you need to reach into that other pocket?

X: I guess I can do it.

E: Just guess.

X: I can do it.

E: Do you suppose you could enjoy finding out just what that great big little fear is?

X: Maybe I could.   Maybe.

> R: You now tell another story which has relevance for her because X also has a fear of planes. The main purpose of this story is getting the courage to know about all one's fears. You then return to X and her fears. You don't accept "tomorrow," but you don't tell her that. Instead you recount a story with the message, "You won't really drop dead." That is, you remotivate her to work through her conscious resistances by telling her the humorous Mutt and Jeff story about our exaggerated fears of self-revelation.

Relocating Dental Pain

E: A forty-year-old man came to me and said that "I was a good hypnotic subject in college.   I have a dentalphobia.   I know you suffer endless pain,   excruciating pain when you go to the dentist.   And I have neglected my teeth, they are in bad shape, and I have got to have dental work done, and going to a dental office means pain.   Can you hypnotize me?"   I said "Why not let the dentist who will be doing the work on you, do it?"   He saw two dentists I had trained, and they worked on him separately and jointly. They couldn't induce a trance.   So I had them bring him to a study group. I told him for the time being to keep his fears, keep his pain, but to go into a trance. In the trance I told him to keep his pain, all his belief in pain, and to go to the dentist and know that all his pain was in his left hand, and hold it away from him.　And tell the dentist by no means to touch that left hand. The slightest breath on his left hand would be excruciatingly painful.　Throughout all his dental work the pain was out there.　If he ever goes to a new dentist, the new dentist will wonder why.　This thing you don't want to know," has it anything to do with your hands or harp?　[Pause]

> R: She continues to pause, so you tell her yet another story.
>
> E: I am giving her a breathing spell but at the same time it is giving her instruction. I told the dental patient to locate his pain in his hand. She can have all the pain of self-realization, but she could know what she really wanted in spite of the pain.

Utilizing Explosiveness to Reach the Unconscious

E: All right, now answer this question explosively. [To R] Would you say a word explosively.

R: Damn it!

E: Can you [X] say a word explosively?

X: No!

E: How do you know the meaning of that word?　You know you don't want to tell the meaning of that word, do you?　Answer this question explosively.　Should you tell the meaning of that?

X: No!

E: Answer this, ought you?

X: Yes!

E: Are you?

X: Yes!

E: When?

X: Later!

E: How much later?　[Pause]

X: In fifteen minutes.

226

E: All right, but you can say it explosively.

X: Fifteen minutes!

[The senior author now occupies her in small talk about her home and family for fifteen minutes. Without her realizing it, he is actually utilizing many female and sexual symbols—fish, box, things coveted, etc.— conversation that will keep her unconscious primed to the task at hand.]

E: Explosiveness is a sudden welling up of the unconscious and everyone has had that experience. Now I'm asking her to have her unconscious mind explode new understandings.

Comfortable Self-Revelation: Altering a Lifetime Identity

E: Now will the disclosure be in connection with harp, your hands, or something else?

X: With the harp and my hands.

E: Fifteen minutes has not yet gone by.   How ready are you?

X: I'm ready.

E: You want to, now?

X: It is not going to seem so bad.

E: That is too bad, isn't it?

X: Should I say it?

E: Sure.

X: I never did want to be a harpist.
[Pause]

E: What do you want to do in relationship to the harp?

X: Play just for myself.

E: And whose idea was it that you be a concert harpist?

X: I always blamed my Dad, but it might have been mine. I think originally it must have been Dad's.

E: Now why did you have wet hands?

X: I know why. So I wouldn't have to play.

E: As an excuse.

> R: When her self-revelation does come, it is surprisingly free of emotional trauma. Not wanting to be a concert harpist seems to be such a simple pragmatic fact, yet for her it is giving up an identity built up over a lifetime. One of her major mental frameworks about herself has been altered.

Insight Therapy to Support the Reorganization of the Symptom Complex

[A fifteen-minute conversation takes place wherein X now experiences a flood of insights about her family's psychodynamics and her symptom of sweating.]

> R: Now begins a flood of insight and conviction about the source and nature of her problems in her family. You are here utilizing the classical means of insight therapy to support the reorganization of her psychic economy so that symptom formation is no longer necessary.

Ideomotor Signaling to Facilitate Further Insight

E: Now why do you think you have claustrophobia on the plane?   Let your unconscious mind answer this question, and you just wait   if you don't know the answer.   Your unconscious mind will answer with a head movement after it has digested my question.   Can you in any way say anything to indicate why you have claustrophobia on the airplane? [Long pause as X closes her eyes]   Either a nod or shake of the head involuntarily.   Do you know what it was?   Does your unconscious mind know it?   [Pause as her head nods "yes" very slowly]   Do you consciously know it?

X: Yes.

E: What was it?

X: When my brother and I were little, we fought like cats and dogs, and one day when I came home from school I was angry with him about something and tore a page out of his stamp collection book. He hauled me

228

into a closet and nailed it shut with a cat inside with me. I don't like cats either.   It was on St. Patrick's Day.

E: There is nothing bad about knowing it, is there?

X: No, I'll beat the hell out of my brother when I go home [laughs].

E: I think it is delightful to know all the good and the bad.   Comb your memory, see if there is anything more you ought to know about yourself.

I was returning from somewhere in New York state by plane in a bad blizzard. [E. now tells an amusing story about an uncomfortable plane trip he once had. He is evidently tapping into her associations about airplanes to give her an opportunity to bring up her fear of flying. She does not pick up the hint, however, so he has her review all her psychodynamic insights and the critical trauma of March 17, 1958, when her brother nailed her in a closet, which Erickson believes may also account for her fear of flying.]

> R: You do not rest content with that major flood of insight about her sweating. Now that she is opened to doing creative inner work, you take advantage of her availability and press on to her claustrophobia with an ideomotor approach to facilitate the flow from unconscious to conscious.

Review of Psychodynamic Insights: Resolving the Airplane Phobia

E: You really concentrated on not knowing. You have had lots of practice having sweating.   Now you can have ahead of you a little practice of being dry-handed and hot-handed.   Now is there any more help that you want?

X: No, right now I have a compelling need to run to the airport and catch the first plane out.

E: It is a nice feeling, isn't it?   Are you going to be completely open and truthful to yourself from now on?

X: Probably not.

E: Well, we aren't perfect you know, but let's make self-concealments as small as possible and not disabling.   How do you feel about it—in two days' time learning all this about yourself?

X: I guess I kind of feel as if I was on the verge of deciding about it, about knowing about it for a while.   I am somewhat relieved that it is out in the open now.

E: Any anger at me for uncomfortness?

> R: Here you have her review all her newly acquired insights so they can be integrated on a conscious level. You are also exploring the possibility that her fear of flying may be related somehow. As a final touch you give a lot of permissiveness regarding sexuality in the form of a two-level communication about hot hands. She then reveals an apparently spontaneous resolution of her airplane phobia when she says she feels "a compelling need to run to the airport and catch the first plane out."

Gradualness of Symptom Diminution: Creative Reorganization of Psychodynamics

E: You are aware that it will take a while before you will get dry hands.

X: Um hum.

E: That isn't so embarrassing to you now, is it?

X: No.

> R: You again make sure she knows that the symptom will disappear gradually over some time. You thereby give her system a fair chance to reorganize itself and forestall her fears of failure. Thus you are not involved in the simplistic notion of "removing a symptom," you are doing vastly more: You are facilitating a creative reorganization of her psychodynamics so that a symptom is no longer necessary. Time is needed for that continuing process of inner adjustment.

The Utilization Theory of Hypnotic Suggestion

E: I hope you have enjoyed this and you are aware of the fact that you are a good hypnotic subject?

X: I don't want to take too much credit for myself being a good subject.

E: You can take all the credit. All I have done is say words and   in so doing   I have stimulated   memories,   ideas   that you already had, and then you acted on those memories. You have memories of the time when you didn't even know your hand was your own.　　And you don't even know when you first knew where your ears were.　　And you don't know how you finally located your ears.　　Parents like to have a child point to the hair, forehead, eyes, nose, mouth, chin, and ears. But when did you really know where your ears were?

X: I don't know.
[Erickson demonstrates knowledge of ear location by touching the right ear by reaching with the left hand behind the head.]

E: One time you didn't know those were your hands, so you tried to pick up your right hand with your right hand. It took you a long time to learn to pick up your left hand with your right and your right hand with your left hand.　　So you have a whole bank full of memories and understandings, and all I do is say something that touches upon those memories.　　Yesterday when I said, *"Try* to stand up,"　　I tapped into your memory bank to a time when you couldn't stand up. And there was a time when you couldn't sit down because you didn't know what "sit down" meant.
There was even a time when you didn't know you were a people.　　All I needed to do was tap into your memory bank and you couldn't talk.

R: That is our theory of hypnotic phenomena.

E: Um hum. [Pause]

R: In these closing remarks you are actually giving a clear outline of our utilization theory of hypnotic suggestion. Suggestion is *not* putting something into the subject; suggestion is the process of stimulating "memories and ideas that you already had" that can be acted on by the subject. Suggestion is simply the process of evoking the subjects' own internal associations and helping them utilize these associations for new purposes. All so-called hypnotic phenomena are actually dissociated bits and pieces of behavior that were once normal in earlier stages of development and the initial stages of learning.

E: Knowing things and not knowing them at the same time. [Erickson tells another of his favorite stories about his daughter Christie, who screamed and carried on for seven days until she finally stood up and took 142 consecutive steps the first time she walked. She just knew she was a people and thus had to prove it.]

Full Disclosure About Hypnotic Phenomena: Control, Freedom, and Behavioral Flexibility

E: Now you don't need to ever let anybody hypnotize you unless it is for your purposes.   And nobody can control you, and you can defy me any time you want to,   or anybody else.   You are a free citizen, and be free with yourself.   It is hell, isn't it, to be tied there to sweating   and to have unpleasant feelings on the plane.

[Erickson now tells an amusing story of how he overcame a lifetime aversion to caraway by simply chewing enough of it until he began liking it. He thus proved to himself that he could change his tastes if he wanted to.]

I did need to know that I could alter my behavior, and you can do the same with your sweating.   Is there anything more?   I have talked to you so extensively.   Should I charge you?

X: No!!!

E: That is wonderful! That is really wonderful!

E: Now will you send me a Christmas card?

X: OK.

E: It has been very, very pleasing to know you.

X: It is very pleasing to know you too.

E: Have a good time in . . . and I hope I see you on the way back.

> R: I've frequently witnessed how at the end of a therapy process you give full disclosure to your patients about the nature of hypnosis. In particular, you emphasize that they actually have control over the process and they can use it for any constructive purpose. You dispel any lingering misconceptions about the process of control by giving control and freedom to the patient. It is ridiculous for the therapist to believe that secrets must be kept from the patient. A full understanding of hypnotic phenomena and the methods of hypnotherapy can only help the public and individuals seeking help. With this final story of how you overcame your distaste for caraway, you send her off with a good model of self-change and behavioral flexibility.

> E: Her "No!" in response to my question about a fee was highly explosive. . . . If she could be explosive with me, she can be explosive with anybody.

R: Here you gave her a social opportunity to use her newly acquired self-assertiveness and at the same time, by not charging her for the sessions, you compensate her for allowing us to tape her sessions and publish them. The request for a Christmas card serves as a simple follow-up device.

A Note on the Creative Nature of Psychotherapy*

Although we have made an effort to generalize the principles involved in this case, we must acknowledge that each psychotherapeutic encounter is unique. Erickson continually comments on the theme that every hypnotherapeutic endeavor is a creative exploration. This is so because behavior, whether in the ordinary waking state or in hypnotherapeutic trance, is not necessarily logical, well-ordered, properly pertinent, or even reasonably appropriate to the situation or conditions evoking it. It may be logical, illogical, meaningless, irrelevant, random, misdirected, nonsensical, metaphorical, humorous or whatever. It is usually impossible to predict with precision just what an individual's response will be in any therapeutic encounter because the simplicities and complexities of behavior and its reasonableness and idiosyncracy derive from many permutations of unknown experiential factors in the person's lifetime of learnings. At the very most, only broad generalizations can be made. All too often, however, these generalizations break down or are lost in a maze of complexities when a particular therapist faces a particular patient at a particular time and place.

Hence, when the problems of distressed, disturbed, and abnormal behavior are encountered, any treatment approach must integrate the individuality of both the therapist and patient. There is no rigidly "controlled" or "scientific" method of eliciting the same behavior from one or more patients under the same conditions at different times. Even when the range of responses seems to be greatly limited, totally unpredictable behaviors may occur. Thus while general scientific principles of psychotherapy certainly exist (this principle of its essentially creative character being one), the utilization of these principles requires a continual appreciation of the unique and exploratory nature of all psychotherapeutic work. Psychotherapists cannot depend upon general routines or standardized procedures to be applied indiscriminately to all their patients. Psychotherapy is not the mere application of truths and principles supposedly discovered by academicians in controlled laboratory experiments. Each psychotherapeutic encounter is unique and requires fresh creative effort on the part of both therapist

---

*The following is an edited version of one of the senior author's efforts to formulate an overview of a half a century of hypnotherapeutic explorations.

and patient to discover the principles and means of achieving a therapeutic outcome.

This individualized and creative approach is particularly important in hypnosis. In seven years of studying the senior author's approach, for example, the junior author has frequently requested the demonstration of a particular hypnotic phenomenon with a particular patient during an ongoing therapy session. Much of the time the senior author rejected such requests with humorous scorn because he felt the junior author should have realized that the request was inappropriate or impossible for that particular patient at that time. Whenever he undertook the requested demonstration, however, the senior author was usually successful in evoking most of the hypnotic phenomenon associated with clinical work such as ideomotor action, catalepsy, dissociations, amnesia, hyperamnesia, time distortion, the alteration of cognition, emotions, and, of course, the modification and transformation of symptomatic behavior that we see in this case.

The most common reason the senior author gave for both his successes and failures was the degree to which he was able to evoke and utilize the particular patient's motivation and repertory of experiential learning. The most remarkable hypnotic effects could be evoked because of the nature of the transference relationship and the importance of these hypnotic responses for the patient's much desired therapeutic outcome. The failures, particularly those involving the hypnotic effects that the senior author was most experienced in evoking in experimental settings, were likewise accounted for by their apparent irrelevance to the patient's real needs. Although the senior author used some standard routines in setting up hypnotic experiences, he was perpetually tuning into and utilizing the patient's own mental frameworks and idiosyncratic association patterns.

A Three Year Followup

On the next three Christmas holidays, X sent the senior author a Christmas card with a bit of family news and some pictures of her newborn children. Each message confirmed her freedom from symptoms, her new life orientation with her growing family, and her pleasurable cultivation of music for herself.

Case 6   Demonstrating Psychosomatic Asthma with Shock to Facilitate Symptom Resolution and Insight

A basic hypnotherapeutic approach to psychosomatic symptoms is to demonstrate clearly and unequivocally how they are controlled and maintained by psychological processes. Such a demonstration breaks

234

through limiting preconceptions about the organic nature of the problem and usually puts the patient in touch with the psychodynamics of the problem. If it is correct that psychosomatic symptoms are more closely associated with right hemispheric functioning (Galin, 1974), an hypnotic demonstration of the psychogenic control of the problem may be making contact with the actual hemispheric sources of the symptom, since trance itself is considered to be a right hemispheric activity (Bakan, 1969; Hilgard and Hilgard, 1975). This helps us understand why it is that "spontaneous" insight into the sources and psychodynamics of the problem frequently follows closely upon a demonstration of the psychological control of the symptom. The trance experience opens up common pathways between the psychodynamics and the sources of control of the symptom. The following case, written by the senior author, is a typical example of how this approach can be used.

Psychosomatic Asthma

Mrs. G., aged thirty-five, married ten years, with one child aged nine, sought a psychiatric consultation. This was in protest to the repeated diagnosis she had received from a half-dozen different allergists to the effect that her chronic asthma, lasting from November through April, of ten years duration, was largely psychological. The pertinent history obtained was that the excitement of her wedding had been followed within two days by the long-expected death of her bedridden mother. The mother had left no will but, as a wedding present for her daughter, had extracted from the father a solemn sworn promise that, when she died, he would dispose of the farm, give the daughter half of the proceeds, and then, if he wished, he could retire on his half.

After the funeral the father told her that his promise to the mother was meaningless and that she would receive only half the yearly income until he died, when she would inherit everything. She and her husband angrily took their departure to live in another section of the country. Within two months the couple became reconciled to the father's actions and initiated a friendly correspondence in late October. The father replied, and his first letter found her in bed with a severe cold. Her recovery was slow, and this was attributed to a pulmonary reaction to atmospheric impurities resulting from the mining industry in that town. Asthma developed as a complication, but with the advent of warm weather this vanished. In June they moved to the San Fernando Valley, but in November, presumably because of the smog, she again developed asthma, which persisted until May. In June they moved to San Francisco, but the following November the asthma reappeared and persisted until May. Further moves were unavailing. Wherever they went, the asthma redeveloped in November and ended in May.

Inquiry about the father disclosed that he had continued farming but in a peculiar part-time fashion. He planted the crops, cultivated them, and harvested them. This done, he turned the entire management over to an employee and spent the winter in a somewhat distant city in ease and comfort. With the advent of spring, he returned to the farm and worked hard until the last harvest was completed. Immediate inquiry about the frequency of her father's letters disclosed that in the summer he was always too busy to write and that he reserved his weekly letter-writing for the leisure of his winter life. The patient failed to recognize any possible connection between her asthma and her father's weekly letters.

She was asked if she were willing to have the writer prove definitely that her asthma was either psychogenic or organic. She emphatically replied that, in either case, she would be tremendously relieved, but added that it was unquestionably organic since it had begun with a cold, had been aggravated by the atmospheric impurities of the mining town, and only occurred during cold weather. Furthermore it always disappeared with the advent of warm weather. Also, it had to be organic, since in ten years she had never had a single attack in the summer, and she was the same person psychologically in both cold and warm weather. She was told that hypnosis would be useful as a diagnostic aid, and she consented readily to be hypnotized.

She proved to be an excellent subject, developing a deep trance easily. She was given rapid training in posthypnotic suggestions. She was then instructed during trance that at a specified cue (when the writer tapped his pencil three times) she would be given a memory task, a most important memory task, which would be defined at the proper time. She agreed to follow all instruction and, also, to go to sleep whenever another specific cue was given (when his cigarette lighter was dropped into his ashtray). She was awakened with a comprehensive amnesia for the trance experience. After a few casual remarks, further inquiry was made about the possibility of summer attacks of asthma. She was most positive in her denials.

Mention was made that the clock indicated the time as 2:17 P.M., and she was reminded that it was a very hot July 8th in Phoenix, Arizona. Then she was asked if she thought she could develop a severe attack of asthma exactly at 2:37 P.M. She declared the idea to be most ridiculous. She was assured that if her asthma were psychogenic, it was both possible and probable. However, if it were organic, she need have no fears. Somewhat puzzled, she waited for further elaboration, but the writer merely directed her attention silently to the clock.

At 2:25 P.M. she was asked if she felt comfortable. She replied that she was merely puzzled, because watching a clock certainly could do nothing to her. At 2:34 the comment was offered that only three minutes remained before she would or would not develop an asthmatic attack. She only smiled in reply. At 2:37 she turned expectantly to the writer. Immediately the writer tapped his pencil on the table three times (this was a cue for the posthypnotic suggestion to remember) and said, "Remember fully, completely, just as if you were reading it, the content of any letter your father has written to you." A violent asthmatic attack ensued.

During it she was told, "The day is hot. It's the 8th of July. It is summertime. There are no fumes or dust or cold. You have not a recent lung infection. You are having a severe asthmatic attack. It began at 2:37, twenty minutes after I said it would, *if it were psychogenic*. It will stop when I say so. It *is* psychogenic! Shall I remove it at 2:45 or 2:47, because I can. Do you see this cigarette lighter? That's all it is. It is neither medicine nor magic. But when I do a certain thing with it, your asthma will disappear. Watch it carefully. Be sure you know, really know, that your asthma is psychogenic. Now watch." Immediately the lighter was dropped into an ashtray. A deep trance state ensued, and she was told to sleep deeply, comfortably, and to awaken free of her asthma and with a full recollection of everything. This she was then to relate to the writer.

She responded fully, and upon awakening she began to verbalize freely and comprehendingly. Her recollections may be summarized as follows: Her mother had long been bedridden because of paralysis, cardiac disease, and accompanying respiratory distress. Her father had never treated her mother or her very kindly, and he was tremendously guilt-ridden. Shortly before her first attack of asthma, she had received a letter from a friend, hinting strongly about her father's undue interest in a woman known to be promiscuous. Her asthmatic attack followed her father's first letter. Thereafter she dreaded from week to week his next letter, but felt duty-bound to answer each letter. His return to the farm each spring gave her a sense of relief because she knew he would be too busy to engage in undesirable activities or to write to her.

When she had completed her summation, she was asked what she intended to do. Her reply was that she would think matters over thoroughly and decide on a course of action. Subsequent reports disclosed that she had visited her father, discussed the situation with him, engaged a lawyer, and intimidated her father into executing legal instruments ensuring her control over and eventual ownership of her share of the farm, and giving him his freedom to do as he wished with his share. Since then the father has handled her property well, but he has been slowly dissipating his share.

He still writes regularly each winter, but the patient has had no further asthmatic attacks since the one induced in the office on July 8, 1949. She was last seen casually in late June 1954.

It will be informative to closely examine the stages of how this case progressed. The five stages of our general approach outlined earlier will be numbered and emphasized in italics, together with the senior author's use of shock and surprise to facilitate a reorganization of her understanding.

There is an initial period during which the patient consults a number of physicians for the organic treatment of the problem. Since this repeatedly fails or results in only short-term placebo effects, the patient is reluctantly told that it must be "psychological."

The patient arrives at the psychotherapist's office with much inner confusion and tension, still protesting that it cannot be psychological. In spite of these protests *confusion* is an indication that *the patient's original frame of reference of the organic nature of the problem has been shaken and depotentiated at least in part.* Confusion is a sign of being lost between having to give up the organic framework and not yet really understanding the new psychological framework. Confusion is thus an important psychological prerequisite for therapeutic change; it signals patient-readiness for change even though they do not always recognize it.

The therapist in his initial survey of the problem ascertains for himself the relevant facts and possible psychodynamics of the symptom. In this case the senior author rapidly found the possible psychogenic sources from the obvious motive for a problem: (a) the patient's clouded inheritance under the particularly trying circumstances of her marriage and almost simultaneous death of her mother; (b) The regular association between the patient's symptoms and her father's letters. When the patient failed to recognize any possible connection between her asthma and her father's letters, the senior author recognized a possible block or dissociation that could be a factor in the formation of the psychosomatic symptom. At this point, when all the facts are clarified, some patients do recognize the connection. They gain insights and work them through with the therapist's help to a final resolution of the problem. No hypnotherapeutic intervention is necessary.

Although this patient could not grasp the psychological associations outlined by the facts and circumstances of her life, this initial inquiry did establish *(1) rapport and a therapeutic frame of reference* on a conscious level. It now remained for unconscious dynamics and experiential sources of recognition and knowing to be activated.

The senior author approaches these unrecognized sources of the symptom with a hypnotic demonstration of the psychological control of the asthma. He first trains her to experience trance effects and to follow posthypnotic suggestions. As is typical of his general approach to symptom problems he *(2) demonstrates with her own experience how her unconscious can control her behavior and thereby indicates that the locus of therapeutic change will be within her unconscious.*

During trance she is given careful suggestions to respond with an important memory when given a specific cue. She is not told what the memory is to be about, since that might only arouse further conscious resistance. Her unconscious, however, will probably respond to the obvious implication that it will have something to do with her asthma by activating its relevant unconscious search programs in that area. Implication is a most effective means of *(3) evoking searches and processes on an unconscious level* that can be precipitated into consciousness when given a specific cue.

Before preceeding the senior author added a safety measure. After giving her training in following posthypnotic suggestions, he instructs her to go to sleep—that is, to enter trance—whenever a specific cue is given. Thus any behavior or symptomatic processes that threaten to get out of hand could be immediately attenuated by having her enter trance.

He then gives her unconscious time, from 2:17 P.M. to 2:37, to align itself to produce an asthmatic attack on cue if the asthma is in fact psychogenic. The unconscious does not work by magic. Time is required for it to do its own work. The senior author judged it would take at least twenty minutes to work through the inhibiting limitations of the patient's conscious sets, which "declared the idea to be most ridiculous." An expectation was given for an asthmatic attack at 2:37.

The senior author then allows expectancy and tension to build for twenty minutes. At the appointed time, 2:37, she turns (1) *expectantly* to him; her readiness is apparent. He then gives the expected posthypnotic cue (tapping his pencil three times) and gives her the critical memory task of recalling "the content of any letter your father has written to you." A violent psychogenic asthmatic attack ensues. She is thus precipitated into a *(2) state of shock during which her habitual mental frameworks and patterns of defense are momentarily depotentiated.*

During this critical period the senior author simply states all the obvious facts regarding the psychogenic nature of her asthma. When one's habitual mental frameworks (the generalized reality orientation) are so shaken by (3) *shock and surprise,* one tends to grasp onto any suggestions or belief system that will reestablish security and comfort. The facts about the psychogenic nature of her asthma are then reinforced through the security and comfort that follow from the posthypnotic cue (lighter-ashtray) to enter a deep and comfortable trance state from which she can awaken *free from her asthma* with a full recognition of everything. The senior author thereby *(4) demonstrates her release from symptomatic behavior* while opening the possibility of *(5) her gaining insight into the sources and psychodynamics of her problem.* She gains these insights and makes her own plans about how to settle her problems.

Case 7   Symptom Resolution with Catharsis Facilitating Personality Maturation: An Authoritarian Approach

This case illustrates how hypnosis can be used effectively even when the patient is a difficult and unresponsive hypnotic subject with whom only a light trance state is possible. Three two-hour sessions were required to achieve even that light trance, but it was enough to present the basic suggestion: "Your unconscious will know what to do and how to do it. You will absolutely yield to that need and give full expression to me. When finally that has been done completely, you can then recover from your present problem." Although the senior author could not evoke any of the classical hypnotic phenomena with this patient, the above suggestion was enough to *assign the locus of therapeutic change to his unconscious.* The patient's unconscious was given time to incubate until the next session, when his *usual conscious frameworks were suddenly depotentiated with the shockingly authoritarian demand* to, "Shut up with your conscious mind and its foolish requests for medicine, and let your unconscious mind attend to its task!"

That was enough to precipitate an unusually violent and prolonged catharsis that proved to be the vehicle for the resolution of the patient's psychosomatic symptom and a striking change and maturation of the total personality. The periods of the patient's intense catharsis could be looked upon as altered states in which personality reorganization could take place. But scientific conceptions cannot do justice to this happening; it is essentially a love story. It is presented as written by the senior author more than a generation ago.

None of Your Lip!

Pietro, in his mid-twenties, had been forced to give up his position in a symphony orchestra because of an inexplicable swollen lower lip. This had developed suddenly after an altercation with the orchestra conductor. The swelling was so severe that his lip was a full two inches thick. During the three years that this swelling had persisted, he had been treated by more than one hundred doctors, and the measures employed ranged from physiotherapy, hot compresses, medication, and bed rest to infrared and X-ray therapy. No benefit was derived.

He was finally sent to a general psychiatrist, who promptly referred him to the writer for hypnotherapy. The salient points in his history are as follows: He was born in Italy, but his family emigrated to the United States when he was four years old. His father, a hard-working baker by trade, had an overwhelming ambition for his son. Since the boy had shown very early a keen interest in music, the father had determined to make a famous musician of him. Accordingly, the boy's training started at the age of three on the piano, while the father explored the field of musical instruments to determine the proper choice of an instrument. He finally selected the flute.

To understand the training the boy received, a brief statement concerning the father is necessary. He was a domineering patriarch, who ruled the family in an incredibly rigid fashion. He ate first, the choicest portions, and his wife and children stood silently at hand, ready to obey his slightest wish. Since he owned his own bakery, he worked on the average of twelve hours daily, seven days a week. Home conversation was essentially a series of reports on the daily activities of each member of the family. His wife reported on her housework, shopping, and the activities of the preschool children. After the children entered school, they reported on their daily work, and during vacation, on their day's activities. He listened intently, discussed their reports authoritatively, was lavish in his praise and encouragement for "good" accomplishments, and equally lavish in his condemnation of "foolishness." Since his education was limited, when the older children entered school, they had to sit in judgment upon each other concerning those matters for which the father felt that he lacked knowledge. As for himself, he too gave a daily report in which he discussed his own accomplishments and his own shortcomings. The father was never wrong in anything unless, unaided, he himself reached that conclusion independently. He had early learned the expression "None of your lip" and its variations, and it had become a standard daily cliché. Nobody ever game him any "lip," a constant boast that characterized every report that was given of the family's daily activities and relationships. He treated his employees in a comparable fashion but was so eminently fair that he had their loyalty.

All home activities were conducted by rule and on a time basis, which he would alter magnanimously as he saw fit. Thus shoes were polished in so many minutes per shoe, and the lawn was mowed in an exact length of time at a set hour. The advent of a rain disrupting this schedule was met by him with a dissertation on the need for meeting reality by adjustment to whatever situation arose through schedule alteration and no sacrifice of obligations. Thus, the time gained by a rain that rendered unnecessary the watering of the flower bed had to be utilized in special tasks reserved for such contingencies. Play was regarded as an essential part of living, but its duration and character were predetermined. Thus, the boys played ball and the girls played with dolls for regular periods. All was orderly, constructive, and systematic.

Since Pietro was to become a famous musician, a special set of rules was established for him. Calisthenics rather than play, biographies of musicians rather than fairy tales, etc. became his lot. Schoolwork had to be average, since there had to be a conservation of energy for his daily after-school music practice. The other children were required to have excellent grades. Next to the father, Pietro received the more choice

241

portions at the table. At first the father supervised the son's musical training, and he was a highly intelligent man with an excellent ear for music. So many hours a day were spent playing the piano, not to play music but to establish "nimbleness" of the fingers, dexterity, and absolute precision of movement. Then a teacher was engaged to teach him to play compositions so that he would learn music. Since the father was profoundly appreciative of music and would discuss it happily and enthusiastically, he succeeded in inspiring his son with equal enthusiasm and love. The first lessons with the flute were supervised by the father, and their character is best summarized by the father's explanation, "You musta feela da flute before you playa da flute."

Taking the flute, an expensive instrument, out of its case and putting it back, lifting it to the mouth, lowering it and again raising it, measuring its length and diameter by finger movements, learning to balance it with utter accuracy and learning the exact distance from his lip to place it, constituted those initial lessons, practiced endlessly until the father was satisfied. Always the father's praise was lavish and his patience unlimited, thereby rendering his otherwise unbearable demands endurable. Then the learning of one note at a time, one key at a time, and the increase and decrease of volume followed in the same rigorous fashion. Along with all this the piano practice continued, so many hours at the piano, so many hours on the flute, so much time for calisthenics, so much time for rest, so much time in discussion "to learna da soula da music." This latter, of course, was the salvation of the patient, and when he was in therapy, it was a thrilling, inspiring experience to have him discuss "the soul of music." Then an excellent teacher was engaged, who stipulated the length and frequency and types of lessons, while the father restricted himself to the stipulation of the amount of intervening practice and other "essential" activities.

After graduating from high school, Pietro spent twelve hours a day for two years perfecting himself as a flutist. Then he was allowed by his father to seek an audition at the age of twenty. His first application resulted in his engagement by a well-known symphony orchestra as first flutist. His father's ambition was satisfied except for certain refinements. His son's position in the musical world had been achieved, but there remained certain additional achievements of a personal nature. His son must now fall in love, marry, and father children, so that he would "learna da feela, da sweetness, da love da woman, da beauty, da laugha da bambino."

The son, as always, acquiesced, and a procession of girls was paraded through the home, but unfortunately, at a concert he met the girl of his choice. His father was in deep despair. The girl was Yugoslavian and not Italian. The son was adamant but did yield somewhat by agreeing to postpone marriage. Partially consoling to the father was the fact that the girl came from an artistic family, was a college student, a trained

242

singer, could paint excellently, and had a brother who was a sculptor of note in Yugoslavia.

For over two years he played in the symphony orchestra. Then a new conductor was engaged, who promptly became at sword's points with most of the orchestra members because of his harshly critical, dictatorial manner. At a practice session he accused the patient of an error, and when the patient attempted to protest, he told the patient that no "lip" was wanted out of him. At the next rehearsal the patient's lower lip was slightly swollen and his playing was faulty. When he attempted to explain, the conductor harshly told him again, "I don't want any more lip out of you or you can resign." His resentment toward this was tremendous, and he dared not express it in any way. Neither did he dare to tell his father. Within a month his lip was so swollen that he was forced to resign, and he explained the situation to his father solely on the basis of his lip condition.

Then began the frantic search for medical help, while in addition, he practiced playing the piano and fingering the flute never less than nine hours daily. During these three years the father watched the swollen lip with increasing anxiety and impatience and finally expressed his feelings with long, bitter denunciations of the medical profession and demands that his son seek a more competent physician. At last he lapsed into bitter, frustrated silence on the subject. The romance with the Yugoslavian girl was terminated. She left the state to complete her college studies and to take additional training in singing and painting.

Clinical Course

The first few interviews were devoted to the securing of the above history. He did not like this and suddenly demanded that history-taking be dispensed with and hypnosis employed without delay.

At the fifth interview an effort was made to hypnotize him, but he proved to be a difficult, unresponsive subject. However, after three sessions of two or more hours' duration, a light trance was induced. This was utilized to suggest, as emphatically and as authoritatively as possible, that his swollen lip was of psychological origin, that it could be cured, that it was an external manifestation of a profound and compelling need for his unconscious mind to manifest and to express behavior which had been repressed, ignored, overlooked, and consciously forbidden over the years. He was told that his unconscious must express itself completely, however terrifying or irrational such expression might seem. Furthermore, his unconscious would know what to do and how to do it, and he would absolutely yield to that need *and give full expression to the writer*. When that had been done completely, he could then recover from his present problem. These posthypnotic suggestions were given with much emphasis and repetition and in the most authoritative, dictatorial manner possible. At the close of the session he was curtly told to ask no questions, to go home, to let his unconscious mind prepare for its task, and then, at the next appointment, he was to appear promptly at the exact hour and to let his unconscious begin its task without delay or any conscious interference. This extremely authoritarian approach was deemed appropriate because it utilized the patient's previous life experience and current expectation that effective guidance always came in an authoritarian form. The senior author was simply utilizing his authoritarian expectation.

At the next interview he entered the office as instructed but immediately asked for some medicine for his lip. He was told emphatically, "Shut up with your conscious mind and its foolish requests for medicine, and let your unconscious mind attend to its task!" His reaction was one of intense, violent anger. He leapt out of his chair and loudly and bitterly denounced the writer as a wretched example of an incompetent, lowly profession, sparing neither profanity nor obscenity to express his opinion. The entire hour was spent in this vituperative attack. Exactly at the close of the hour he was told sternly, "Your unconscious can now shut up, and at the next hour it will continue, exactly on time, and do a more thorough and better job. Leave the office at once."

He appeared exactly on time for the next appointment and launched into another diatribe, even as he closed the door behind him. The interview was terminated in the same manner as the previous one, and this pattern was followed essentially throughout the course of therapy. For nine months, two hours each week, this procedure was followed, except that about once a month he would arbitrarily be told that the next immediate appointment would be different, but no further information would be given. However, as he entered the office on such occasions, he would be greeted with the demand that he give a good discussion of such separate topics as the meaningfulness of music, how the members of an orchestra feel and sense during and after a concert, how the individual expresses his emotions and his life experiences, hopes and fears, in his own playing. The patient entered into these sessions with the same intensity and enthusiasm manifested in the hostile behavior, and he was truly inspiring in his discussions.

At first the denunciations were primarily of the writer as a member of the medical profession and then as a medical man in a specific field. This led to a denunciation of the writer as a member of the human race, particularly as a descendant of the Norsemen, who ravaged and pillaged every land to which they could sail their ships. He seasoned these vituperative comments with many choice Italian phrases, which he kindly translated for the writer. This developed then into a vituperative description and vilification, both collectively and individually, of all of the writer's progenitors, with the exception of the writer's parents and grandparents, back to the beginning of time. Should his discussion be

244

broken off in the midst of a sentence at the close of the hour, the next hour would be marked by a completion of that sentence and a continuation of the topic. Also, his trips home on the bus were usually devoted to a study of what better insults he could offer at the next interview. From the writer's progenitors he turned to the topic of the writer as a man, first as a physiological creature. When this was exhausted, he turned to the topic of the writer as a member of society in general but with an inheritance only of pillage and rapine. Having treated this topic exhaustively, he progressed to the writer as a family man. As he developed this topic, there occurred a marked change in his motor behavior. Previously he had paced the floor agitatedly and gesticulated violently. Upon developing this topic, he added to his motor behavior by leaping at the writer to shake his fist underneath the writer's nose, and explained how he would like to strike and hurt the writer and to inflict all manner of mayhem upon the writer's body. At each demonstration he demanded the writer's close attention while he pantomimed how he would like to gouge out the writer's right eye, his left eye, etc. Additionally, he gave emphasis to his utterances by expelling flatus, belching and spitting.

As he developed the topic of the writer as a family man, he took up, item by item, the various things he had told about in describing his father's home. Thus the writer's table behavior, his attitude toward each of his children, his demands regarding home activities and work, and other habits and characteristics were speculated upon extensively, unfavorably, and with intense bitterness and hatred. Hour after hour was spent on this general topic with an increasing outpouring of hatreds and resentments and extravagent declarations. Finally one day, near the end of the hour, he made the first mention of his father in any of his tirades by declaring, "If you were my father . . ." Immediately he paused in a frightened fashion, sat down weakly, and gasped, "But you aren't my father, you aren't my father, you aren't my father." In a friendly tone of voice, he was told, "No, I'm not your father. Your unconscious has been talking to me, saying things that would help you to understand your feelings toward your father. Now that you have said all the things that have piled up in you for years and years, your lip can get well. You have given me all the lip you did not ever dare to give anyone, and which you kept to yourself. You are free, your lip will now heal. The only thing you need to do is to look at your father and see him as one man looking at another. You are grown up now. Tell your father simply what you want and feel and wish, limiting yourself only to those things he can understand. Things he can't understand do not need to be said." His reply was, "I'll have to think. I'll talk to him tonight."

His report at the next interview was that that evening, at the usual gathering for the day's report, he had told his father in effect that he was a man, that he knew what was right and good, that thenceforth he would be answerable only to himself, and that he was now ceasing to take parental orders. To this he added that his lip would be healed shortly. His father's response was typical. After a long, thoughtful silence the father arose, walked over to the patient, shook hands with him, and in Italian said simply, "My son, I'm an old man. I forgot that you are grown up. Please forgive me."

Within a month the patient's lip was normal. While he practiced daily, there were no longer nine-hour stints. He announced his intention to his father of going east to some large city, and he chose the one where his former fianceé was studying. He secured employment as a waiter until an opportunity arose a few months later for an audition. He was engaged as a flutist in a large symphony orchestra. He renewed his engagement and sent his fianceé on a visit to his parents and the writer. She was a most charming girl but most unhappy about the growing unrest in Europe. She told of her plans to return to Yugoslavia to see her family. She was not seen again until 1947. The outbreak of World War II had trapped her in her native land. She had joined a guerilla force and fought the Nazis under most difficult conditions throughout most of the war. Then she had been captured and put in a forced-labor battalion and brutally treated. Finally she had escaped and managed to get back to the United States. She was no longer a charming girl. She was an aged, stooped, gray-haired woman, scarred badly on the face, arms, and legs. She inquired about Pietro, but could only be told that, although he had written repeated enthusiastic letters to the writer, the entrance of the United States into the war had ended the correspondence. Also, his father had given up the bakery and had gone into war industry, and thus all contact had been lost. She accepted this information resignedly and bade the writer farewell.

Case 8   Sexual Dysfunction: Somnambulistic Training in a Rapid Hypnotherapeutic Approach

A retired professional man who greatly respected the senior author's reputation telephoned for an interview to deal with a personal problem. In the first part of this single, one-hour interview the senior author illustrates his typical approach in facilitating somnambulistic behavior. He establishes a therapeutic frame of reference and then deftly utilizes many of the indirect forms of suggestion and a series of posthypnotic suggestions to initiate the close rapport and following behavior that is characteristic of somnambulism. He illustrates how two-level communication and a continual discharging and displacement of resistance are of primary importance.

In the second part of this session he illustrates how a classical hand levitation approach to trance induction can be used as a rich context for introducing many therapeutic suggestions in a symbolic as well as a direct form. Therapeutic suggestions are introduced during those first moments of initiating trance experience when patients' attention and expectancy are frequently at their highest pitch. In this unusually rapid approach the patients receive therapeutic suggestions before they realize what is happening. Their consciousness can be so fixated on the novel experience of hand levitation that they do not notice the therapeutic suggestions. The therapeutic suggestions are, therefore, received by the unconscious in a way that bypass some of the patients' conscious, habitual attitudes and learned limitations.

If we translate the terms "conscious" and "unconscious" into "dominant" and "nondominant" hemispheres, we may have the neuropsychological basis for describing a new hypnotherapeutic approach. Occupying the dominant hemisphere with a trance induction such as hand levitation which can be easily lateralized can release the nondominant hemisphere to receive therapeutic suggestions phrased in the symbolic language of the nondominant hemisphere. Part Two of this session is a demonstration of this approach which utilizes hemispheric interaction in trance induction and suggestion in an unusually clear form.

Part One: Facilitating Somnambulistic Behavior

E: Tell me what your problem is.

P. I lost my wife a few years ago. She had been ill for a couple of years. We always had a normal sex life. But after she died, I seemed to be absolutely impotent and I couldn't get an erection. That did not bother me because I did not plan to remarry. Now I've met a woman I want very much. I want to marry her. I did all the pushing. She thought we should wait longer. I could have lived with her, but I didn't want to. I want to marry her. But I found in the love-making process with her that I didn't get the sexual feelings that I knew I had. I realize I'm older and those things don't happen so frequently. I'm sixty-eight. Since I called you a few days ago, this has changed. I haven't had intercourse, but I've had erections during the love-making. I just want to feel secure in this. We are planning to marry in about five weeks. I want to feel secure for her as well as for myself.

E: Have you an interest in archeology?

P: No, not very much.

E: You know that seeds found with Egyptian mummies have sprouted after 5,000 years.

P: Yes, I know that.

E: Now is there any reason for you to think that your penis located in a vagina won't become tumescent?

P: No, not now there isn't. It's changed in the last few days, but that was my worry when I called you.

E: Why should you ever worry about your heart function or your pancreas function, your salivary glands?

P: Well, I never worry about those things, but this was a personal relationship. That was the thing that worried me. I wanted to be sure. And I think she wanted to be sure, too.

E: All right, from the physiological point of view you really shouldn't have a worry.

P: I don't think so.

E: You don't think so?

P: No, I should say I'm sure.

E: From the psychological or emotional point of view you can have a worry.

P: Yes.

E: Do you think from an emotional and psychological point of view that you can have any doubt when she is nude?

P: No, I don't think so now, but three or four days ago I did.

> E: You never forget the problem at hand, but you translate it into many other avenues of the patient's experience. You utilize their other experiential learnings to deal with their current problem.
>
> R: That's what you do right in the beginning of this interview. He states his problem and you immediately ask about his interest in archeology. This enables you to bring up the idea of seeds sprouting after 5,000 years which, of course, it a humorous but meaningful analogy with his problem. You're immediately using another modality of his knowledge to establish that it is possible to regain a life function that has been unused for some time. This is your first approach to facilitating a therapeutic frame of reference. You then ask a *question* about the functioning of the heart, pancreas, and salivary glands which leads to the *implication* that he does not have to worry

about penis erection because that's also an automatic function. You're thereby introducing another therapeutic frame of reference: Unconscious processes within the body will regulate penis erections just as they do other functions once he gives up the limiting and inhibiting effects of his conscious worry about it. The patient objects by saying a "personal relationship" is involved. You then utilize this to confirm that "from the physiological point of view you really shouldn't have a worry." This resolves the physiological aspect of the problem and enables you to define the problems as "psychological or emotional" in a manner that he can easily accept. Then with your hypothetical question about "any doubt when she is nude" you help him acknowledge that even this psychological aspect of the problem is resolvable. Thus in the first few minutes of the interview you have facilitated series of acknowledgments from the patient that structure a very strong *therapeutic frame of reference* for the hypnotic work that will follow. In his last remark the patient is already placing the problem into the past. He approaches trance with a very high *expectation* that his now very limited problem can be resolved with ease.

Trance Induction: The Early Learning Set

E: Now sit with your hands on your thighs like this. And just look at one spot there. And just look at it continuously.

You do not need to talk.

You do not need to move.

You actually do not need to move.

Just look at that one spot.

And many years ago

you went to kindergarten,

first grade.

And you were confronted

with what seemed then

an insurmountable task

of learning the letters of the alphabet

in all their many forms.

And it seemed an insurmountable task.

But you did form mental images

for every letter of the alphabet.

And you formed mental images

of the numbers.

And you formed those mental images
to remain with you for the rest of your life.

> R: Here you induce trance without any initial introductory remarks because this professional man already knows its therapeutic possibilities and he has a positive expectation about it. This early learning set induction (Erickson, Rossi, and Rossi, 1976) tends to facilitate age regression by *indirect ideodynamic focusing* that evokes early learning experiences. This activation of early learning experiences is a foundation for the hypnotic phenomena you will later evoke.

Ratifying Trance: Body Language in Trance

While I have been talking to you
your respiration has changed,
your pulse has changed.
Close your eyes N . . . O . . . W.
[Pause as the patient's eyes close and his head bows down very slowly, bit by bit, until it almost touches his chest]

You go deeply into a trance
and enjoy the feeling of comfort
and satisfaction *all over*.

[Pause as patient's body tips forward a bit precariously]

You can lean back in the chair.
[Pause as patient's body reorients back comfortably in the chair]

> R: You begin your process of vocal conditioning with your slow drawn-out N . . . O . . . W and then emphasize that in a deep trance one can enjoy feeling comfort and satisfaction all over. This is a form of indirect suggestion because we know that such comfort is a characteristic of trance.

> E: My emphasis on "satisfaction *all over*" includes his scalp, nose, buttocks, and penis.

> R: The patient does not recognize this as an *indirect suggestion by generalization:* Since his penis is the "problem" his unconscious will tend to automatically focus some of that suggested satisfaction there.

> E: The fact that his body tips forward may be an indication that

he is leaning toward the light of love; he had been leaning away from it after his wife died.

R: Leaning forward may be an indication of a positive rapport. Does that mean that a leaning backward or pulling in a direction away from the therapist is an indication of a negative transference reaction or a problem between therapist and patient?

E: It can indicate a difficulty with the ideas being presented.

Posthypnotic Suggestions Initiating Somnambulistic Training: Being in Trance Without Knowing It

And now I want you
to realize something.
Shortly after you awaken
I'm going to say something to you.

R: This posthypnotic suggestion is a way of initiating somnambulistic training. It is a very easy suggestion to accept because after a patient awakens he naturally expects you will say something. He doesn't realize, however, that when you do say something, you're actually giving a posthypnotic cue that will initiate another trance. Your earlier research (Erickson and Erickson, 1941) indicated that subjects reenter trance when receiving posthypnotic cues and carrying out posthypnotic suggestions. When you begin to say something after trance, they will tend to reenter trance even though their eyes may be open and they may act as if they are awake. This is your definition of the somnambulistic state: A person acting as if he is awake but capable of following the therapist's hypnotic suggestions.

E: Yes, with hypnotic training you want them to be content with the thought that they are awake.

R: Even though they are really not. Do you define that as the somnambulistic state? The patient thinks he is awake, but he is following you so closely and is thereby capable of carrying out so many hypnotic responses that we say he's actually in an altered state called trance. He is not critical and initiating his own behavioral directions; he is waiting for your suggestions. He is in trance without being aware of it.

E: I once told a subject to act as if he was awake with all of us who were in the room. But when a totally unexpected person came in the room, the subject could not respond to his presence. He never heard the newcomer speaking to him.

R: Indicating that there was a special rapport with those already present in the room that excluded any strangers. Such an intense state of rapport is characteristic of somnambulistic trance. I'm beginning to believe that patients are frequently in somnambulistic trance without the hypnotherapist recognizing it or knowing how to use it.

E: I certainly agree! Most have such fixed and rigid ideas of what somnambulistic behavior is. [The senior author goes on to point out how subtle changes in behavior that indicate the presence of therapeutic trance are frequently missed by many therapists. See Erickson, Rossi & Rossi, 1976.]

Utilizing Patients' Motivation to Reinforce Suggestions

And you can be surprised
that you ever really have doubted
yourself.
[Pause]

R: You throw in a therapeutic suggestion here?

E: To reinforce the preceding posthypnotic suggestion.

R: You utilize the patients' own motivation for therapy to reinforce your suggestions.

E: All your suggestions in therapy should be a connected whole.

Hypnotic Amnesia Facilitating Somnambulistic State

Now it isn't necessary for you to remember
what I say to you in the trance state.
But your unconscious mind
will remember.
But all of us know very little
about what the unconscious mind knows.

R: This is a permissive suggestion for amnesia. You don't command amnesia—that might only arouse conscious resistance. You are apparently letting the patient do something easy: "It isn't necessary for you to remember." This implies that it's too hard to remember (as we all well know from many experiences in everyday life.)

E: If you tell anyone they *have to* do something, they invariably come back with they *don't.*

R: You then admit "Your unconscious mind will remember. But all of us know very little about what the unconscious mind knows." This tends to reinforce amnesia and the role of the unconscious while *depotentiating the importance of his more limited conscious mental sets.* This emphasis on conscious amnesia and the significance of unconscious functioning is another way of facilitating the somnambulistic state.

Deepening Trance by Rehearsal

I'm going to arouse you
and put you back into trance.

E: Awakening and putting a patient back into trance repeatedly is a way of deepening trance (Erickson, 1952).

R: Is it also a way of further depotentiating his conscious orientation, a sort of confusion approach to somnambulistic training?

E: Yes, you're training the patient to respond in a therapeutic way.

R: You're training him to respond to you.

E: And you base your therapeutic suggestions on his own patterns of behaving.

R: By deep trance you mean that the patient is following you very closely in accord with his needs.

Questions as Direct Suggestion in a Permissive Manner

And you are going to do everything I ask you to do.
Can you be surprised
at your ability
to make true whatever I say?
[Pause]

R: Your first sentence here seems to be a shocking authoritarian demand for obedience.

253

E: "Everything I *ask* you to do." I did not say, "Do what I tell you to do."

R: When you "ask," you are actually making a permissive request that the patient could refuse. Then you follow it up with a very innocuous-sounding but strongly reinforcing *question* about being "*surprised* at your ability to make true whatever I say?"

E: Even infants like surprises.

R: A surprise also implies that the unconscious will be active and surprise the conscious mind.

E: Too many therapists tell their patients to do this or that rather than ask. That's an iron hand covered with a lot of velvet.

Discharging and Displacing Resistance: Use of the Negative

And you will make true whatever I say,
vill you not?

E: You will, will you not? If anybody is going to use the negative, it had better be me.

R: If the patient has a resistance in the form of a "no" within, then your use of "will you *not?*" tends to displace and discharge the "no." Beginning students in hypnosis are usually trained to express suggestions in a positive manner. That is a valid approach. You assume, however, that resistance in the form of contrary trends is always present. You therefore use negatives in this rather curiously concrete way to pick up the patient's negative and convert it into a constructive direction. This does not make sense from a rational, left-hemispheric point of view, but it may be effective because trance is a right-hemisphere phenomenon, where such concrete transformations are easily possible.

Hypnotic Poetry Bypassing Conscious Resistance

In spite of any thinking you do,
what I say will be true.

R: This poetic couplet is another way of dealing with resistance. Many patients fear that if they have contrary thoughts during trance, the therapeutic suggestions cannot be effective. Your couplet reassures them on this point. The smooth pattern of sound and stress in this couplet suggests it may be an example of Snyder's Hypnotic Poetry (1930), which bypasses the critical, intellectualistic left-hemisphere so it can be accepted by the right.

E: I'm bonding my therapeutic suggestion to whatever resistance he may have within.

R: In this case you don't necessarily eliminate resistance but rather add your therapeutic suggestions to it. It's a way of utilizing the patients' resistance so that whenever they express it to themselves, they find themselves also expressing the therapeutic suggestion. This is especially important for this type of patient, who seems so cooperative in his manifest behavior. Since he is so cooperative on the outside, his resistances must be hidden within. You therefore utilize this inner resistance by adding a constructive suggestion to it without even having to bring it up with the patient.

Apparent Trance Awakening and Spontaneous Reinduction: Individual Characteristics of Somnambulism

Take your time
and mentally, silently,
count backward from twenty to one.
Awakening one-twentieth of the way at each count.
And begin the count now.
[Pause as P appears to awaken in about one minute]
Pretty hard to awaken wasn't it?

P: Um-hum.
[E answers the phone, and as he does so P closes his eyes and evidently goes back into trance.]

E: And it's hard to awaken,
but you can awaken again.
[Pause as P opens his eyes slowly. He does not reorient much to his body, however, so we may presume he is still in trance.]
And awaken with a very comfortable feeling.

P: I feel comfortable.

E: Why did you go back into trance the second time?

[Pause as P looks perplexed]

Your unconscious mind understands a lot more than you do.

R: It's an indication of his intense somnambulistic rapport with you that he closes his eyes and goes back into trance when you remove your attention from him by answering the phone. He is now following your earlier posthypnotic suggestions that he would go back into trance after awakening. If he were really awake, he might have moved about a bit or related to me since I was right next to him. But he completely ignores me and all the recording equipment. Deep trance does not mean a patient is stuporous or unconscious; it does mean that a patient's attention is intensely focused on what is relevant, so that everything else is ignored. You ask him to awaken again, but he only opens his eyes. When you tell him to "awaken with a very comfortable feeling," he responds in an *almost exact* paraphrase, "I am comfortable." This exact following of your words is another indication of the somnambulistic state. Why is he perplexed when you ask him why he went into trance the second time?

E: There is a *retardation of intellectual processes* that easily leads to perplexity in the somnambulistic state.

R: So here we have three characteristics of somnambulism: (1) the intense rapport; (2) the exact following of the therapist's remarks that are in accord with the patient's own needs; and (3) the lack of mental initiative. The somnambulistic state does not mean the patient is an automaton but that he is extraordinarily well related to the therapist.

E: It's his conscious mind that is perplexed. I verify that by adding that his unconscious understands a lot more than he does. I keep out of the situation; don't say, "I know what's going on." I say, "*Your* unconscious knows."

R: Are there any general characteristics of somnambulism, or do we have to pick them out as highly individualized manifestations in each person?

E: You have to pick them out for each individual; they will vary depending upon the purposes of the patient.

R: This patient showed little initiative in his somnambulistic state, but other persons might show a lot—expressing their fantasies, etc. Is there a general difference between an active and passive somnambulism?

E: This patient did not like what he was receiving from himself, therefore he remained passive in order to get what he could from me. That's why I worked for amnesia and perplexity to depotentiate his conscious sets.

R: Those were ways of depotentiating his habitual conscious attitudes so that an unconscious search and process could be initiated to facilitate a therapeutic response. Thus, even when the patient is in a very passive and receptive state, you do not resort to directly programming him with what he is to do. Rather you make an effort to help him sidestep his own conscious limitations so his unconscious potentials can become manifest.

E: The patient had better believe in his own unconscious.

Hypnotic Phenomena as Early Patterns of Behavior: Implication Evoking Early Psychomotor Patterns? Two-Level Communication for Therapeutic Suggestion via Metaphor

E: And all of your life
since the age of one
you have known you could stand up.
Right?

P: Um-hum.

E: And now you know you can't.
Try it. *You can't.* [Said very quickly and softly]
[Pause as the patient makes a few slight abortive movements with the upper part of his body and looks about, a bit distressed]

E: "Since the age of one you have known you could stand up" implies that before the age of one you could not. At the same time this is a two-level communication dealing with his problem in a metaphorical way: Not being able to stand up is like not being able to get an erection.

R: You choose a hypnotic phenomenon that has an unconscious connection with his psychological problem, so that when you later resolve the hypnotic phenomenon (allow him to stand up) you may also be resolving his sexual impotence to some degree. This is an unusually clear example of indirect therapy being done on an unconscious level. This also appears to be an unusually clear example of your utilization approach to hypnotic phenomena. Do you believe that you are actually evoking an early psychomotor level of "not being able to walk" and then utilizing it as the basis of this hypnotic phenomenon? Hypnosis is not just imagination; it is based on the activation of the relevant neurological circuits—very often those from infancy and early childhood.

E: Yes. Those infantile and early childhood patterns have a long history.

R: Because of their long history they have a certain prepotency within us; they have never been really extinguished, and when properly activated they can be expressed in behavior. It is usually more effective to activate such early psychomotor patterns by indirect means such as implication, because a direct command could evoke the doubting attitudes of consciousness that in turn block the hypnotic response.

E: You deal with the patient as a total historical being. You can rely on those neurological tracks and memories of long duration much more than you can on the very recent ones.

R: It would be well for the hypnotherapist to study early childhood development to gain a more adequate understanding of the type of phenomena he can evoke as well as hints about how they may be evoked. Most if not all hypnotic phenomena are actually early patterns of functioning. This is a distinctive aspect of your work: you believe you are evoking real mental mechanisms and unconscious processes in hypnotic phenomena. It is the utilization of an individual's early experiential learning rather than hypersuggestibility or imagination per se that is the basis of hypnotic phenomena.

E: Patients can only respond out of their own life experiences.

The Creative Process of Therapeutic Analogy

E: And now you *truly* know
how an idea can take possession of you.
[P closes his eyes and appears to lapse deeper into trance]

E: In mentioning that he now "truly" knows how an idea can take possession of one, you are by analogy referring, of course, to his problem: Just as an idea can prevent him from standing up, so can an idea prevent his penis from standing up.

R: He probably closed his eyes again because of a sudden realization of "standing up" having those different meanings?

E: Closing his eyes probably corresponded to the *inner search and unconscious processes* that actually create that meaning. To grasp such an analogy requires a creative effort on his part. Because it is his own creative effort, he is less likely to reject it than if it was simply thrust upon him as a direct statement.

Two-Level Communication: Further Somnambulistic Training

E: And rouse again
and feel very comfortable all over.
[Pause as P opens his eyes again]
How do you feel about not being able to stand up?

P: Well, it didn't bother me. I didn't want to stand up.

E: And now you can't remain seated.
[P looks around and stands up, seemingly a bit embarrassed for a moment or two]
Now you can sit down.
[P sits]

E: When he said he didn't want to stand up, that implied he had a choice. On an unconscious level it also means he has choice about his penis not standing up.

R: I see—he may want to make that choice at times. He may be using two-level communication here without quite realizing it. The further suggestion that he "can't remain seated" in this context now has the symbolic meaning of not being able to keep his penis down and may account for his apparent embarrassment at this point. It is also a means of further training in somnambulistic behavior wherein he follows your hypnotic suggestions even while acting as if he's awake.

E: To say that he "can't remain seated" is therapeutic on an unconscious level. Notice that I carefully avoided saying "You have to stand up." I wanted to avoid the "stand up" issue because he had such difficulty with his penis standing up that it could have defeated the hypnotic suggestion on an unconscious level.

Part Two: A Rapid Hypnotherapeutic Approach Utilizing Therapeutic Symbolism with Hand Levitation: Hemispheric Interaction in Trance Induction and Suggestion

E: I want you to enjoy this experience.

One or the other or both of your hands will lift up toward your face. And no matter how hard you try to press down, it's going to lift up toward your face.

[Fingers of the patient's right hand lift tentatively, and then the whole hand lifts with a gentle, bobbing motion]

And you can't stop it.

[Pause as P's right hand slowly approaches his face]

And there is nothing you can do to stop it.

[Pause as the hand bobs up toward P's hairline]

A little bit higher.

There is nothing you can do to stop your hand from feeling hair.

[P's hand approaches and finally touches the hair on his head]

The feeling of hair,

and you can't stop your hand from doing that.

And now you know

that whenever you wish

your penis can stand up and feel hair.

[Pause]

R: You now undertake a classical hand levitation, but your words have another level of meaning where hand levitation becomes equivalent to penis levitation. Several times you mention "You can't stop it." Are you thereby attempting to symbolically depotentiate his conscious mind's ability to stop a penis erection?

E: Yes.

R: It is fascinating to hypothesize that his left hemisphere may be so preoccupied with levitating his right hand that it leaves his right hemisphere more available to accept and act upon your therapeutic suggestions given in the symbolic language of the right hemisphere. Recent research (Smith, Chu, and Edmonston, 1977; Diamond and Beaumont, 1974; Kinsbourne and Smith, 1974) indicates that preoccupying the dominant cerebral hemisphere with one activity does tend to leave the other hemisphere free to deal with other data. This may be the neuropsychological basis of your common practice of interspersing therapeutic suggestions in the symbolic language of the unconscious (or non-dominant hemisphere) along with hand levitation or any other approach to induction that occupies the attention of the dominant cerebral hemisphere. A great deal of systematic research is now required to test this hypothesis of hemispheric interaction in trance induction and suggestion in order to ascertain the parameters under which this therapeutic approach could be maximized.

Posthypnotic Suggestion Contingent on Inevitabilities

E: And you can enjoy it.
It won't be your hair.
It won't be your hair.
It will be the feeling of hers.
And you can't lower your hand
until you've enjoyed
sensing the feeling of hair
sensing a warm body.
[Pause]
And nothing can tell you
that your penis won't stand up.
Nothing can tell you that.
[Pause]
And nothing can prevent it from feeling hair and a vagina for as long as you
want.
[Pause]
And I want you to notice
your hand doesn't feel as if it's touching your hair,
it feels as if it's touching
that lady's hair.
[Pause]

E: I initiated the process of lifting toward his face and hair. Once that was well under way and could not be stopped, then I could shift it to the issue of vagina and pubic hair.

R: Having accepted the initial condition, he is carried on by its momentum to accepting the therapeutic suggestion.

E: Now he can't avoid sensing a warm body when he is with her; that's inevitable and I've symbolically tied an erect penis to her warm body when I say "You can't lower your hand until you've enjoyed. . . warm body."

R: This is a basic principle of posthypnotic suggestion wherein you always make a suggested behavior contingent on an inevitability.

Further Posthypnotic Suggestion

And I want you to have the surprise of your life
because sometime today
or tomorrow
your hand will touch the hair on her head,
and you'll find
what your penis will insist on doing.
And you're going to let that be a surprise
are you not?
[P nods his head yes]
[Pause]
And you're going to be so delighted
with the forcefulness of your desire.
But you will not offend the lady.
But you will be pleased
with the very forcefulness of the desire.
[Pause]
And philosophers
of old have said,
"As a man thinketh, he is."
And you'll never forget that, will you?
And now think this question over well,
are you willing to tell us something about the lady?
[P nods head yes]

E: "Sometime today or tomorrow" actually means anytime. It could be next month and still fall within the generalized time range of this suggestion.

R: Here you again make a posthypnotic suggestion about penis erection contingent on another inevitability (touching her hair).

E: How do you "offend the lady?" By either being too forceful or not forceful enough. I've covered both possibilities there while emphasizing "forcefulness of your desire." When I then ask him if he wants to tell us "something about the lady," it implies he has choice, and if he tells us something he also has the right to hold back other things. The right to hold things back gives him potency and power.

Preparation for Awakening

**All right, take your time and awaken
and just spontaneously tell us something about her.
[Pause as P opens his eyes and focuses as if he is awake. His hand remains at his head, however, and he does not reorient any other part of his body]**

**P: Well, she is beautiful.
She is the same age as I am.
And I never loved anyone like this before in my life.**

> E: I've just given him the implied posthypnotic suggestion to hold back and he responds with the generalization "Well, she is beautiful." He is actually holding back. He's following a posthypnotic suggestion without even realizing it.
>
> R: In having him hold back you're returning him to his normally awake ego controls and are thereby preparing him for a full awakening.
>
> E: Yes, when he admits loving her more than anyone else in his life, he is volunteering that on a more conscious awake level.

Symbolically Displacing and Discharging a Lack of Confidence

E: What did you just learn about yourself?

P: More confidence, for one thing.

E: There is something lacking in your confidence?

P: Yes, there was doubt.

**E: There is something now lacking in your confidence. I'll tell you what it is.
You can't put your hand down.**

P: Hum!?

> E: When he talks about confidence here, he's implying a lack of

confidence, so I displace it onto the hand. Put the lack of confidence in a harmless place.

R: This is a way of displacing and discharging a lack of confidence in a symbolic manner.

Two-level Communication with True Trance Awakening

E: **And you can't push it down until you have a feeling of intense satisfaction.**

[Long pause as P closes his eyes. He finally opens them again, puts his hand down, and adjusts his whole body slightly, as is characteristic of patients awakening from trance.]

P: **Yeah, I feel pretty good now!**

E: **And what are you going to need?**

P: **Uh?**

E: **You don't have to tell us.**

P: **No.**

E: **But you think it over.
She's got two beautiful twins,
and both deserve a name.**

[Pause]

P: **Yeah.**

E: After a pleasant sexual intercourse what happens?

R: You relax and your penis goes down. So your suggestion that he can't put his hand down until he has a feeling of intense satisfaction is another bit of two-level communication that he receives just as he is waking up. This tends to build a bridge between the therapeutic suggestion on the unconscious and conscious levels.

E: He then responds with, "Yeah, I feel pretty good now!" A two-level response without his quite realizing it. I now continue with remarks about her "two beautiful twins," which he recognizes as a reference to her breasts. If he is to make love to her, he had better appreciate her breasts.

Indirect Ideodynamic Focusing

E: Someone who liked mountain climbing was asked on a social occasion, "Do you intend to do any mountain climbing this weekend?" And he said, "Oh, yes," but he didn't name the mountain. That was a secret between him and his wife.
And every couple should have a language of love.

[Pause]

P: I feel better now.

E: And another friend of mine
was asked at the dinner table,
"Would you like to have a cup of soup?"
He answered, "Yes, I always like a cupful."
What he really meant was, "Yes, I always like a cup full of life."

P: Yeah.

> R: You're here emphasizing the two-level communication about love play in everyday life.
>
> E: Yes, these two-level communications are like the secret language of childhood.
>
> R: Since they come from childhood, they are rich in the sort of ideodynamic responses he will need in his new love life. You are thus activating these processes by talking about them. This is another example of indirect ideodynamic focusing for a therapeutic response.

Therapeutic Restructuring of a Former Symptom

E: Now, I always tell young men,
"Sometime in your lifetime you're going to lose your erection.
And what you don't know
is that your unconscious mind
is telling you that the beauty of your wife's body is overwhelming."
And to enjoy that fact.
Because that's the greatest possible compliment you both can receive.
If on some occasion unexpectedly you lose your erection,
it's a very profound compliment,

because as soon as you realize you
have complimented her in the most ultimate fashion,
then your erection comes back.

[Pause]

> R: Do you actually believe that a loss of erection could really be a compliment, or is this just a rationalization you're offering him?
>
> E: He's placed a bad interpretation on a loss of erection. Why should he keep that forever and ever? Life is much better if sometimes it rains and sometimes it doesn't. I've seen many cases where it really was a compliment.

Further Therapeutic Analogies

E: How long did you practice in X city?

P: Since Y. I retired a few years ago. [A general conversation now takes place about P's medical practice and his use of hypnosis on his patients.]

E: How many Ginkgo trees are there in X?

P: I don't know.

E: I was given a drive through X and passed an intersection and I said to my friend who was driving, "Didn't we just pass a Ginkgo tree up that side street? I've never seen one, but I'm sure it was a Ginkgo tree." He said, "You're right." Later he showed me some petrified Ginkgo wood.

P: Oh!

E: [To R] Do you know the Ginkgo tree?

R: Oh yes, very well! They have live motile sperm!

P: Yes.

E: One time when I was in X, I ordered oysters. The waiter said, "You're lucky, we have just two orders left." I said, "I'll take them both."

[A round of laughter at the implied association between eating oysters and sexual potency. The conversation then drifts to seafood in general and P's hobbies, one of which has to do with working with fine grains and textures of wood.]

266

What more would you like to say to me?

P: I don't think there is anything. I just feel entirely different. I feel as if a load has been lifted off my shoulders. I just feel that I have confidence in myself that I did not have before.

E: Now I'm not able to travel, but will you send me a wedding invitation?

P: Yes, I'll do that. It's a wonderful feeling. It's a good feeling.

E: How do you like this?

[The senior author shows P a fine sculpture of a bird emerging from a branch of wood. The front part of the bird is carved very simply and elegantly, while the latter part of its body is not sculptured at all; it simply merges into the natural form of the wood.]

P: I've never seen anything like it.

E: Like a butterfly emerging from a cocoon. Only this time it's a bird.

P: Did you carve it?

E: No, I used to carve. Do you like wood-carving?

P: I've never done any, but I like it.

E: Would you like to see the world's largest private collection of ironwood carvings?

[The therapy session thus ends with P being shown the senior authors collection of ironwood carvings made by the Indians of Central Mexico.]

R: You terminate the interview with these further therapeutic analogies that now shift the relationship from doctor-patient to friends as you invite him into your home to look at your collection of carvings.

E: He knows I like oysters and he likes wood carvings and so do I. We share likings.

R: Since you like sexuality, then he must like it, too. This aspect of your work is essentially a "transference cure" as well as a way of resolving the transference, since you become just another human being with your personal tastes, etc.

Case 9   Anorexia Nervosa*
Paradox and Double Bind

E: In all cases I have known of anorexia nervosa in children (about fifty, and all girls from ages nine to fifteen) there has always been a peculiar emotional relationship between the parents and the patient. It is one of concealed, repressed anger, resentment, and extreme frustration together with anxiety, concern, and fear on the part of the parents. For the patient the emotional behavior is most difficult to describe. There appears to be an underlying state of fear of all emotional involvement manifested by a submissive passivity, total lack of self-concern, the rejection of food to the point of death by starvation, a concealed fear of the parents, particularly of the mother, and repression of hunger feelings and all autocritical faculties. Underlying all of this is a vaguely conceptualized religiosity suggestive of a poorly formed and often not verbalized identification with a messiah or a messianic purpose.

The problem of anorexia nervosa, to the best of my knowledge and experience, is emotional in character with resulting physical symptomatology. An approach I used effectively in a short period (February 11 to March 13) is as follows. I saw the fourteen-year-old patient with her mother during the first two interviews. As is typical of many mothers of anorexia nervosa patients, she answered all questions put to the daughter in a protective fashion. Having secured a thorough demonstration of the mother's interest, I told the mother politely but emphatically, "Shut up and let your daughter answer the questions." I then proceeded to get general information from the girl. Then I told her most emphatically that her parents sent her to me to have me tell her to eat, but I had no intention of doing so; eating was her own problem, and she could do as she pleased.

> R: In this initial approach you immediately establish rapport with the patient by telling her mother to "shut up." You then facilitate the developing of a yes set by adapting yourself to the patient's own frame of reference, as you tell her you have no intention of telling her to eat. You then place the *locus of therapeutic control* within the patient by saying that eating was her own problem and she could do as she pleased. You apparently allow the patient to keep her resistances and you see to it that she has no need to defend herself against you. There is a paradox in all this and a subtle double bind. The *paradox* is that you are apparently on her side and doing the opposite of what you're supposed to be doing—making her eat. The *subtle double bind* is that by the very approach of not trying to control

---

*The senior author originally wrote this case; the junior author has added commentaries for its current publication.

268

her behavior, you are actually establishing a rapport and relationship that will eventually bind her to therapeutic work you will soon suggest. The paradox and double bind together undoubtedly have the effect of *depotentiating some of the conscious frames of reference* so that she is now more available for whatever you suggest.

Distracting Conscious Frames of Reference

E: I then pointed out that as a medical man I could give proper and competent advice about oral hygiene. I explained to the girl that regardless of whether one eats or does not eat, using the toothbrush on the teeth and on the gums is important, and that in a proper method of oral hygiene you use a toothpaste with fluoride with the understanding that there should never be swallowing of any of the paste. After the child agreed to this, I pointed out that there was further oral hygiene which, as a medical man, I was entitled to prescribe. This was the use of a mouthwash to be used before brushing the teeth to loosen the detritus on the teeth, and the brushing of the teeth should be followed by a second application of mouthwash with absolute instructions that there should be no swallowing of any of the mouthwash. I exacted a promise from the child that my instructions about oral hygiene would be followed.

R: You now further detract her conscious frames of references by this indirect approach of focusing attention on what is actually an irrelevant problem—oral hygiene. You utilize her character structure of passive obedience to get her to follow some rather absurd and practically impossible suggestions.

Depotentiating a Messianic Complex

E: In patients with anorexia nervosa, the messianic complex and their own religious demands compel them to keep the promises made. I prescribed as a mouthwash cod liver oil, emphasizing that not a single drop be swallowed. The child rebelled by whimpering at night and keeping the mother awake. After this happened a few times, I delivered a dispassionate sermon on the wrongness of offenses against others. I described it as bad behavior requiring punishment, and since the bad behavior was not against me, but against the mother—the mother being the offended person—she had the right to prescribe the punishment. The child agreed and privately I told the mother that nocturnal whimpering is not desirable, and might be punished in any way that she chose so long as it was reasonable. The mother decided that scrambled eggs could be used as punishment. That removed food from the area of nonacceptability of the self-imposed ritual of rejection of food. Also, her body received nourishment, which, coupled with the taste of the cod liver oil, created a disruptive situation for her self-imposed passive self-destruction. Her

269

passivity compelled her to accept food as punishment, and her messianic complex also required her to do so. Additionally, the bad taste of the cod liver oil aroused strong emotions of revulsion with consequent temptation to avoid using it, something her messianic complex and passivity precluded. Her only recourse was to rationalize or to "forget" something that would give her both satisfaction and guilt, all of which were destructive of her passivity and messianic complex.

She was queried just once about having secured the cod liver oil and her use of it. The mother had been instructed to oversee only the first occasion of its use, and I asked about it only once. The mother was instructed to remind the girl only once, and that was on the first overnight sightseeing trip in Arizona, to be sure to pack her cod liver oil, that it should not be forgotten for the trip.

Near the end of the treatment private inquiry of the mother disclosed that she had reluctantly purchased, in the company of her daughter, only a small bottle of cod liver oil (under 16 ounces), that she had become nauseated watching her daughter's first use of it, and that after the first two days the content level of the bottle changed very little; sometime later the bottle disappeared.

> R: You accomplished a number of fascinating psychodynamic alterations at this point. Your practically impossible demand of using cod liver oil was accepted by her because her passive, messianic complex required that she accept unpleasant suggestions to assuage her guilt. Yet, since she could not follow the cod liver oil suggestion, the egosyntonic aspects of the messianic complex are shattered (Rossi, 1973b). She can only follow the cod liver oil suggestions minimally, and then apparently she engages in an outright deceit by making the bottle of cod liver oil disappear. In doing this she has to give up her messianic "all good and obedient" identification and begin to mobilize her own will to survive through different patterns of behavior. The impossible task thus shattered her messianic complex (depotentiated that frame of reference) and initiated her into an unconscious search for new and potentially therapeutic responses. The other marvelous twist in all this is that you manage to keep the mother as the dispenser of punishment—you still remain the patient's sympathetic supporter. She has been disobedient and requires punishment. Food, which was formerly a reward, is now changed into a punishment that she has to accept. This is all so difficult to follow that I almost get vertigo even trying to untangle the psychodynamics in an objective fashion. I can imagine how confused and helpless the patient's conscious mind must have felt trying to sort it all out. Obviously it could not, so she was simply open to follow your suggestions.

Depotentiating Conscious Sets and Unconscious Search

E: Then to meet the child's emotional needs further, I proceeded to talk to her, telling interesting things, boring things, exciting things, mildly offensive things, ridiculous things, highly intriguing things. I bombarded the child with a great wealth of opportunities to react to on an emotional level. As one doctor who sat in on one such interview remarked after it was over, "You ran that poor girl up and down the whole gamut of emotions, and so far as she could see, you were just talking about things of interest to you."

> R: You are engaged in one of your typical approaches of *fixing her attention* with your talk of interesting and intriguing things. You thereby also further *depotentiate her own frames of reference and provide her via indirect associative focusing* with many opportunities for *unconscious searches and processes* to stir her emotional life. Hopefully, this will enable her to realign her inner psychodynamics so that she can come up with a new, more adequate frame of reference for a better self-identity and more fulfilling behavior. You don't know what this more adequate frame and pattern of response will be at this point. You are simply shaking up her psychodynamics with the expectation that her unconscious will find its own way.

A Therapeutic Double Bind

E: Now the mother of this particular anorexia nervosa patient liked to travel, and I had her see as much of Arizona as possible so that in the period of February 11 to March 13 I saw the child for only a total of twenty hours. During the first two weeks she gained three pounds, lost one, and gained one back. She had lost five pounds in the month that she had been in the hospital, and her weight when she arrived was sixty-one pounds. Otherwise she was a well-built fourteen-year-old girl. After she had gained the three pounds, the mother, who simply could not understand my handling of the child, was told to stand up and to tell me her height, her weight and age, and the number of her children. She told me she was past forty, mother of five children and an M.D., that she was married to an M.D., and that her height was five feet six inches and her weight was 118 lbs., even as it had been when she had married her husband nineteen years previously. I put on a fairly good semblance of shock at her underweight state. (Actually her height appeared to be around five feet eight or nine inches, but I did not dispute this statement.) I pointed out quite emphatically that a mother of five at that height and that age should weigh 130 pounds; and did she not consider her behavior shameful in bringing her daughter to me in a state of malnutrition when she herself was undernourished? I told the patient, "I want you to see to it that your mother gains weight, and I want you to tell me of any failure by your mother to eat adequately.''

> R: Since the mother may have been about to interfere with her daughter's therapy, you begin to involve the mother with what may have been an indirect induction of therapeutic trance. By asking her to stand up and answer a series of standard medical questions you were actually *focusing her attention* very fixedly on herself. She was naturally in a state of wonderment, confusion, and perhaps a bit of shock about this rather unusual treatment at this stage of the game by a fellow physician. Her *habitual mental sets* were therefore *depotentiated*, and your series of *questions* evoked a set of many problems of *unconscious search*. Your questions were all easily answered, so you thereby very indirectly evoked a *yes set*. She could easily answer your questions even if she was mystified about why you were asking them. She is thus in a mood of heightened and positive *expectancy* about what is to come next. Your denouement is swift in the form of a *double bind* operating simultaneously on mother and daughter.
>
> The double bind is operative in the daughter as follows: 1) certainly she would like to control her mother for a change; 2) yet as she controls her mother by seeing to it that she eats adequately, the daughter is thereby setting into motion a similar pattern of *adequate eating* in herself on an unconscious level by a process of *indirect ideodynamic* focusing; wanting mother to eat adequately sets up an involuntary process of *eating adequately* that cannot help but become activated within the daughter.
>
> The mother may also experience something of a double bind in this situation: 1) she wants her daughter to get well but 2) the daughter can only get well if the mother gives up her pathological overcontrol of the daughter. Since the mother's *habitual attitudes are depotentiated,* at this moment she tends to yield to your apparently paradoxical suggestion because she simply doesn't know how to cope otherwise. But you are not content with only this, so you add more to *overload the situation* further.

Emotional Catharsis

E: The next important procedure was to insult the girl thoroughly by accusing her of being a liar and a coward, and asserting my ability to prove it. Naturally the girl protested my accusations, whereupon I told her, ''Hit me on the arm.'' She was obviously angry, and she tapped my arm lightly. I took her to task for giving my arm a light tap and implying it to be a blow. I told her that she was a coward if she didn't hit me and that she was a liar when she tried to make me believe that a gentle tap was really a blow. The girl did indeed become angry and actually did hit me, though lightly, on the arm, but immediately turned and rushed into the waiting room and shortly returned, dry-faced and dry-eyed, and took her seat. I accused her again of being a coward and a liar, my proof being that she ran away from the consequences of striking me and went into the waiting room because she did not want me to see the tears in her eyes, and that she was a liar by returning dry-eyed and with a tearless face since I saw her tears as she left the room. Thereupon I continued to run her up and down the gamut of emotions, and I did tell her interesting, pleasing, and intriguing things also.

> R: You are again attacking her messianic complex with your accusations and "proofs" that evoke emotional turmoil and conflicts that make evident the contradictions contained in the all-too-pious and passive view she has of herself. You have certainly focused her attention and depotentiated the false persona she has tried to maintain. It is acceptable to her because it's actually interspersed within the positive context of "interesting, pleasing and intriguing things" which keeps her open with a yes set and permits an emotional catharsis.

Reversals Depotentiating the Symptom Complex

E: On one occasion the mother failed to eat all of her hamburger and had wrapped part of it in a napkin, explaining to her daughter that she was going to make it a midnight snack. The patient did not report her mother's misbehavior until two days later. I took the mother to task for setting a bad example for her daughter and told the mother that she had offended against me in not obeying my medical orders. I told the girl she had offended me by shirking her duty to report her mother's behavior, and therefore, since I was the one offended, I would punish both of them, and I would choose the way I would punish them. I then instructed the mother to bring bread and cheese to my house (which adjoins the office), and she would put a layer of cheese on top of two slices of bread, place them under the broiler, and melt the cheese. She was to withdraw the bread, turn the slices over, cover the other side with cheese, and replace them under the broiler. Then each would eat a cheese sandwich under my watchful eye.

> R: Now both mother and daughter are on the hot seat. Both are guilty and therefore open to your surprising punishment of making them eat. Since food is a punishment rather than a

reward, they can now eat to assuage their mutual guilt. Since it's such an odd and funny sort of cheese treat, they can also accept it with good humor. They were both caught in not obeying medical orders and are now "partners in crime." This brings mother and daughter together with a common "enemy," which they now transfer onto you. Mother and daughter are no longer struggling against each other; therefore the basic psychodynamics underlying the symptom of anorexia nervosa are depotentiated.

Therapeutic Binds and Paradox

E: I then took up with my patient the fact that I didn't mind seeing her now and then, but that I really thought she would much prefer to return to her home 2,000 miles from Arizona. I also told her that I might want her to weigh 85 pounds when she returned home, but that she might want to weigh only 75 pounds. I also stated that I thought the mother should weigh 130 pounds, but that the mother might want to weigh 125. I then explained about the daily weight variance of a pound and a half, and that while they could choose their departure weights, they better be sure those weights were at least a pound and a half more than the chosen weight. I also stipulated to the girl that after she went home, she had to gain five pounds in the first month. I then turned to the mother and said, "If she does not gain five additional pounds in the first month she is home, you will bring her back to me in Phoenix where I will further supervise her."

> R: You now place them in a number of simple binds that allow them to choose their own weight but always in a therapeutic direction. You then unashamedly use a paradoxical bit of negative reinforcement in your threat of having the daughter brought back if she did not gain an additional five pounds the first month at home.

Shock and Utilizing an Ethical Value System

E: The mother had kept in constant telephone communication with her husband, and he too came to Arizona with the other four children, two of whom were older than my patient. After meeting him, in a separate interview I demanded to know what age and weight he was, and he stated that he was probably five pounds underweight as a preventive measure against diabetes mellitus. I asked him if there were any family history of diabetes and he said, "No, it is simply a preventive measure." Then in an impersonal, denunciative fashion I read the riot act to the father for gambling his daughter's life by setting an example of being underweight. I told him he could not leave Arizona until he gained five pounds, advising him to make allowance for weight variance.

274

I then had a separate interview with the seventeen-year-old brother and sixteen-year-old sister. I asked them how long they had been aware that their sister had not been eating enough and what they had done about it. They explained that the loss of weight had been noticeable for nearly a year. They had always offered her food, candy, and fruit, but their sister had always refused it, saying, "Keep it for yourself. I don't deserve it." I then read the riot act to the brother and sister for depriving my patient of her constitutional rights, the right to receive presents from her siblings. They were so taken aback by my impersonal riot act that they had no opportunity to recognize its specious character. After dismissing them, I called my patient in for a brief interview and read a most emphatic riot act to her about depriving her siblings and her parents of their constitutional rights to give her presents of any kind they wished.

> R: The father, brother, and sister are all "taken aback" by your impersonal riot acts, which so shocked them that their habitual mental sets were depotentiated and they had to search for new and more adequates responses, which you supply with your direct suggestion about "constitutional rights." You are actually *utilizing their highly ethical value system* in a way that shocks them and initiates a therapeutic change in their behavior. If they did not all have a tightly organized and rigid value system, your "riot act" would simply not work.

Conscience as a Metalevel

E: The mother and my patient attended my daughter's weeding, and my patient helped herself to a piece of wedding cake, although I made sure that she did not think that I knew about it.

On the day of departure the mother weighed 126½ and my patient, 76½ pounds. Before they left, my patient asked if I would permit her brother to take a picture of her sitting on my lap in my wheelchair. I agreed to this, and the brother took two Polaroid pictures. Shortly after her return home she had her father enlarge one of those pictures into a poster for her bedroom. I then reiterated to my patient that I was ordering her mother to bring her back to Arizona if she did not increase her weight by five pounds in the first month that she was home. As a parting gift I gave the girl a recipe for cinnamon pie, which my mother had invented years before I was born while running a boarding house for a mining camp in the Sierra Nevada mountains. When my patient reached home, she found a letter from me stating that I would like to have a copy of her school picture next September. There was also a very concise but emphatic statement that the question of her weight was one that belonged properly to her and her conscience, and nobody else need know it.

R: When the patient requested a photo of herself sitting on your lap, the nature of her parental transference onto you becomes obvious. Temporarily you become parent to this entire family. Your parting gift of a recipe for cinnamon pie is actually a kind of posthypnotic suggestion for a continuation of the pleasures in eating. Your immediate letter to her when she returned home requesting her school picture next September is an obvious way of extending your therapeutic influence over her for a more extended period of time, to reinforce her new eating behavior. At the same time you place her in a double bind by telling her that her weight was a matter of "her conscience, and nobody else need know her weight." You are again utilizing her strong conscience as a metalevel controlling her own behavior, even though you have had a hand in initiating it.

Six-Month Followup

E: I received the school picture in September, and she was a reasonably well-nourished fourteen-year-old girl. I received a Polaroid picture of her in a bathing suit, vacationing in the Bahamas at Christmastime, and she appeared to be a very attractive, well-nourished, strong, athletic girl. I still receive long, well-written letters from my patient, and there is always an indirect mention made of something edible in her letters. On the last occasion she stated that she thought my idea of having friends plant a tree as a way of noting my seventy-fifth birthday was an excellent one, and that she was going to plant a plum tree in the family garden in honor of my seventy-fifth birthday.

In the summer of 1974 she wrote a long, detailed account of the family's month-long trip around Europe, and she sent me a Christmas package of cookies which she said was traditional in her family.

I know of no other way of treating anorexia nervosa patients satisfactorily and rapidly. My first measure, of course, is to make clear to the mother or father, or both, that the therapy is going to be socially oriented, that the emotional and social needs will be the prime consideration, and that while I may be seemingly offensive, there is a worthy principle involved.

To initiate this type of therapy you have to be yourself as a person. You cannot imitate somebody else, but you have to do it in your own way.

Selected Shorter Cases: Exercises for Analysis
An Itch for Life

R: I have a patient who appears to be a deep-trance subject. As soon as I begin an induction, he immediately falls into a deep trance—so deep that he drools and shows no evidence of being able to give ideomotor signals until I begin to wake him up. He has an itching problem. He is a very successful young attorney who just wants to resolve that one psychosomatic complaint. He wants "fast therapy." He does not want to "fool around with a lot of insight," he says.

E: He goes so deeply in a trance that you can't do anything with him. So what part of the itch does he want to keep?

R: You feel the patient is afraid too much will be taken away?

E: Yes, he is protecting himself by going so deeply into trance. So you must not make the mistake of trying to take too much away. He's come to you with the problem of his itch, but he does not want it all removed.

R: How would you approach this problem, then? By letting him have a smaller itch over a more circumscribed part of his body or a less bothersome itch?

E: I'd say, "You're troubled by this itch. Naturally I don't know exactly what it is. I'm certain that you want *your itch for accomplishment to be kept. Your itch to do things can be kept. In fact, there are a number of itches that you want to keep. Any itch that you want to keep—be sure to keep it! Also let's be sure that you get rid of any itch you are willing to lose but no more than you are willing to lose.*"

R: What itches could he possibly want to keep?

E: An itch for political power, political position, for wealth, for sex! "Itch" is a folk word with many connotations about human desires and motivations.

R: I see! If I try to take away his "itch," it could be taking away an important aspect of his personality. He is a dynamo who works sixteen hours a day!

E: He has a big itch! Never forget folk language! You should always recognize how the folk language is related to symptom formation.

R: That's fascinating. He was actually referred to me by his girlfriend, whom I'm also treating for a similar problem of itching. She is a dynamo type also.

E: She must be another "itch" he has.

R: It may be that the folk language of "itch" is treated

literally by the right hemisphere, which then translates it into a psychosomatic process.

Folk language and the unconcious; Need for an individualized patient-centered approach; Structuring a therapeutic frame of reference.

Symptom Resolution Within the Self

A ten-year-old girl was brought to a lecture that the senior author was to present to a medical group. The parents requested that he use her as a demonstration subject for hypnosis, since that was the only way she would agree to see a physician. Noting that the girl was excessively clothed and that she was wearing gloves over her gloves, the senior author asked this girl if her parents had stated matters correctly. She stared at him intently for some moments and then nodded her head. She was told that the senior author did not understand the situation. Her explanation was most informative of her attitude: "I'm afraid. I don't want you to know what I'm afraid of. If I go to a doctor's office, he will try to make me tell or he will make my parents tell. I'm not ever going to let anybody know." She was instructed, "Without telling me what, just tell me how, so I will know if you are afraid of something you see, or hear, or think or whatever you can tell me." After some thought she answered briefly: "I don't want to get dirty." The general assumption was that the problem concerned a fear of contamination or a misophobia.

Because of such guarded behavior on her part the conclusion was reached that it would be well to inquire "in what manner" she would be willing to accept therapy. On that, too, she had remarkably restricted ideas. Her demand was that therapy be done by hypnosis (whatever that word meant to her), that the senior author was in no way to know the informative details of her problem, that therapy had to be done in such manner that it would not be recognizable as therapy—that is, there would be "no talk like a doctor who takes care of crazy people, just talk like when you visit"—and that to ensure this she would act as a demonstration subject "because a good doctor doesn't tell people anything about patients, not even that someone is a patient." (There was no opportunity to ascertain how she had devised her plan or what ideas had been presented to her before meeting the senior author.) Her parents did explain in her presence that she had forbidden them to give any information. She was asked how this help could be possible, dressed as she was, so carefully. Most earnestly she answered that she would go immediately to her hotel room and dress appropriately for a public appearance if the senior author agreed that she could have a chair that had not been sat on that day and if he agreed not to touch her dress. She was told that her wishes would be respected.

At the time of the lecture she came to the speaker's platform demurely, with her arms rather awkwardly held so that her hands did not touch her dress. Noting this, an available armchair was indicated to her, and she sat down and faced the audience with her arms resting on the arms of the chair. A discussion of hypnosis for children was presented, and then the senior author turned to her to induce hypnosis. The technique employed was exceedingly simple. The lecture and the audience provided a background of prestige for her. She was told to extend her left arm at shoulder level, with a slight dorsiflexion of her hand so that she could see her thumbnail. She was instructed to fixate her gaze on it, to see it seem to get bigger and bigger until it filled her visual field, and then, as it grew in size, she was to bend her elbow very, very slowly, bringing her hand ever closer to her face. As her hand came closer and closer, she was progressively to go into a deeper and deeper sleep until finally, when her hand or fingers touched any part of her face, she was to be completely sound asleep with her eyes open, seeing nothing, feeling nothing, hearing nothing, except the senior author.

Within a few minutes she developed a profound somnambulistic trance state, and the various phenomena of deep hypnosis were systematically demonstrated.

During the entire time after first seeing the girl, before the luncheon and during the lecture, the senior author had been frantically searching mentally for some kind of a therapeutic approach. Since the month was September, the thought of Thanksgiving, Christmas, and New Year's Day came to mind, and these suggested the possibility of a birthday. Hence, as she sat before the audience in a deep trance, she was asked if she would be willing to tell the senior author her birthday. She nodded her head affirmatively and said, "Yes." She was asked to name her birthday, and she gave the date as December 29th. This date immediately suggested a feasible plan.

The simple statement was made that while she might have hopes, she did not, at so early a time as September, know what birthday gifts she would receive. She could hope and hope, it was conceded, but she could not possibly know what her birthday presents really would be. Yet there could be something awfully nice, just wonderful, something that she wanted very badly, something that would be very special, even too important for her as a person to be just a Christmas gift. It would have to be a birthday gift. Of course she might not get it because she would have to do a lot of awful good thinking so she would know what she surely wanted most of all. And what might this present really be? It might be something she could do herself, that she could learn, like the best marks of all the students in her school, or learning so slowly and carefully to knit a whole dress for herself, or how to sew a complete dress for herself. But it could be any special, special thing that she wanted, wanted awful bad. Certainly the senior author couldn't know—in fact, all that he knew was that he was very certain that her birthday would be her eleventh and that she would be leaving the little girls and becoming the kind of a big girl she wanted to be.

Then, under the guise of merely presenting to the audience the topics of hypnotic amnesia and posthypnotic suggestions, a series of statements was made to the effect that posthypnotic suggestions, if there were a purpose to be served, could be given to a subject to effect a total amnesia for all trance events and experiences; that one could tell the subject who wished to achieve some particular goal of psychological or emotional importance that there could be an ever-increasing feeling of conviction, of certainty that the desired achievement would come to pass; that day by day, week after week, there could be a mounting feeling of unidentified expectancy, a feeling of intense, pleasurable tension to the effect that some change was slowly, progressively taking place within the self which would become known and fully realized at any chosen time or on the occasion of some special event. All of these statements were presented as seemingly explanatory remarks to the audience, but to the subject's ears they were posthypnotic suggestions. Yet even her father, a professional man, and her mother, a college graduate, sitting in the audience expectantly awaiting some definite therapeutic suggestions, did not grasp the pointedness for their daughter of what was being said. After the lecture, with much concern, the father—in the absence of his daughter, who had been rather quickly dismissed following the remarks on amnesia and posthypnotic suggestion and who had left the auditorium in the company of her mother—asked worriedly when the senior author proposed to do the therapy. He was urgently admonished that the therapy had been done, that he must warn his wife not to discuss anything at all about the lecture or the meeting of the senior author by the daughter. Instead they were to follow a program of silent, watchful waiting.

As was learned later, one month after her birthday, the girl gave her father permission to write to the senior author to tell him that she was no longer afraid, that after the lecture she got a "funny feeling" everytime she "was afraid" that "something nice was going to happen to her." This feeling grew progressively stronger until her birthday on which day she awakened early and aroused the entire household with almost hysterical shouts of "It's gone, it's gone," whereupon she had put herself to test in a great variety of ways. He went on to explain that she had forbidden him to write the news to the senior author but that when a month had elapsed, she gave permission but forbade him to give any description of her problem. She insisted that, since it was "over with, all gone," there was no reason even to think about it, that the only important item of news was the fact of her recovery. He pleaded with her to let him write more but she was adamant until he raised the question of telling the senior author a bit about her behavior from September to her birthday. After considerable thought she agreed but stated she would want to see the account before it was mailed. He began with the above account, stating that he and his wife had noted a slow progressive change in the girl's behavior. Her depressive behavior, her outbursts of anger, her general impatience and her tense anxieties progressively diminished. She began crying less until by December she had ceased entirely to cry at frequent unexpected intervals. Her extreme caution about clothes diminished and she began running to the door every time the doorbell rang or the postman came as if she expected something. They also noted that more and more frequently she would pick up chair cushions and look under them, feel behind the books in the bookcase as if looking for something. Whenever she was asked by her siblings what she was doing, she would answer, "Oh nothing, I just thought maybe something was there."

Her school behavior also changed progressively. She no longer had violent emotional outbursts if the other children accidentally violated her taboos—they had learned to avoid her through distressing experience ever since the sudden onset of her trouble, which had been in April of the year the senior author saw her.

Three years later a pert young lady approached the senior author at a medical meeting and asked, "Do you really think you can hypnotize me?" The reply was made, "I think you can learn to go into a trance." To this she answered, "That's just about what you told me before," and laughed merrily as the senior author scrutinized her face unrecognizingly. Then she added, "I only wear one pair of gloves now when I do wear gloves. Now you know me." The senior author immediately agreed and inquired about her father and mother and waited hopefully and silently. She studied his face, then remarked soberly, "No, really, I can't tell you except to say it's all gone and many, many thanks." She seemed genuinely regretful not to be more informative. Her father was encountered and, after greetings, shook his head, stating that the taboo of disclosure still held, but that her recovery remained a pleasurable fact.

Interspersal approach; Indirect ideodynamic focusing; Initiating unconscious searches and processes; Expectancy; Hypnotherapy without the therapist knowing the patient's dynamics; Indirect hypnotic amnesia and posthypnotic suggestion; associating fears with positive expectation; Progressive therapeutic change.

CHAPTER 7

Memory Revivication

Case 10 Resolving a Traumatic Experience

Part One: Somnambulistic Training, Autohypnosis, and Hypnotic Anesthesia

Mrs. F. gave birth to her first child with caudal anesthesia so that she could participate as consciously and as actively as possible. She felt, however, that she had still missed an important aspect of participation in the birth process. For some reason she could not remember much of what had happened. Three months after the child was born she came to Dr. Erickson with a request that he use hypnosis to help her recover her memories of giving birth to her child. Dr. Marion Moore (M) was a participant-observer in this session. The senior author begins this first session by facilitating a therapeutic frame of reference for memory recall as follows.

Suggestions for Recovering Memories: Truisms Covering Many Possibilities of Response

E: To uncover that memory and return it to you is not likely to occur all at once. What is likely to happen is that you'll remember a little bit here and next week a little bit there. The following week some more of the first part. The following week it slowly builds up in a regular fashion. And then some day the whole thing will straighten out.

> R: You begin with a series of psychological *truisms* about how we do in fact tend to recover memories piece by piece over time. These suggestions, given in the form of educational directions, are actually so general that they cover *many possibilities of*

response. You are giving her unconscious the freedom to work in its own optimal manner.

F: Could you explain simply why the mind works like that?

E: It's like other learning processes. Why is it that babies tend to learn certain words first, yet they always learn other words in different orders? In your own experience: Why are there always certain sentences in a chapter that you clearly remember after the first reading? You select certain things. Next time you read it you get a lot more, but your first reading was highly selective. You can't know and I can't know—nobody can know—just how *you are going to remember any one.* **[The senior author gives a number of examples of the disorderly way people go about recalling memories in everyday life. He illustrates this further by asking her to recall what she had for dinner last night, thus validating within her own immediate experience the fact that her recall comes out in a piecemeal, out-of-sequence order.]**

> R: You answer her question about why the mind works like that with what appears to be a straightforward lecture about the process of learning. You carefully insert a rhetorical question or two about her own early learning and memory processes to evoke her own unconscious associations, and then add a series of examples of how memory works in others. You are not making any demand on her at this time. You are, rather, engaged in a process of ideodynamic focusing. Your general discussion about early learning and memory is automatically evoking ideodynamic responses within her on an unconscious level. Some of these ideodynamic processes may be already intruding into her consciousness in the form of her early memories, or they may remain on an unconscious level at this point. Your simple discussion of these processes, however, tends to evoke or prime them for a vivid conscious experience if you ask for them later during trance. Otherwise, as you have already suggested, the memories she wants may appear piece by piece over time.
>
> E: Yes, I'm emphasizing her own natural memory patterns,— rather than having her rely on some way of remembering she was artificially taught—when I say she can't know and I can't know. Notice the interspersed suggestion, *"you are going to remember."* Consciously she does not hear that direct suggestion because her conscious mind is focused on the "how" that precedes the direct suggestion, *"you are going to remember."*

283

Indirect Hypnotic Forms Preparing for Trance Induction

E: All right, how do you think I will induce a trance in you?

F: Well, I know there is a way by counting one to ten, I believe. I know very little about it.

> R: You begin this trance induction with an indirect form of suggestion: the question, "how do you think I will induce a trance in you?" This question already *implies* that you will induce trance; it's now only a question of how. The question tends to evoke whatever understanding she may have of trance induction so you could possibly utilize it. The question also respects her life experience and individuality; she has an opportunity to express her knowledge and possible preferences. As such, this question tends to mobilize her good will and an *acceptance set* for whatever follows.

Trance Induction via not Knowing and not Doing: The Early Learning Set Induction: Unconscious Conditioning

E: Will you sit back in your chair with your feet flat on the floor and your hands on your thighs. The hands not touching each other, and just look at one single spot here.

You don't need to talk.

You don't need to move.

You don't even need to listen to me.

Your unconscious mind is close enough to me

to hear me.

And that's the only important thing.

Now there are various changes

that take place in you.

Your heart is beating at a different rate.

Your breathing has changed.

Your reflexes have altered.

And you are doing the same thing

now that you did when you first went to school.

You looked at letters of

the alphabet.

They seemed impossible to learn.

But you did learn them.

And you developed a mental image
of the letters
and the numerals.
And you developed a mental image of each of them in various forms that
stayed with you for the rest of your life.
You have looked at that one spot long enough so you have a mental image,
and you do not know where it is in your mind.
You can close your eyes
N . . . O . . . W

E: When she responds initially by sitting back in her chair with feet flat on the floor, she is saying to herself that she will *go into trance*. These initial adjustments allow her to make that important suggestion to herself rather than my telling her. It's always much better to have patients make the important suggestions to themselves.

R: You now embark upon your favorite form of trance induction via eye fixation and a number of indirect hypnotic forms that are effective precisely because no one could really argue with anything you say. The patient is lulled into *not knowing and not doing* (need not talk, move, or even listen) to *depotentiate her conscious sets*. A *dissociation* is facilitated by your emphasis on her unconscious functioning as a subtle form of the conscious-unconscious double bind.

E: Not needing to listen to me is an indirect way of emphasizing that it's her own personal experience, not mine.

R: You then *ratify* the process of trance experience as an altered state by pointing out how physiological changes have taken place (heartbeat, breathing, and reflexes). You conclude this initial stage of trance induction with the early learning set (Erickson, Rossi, and Rossi, 1976) that tends to evoke ideodynamic aspects of early childhood learning, when so much was absorbed on an autonomous or unconscious level. These early learning patterns may now be activated for learning trance experience, which must also proceed on as much of an autonomous level as possible. You then precipitate eye closure with the direct suggestion to close her eyes "N . . . O . . . W" said in a slow but quietly emphatic and insistent manner. This particular vocal emphasis now acquires the value of an unconscious *conditioned stimulus*. The next time you use that low tone of voice with similar emphasis and insistence, she will tend

285

to enter trance but not really know why. If you later use the word "now" to awaken her, you will use a clear, quick, bright, and louder tone of voice that will acquire the value of a conditioned stimulus for awakening.

Trance Deepening via Contingency Suggestion: Pause as an Indirect Suggestion

E: And with each breath you go deeper and sounder   in the deep hypnotic sleep.
[Pause]
Now you know why
you want to go into a trance.
You do not fully understand why some of that memory escaped you.
[Pause]

R: You are using a contingency suggestion when you now facilitate trance-deepening by associating deeper trance with an inevitable behavior—breathing.

E: I pause after telling her to "go deeper and sounder" because that does take time. The pause itself is an indirect suggestion to do that now.

R: You then further motivate her for deepening trance by reminding her of her purpose in seeking hypnosis. You thus utilize her own motivation for deepening trance.

An Associational Network Facilitating an Unconscious Search for Lost Memories

E: But the mental images that you formed
in kindergarten
are still within your mind.
Things long forgotten
still have
their mental images in your mind.
You can lose learnings by the loss of brain cells.
But you haven't lost the brain cells concerned with your delivery.
[Pause]
And those mental images belong to you,
and you can enjoy getting them back.
And I think the best way of getting them back

286

is doing so by getting one small one and being completely delighted by it.
Not asking for more,
but just enjoying the pleasure
and delight of that one little memory.
And the next thing you know
you'll get another little memory that will give you a great deal of pleasure
and delight.
And doing it this way
you will build up your pleasure and comfort and ease
very rapidly.
Not rapidly in time but rapidly in force,
in strength.
And then some day you'll realize
you really do have all of it.
And when one uses the unconscious mind,
one does it
at the rate of speed that belongs to the unconscious.
Your unconscious knows how fast it can work,
how fast your conscious mind works.
And your unconscious will know how to feed that memory back to you.

E: I now follow up on my earlier remark about "that memory escaped you" by pointing out how even earlier mental images are "still within your mind." This implies that the escaped memory is still within and available to her.

R: You are now building up an associational network wherein you utilize the early learning set you evoked earlier as an *analogy* or *ideodynamic process* that could facilitate her conscious mind does not know how to do it (that's why she came to therapy). Analogy and/or ideodynamic processes thus function here as indirect hypnotic forms to facilitate that search on an unconscious level. You then leave it to her *unconscious to mediate the process* in a manner that is most suited to its own functioning (fast or slow, a lot at once or a little, and so on).

E: I admit to her that there is a way of losing memories by a loss of brain cells, but I affirm that is not the case with her.

R: You thereby pick up some doubts she might have about being able to recover her memories, and depotentiate them.

E: When I affirm that the "mental images belong to you and you can enjoy getting them back," I'm referring back to my earlier remark about how they "escaped you" and the implication that she deserves to get back what belongs to her. I then emphasize the delight one little memory can give her.

R: That can reinforce her so that she will tend to have more and finally a chain of recovered memories.

E: "Someday you'll realize you have all of it" implies a *noncritical acceptance* of each small bit of memory as it comes. I'm attempting to rule out self-criticism.

R: That conscious self-criticism can so limit the spontaneous creativity of the unconscious.

E: Yes, I say it "belongs to the unconscious" and the unconscious knows how fast it works. I then contrast that with "how fast your conscious mind works," thereby separating the conscious and unconscious.

R: You emphasize the separation of conscious and unconscious to make sure she leaves it to the unconscious rather than try to work on it with the more limited means of her conscious processes. That is the essence of your hypnotic approach: *depotentiating the conscious mind's limited means and reinforcing unconscious processes with their greater potentialities*.

E: Yes, and the separation is stated in such a way that it has to be accepted because what I'm saying is true.

R: Hypnosis is not a means of directly programming people to do things in one way. With billions of neurological connections in the mind it is terribly presumptuous to try to program people.

E: It is a very uninformed way.

R: We are allowing the infinite diversity of the unconscious to come forth rather than trying to program one idiotic idea or point of view we may have. There are infinite patterns of learning and ways of doing things. Our approach helps people unlearn their learned limitations.

Surprise and Pleasure to Reinforce Unconscious Functioning: Safety Suggestions

E: Many times in the past you have been taken by surprise.
And before you could think of what to do,
you just did it
because your unconscious knew

before you did.

[Pause]

And this is a situation for you

to be willing to let your unconscious mind

return that memory to you

in the way it knows you should get it back.

There is no hurry.

But there is a pleasure awaiting you.

[Pause]

R: You use surprise as another indirect hypnotic form that will tend to *depotentiate the limitations of her conscious sets and habitual attitudes* that may be blocking her memories. You reinforce this by again emphasizing the central role of the unconscious being allowed to work in its own. You continually suggest that "pleasure" and "enjoyment" will accompany the *unconscious search and processes*. This is in part a truism and in part a means of motivating her further. It would be a significant research problem to determine if, in fact, such suggestions for pleasure are ideodynamically mediating further reinforcement by activating the positive reward centers of the limbic system.

E: If there are any resistances or hidden trauma associated with these memories, I'm using a safety factor by suggesting that her unconscious will "return that memory to you in the way it knows you should get it back." I then balance a negative and a positive in the next suggestion, "There is *no* hurry . . . there *is* a pleasure awaiting you." The negative emphasizes the positive.

Separating Conscious and Unconscious Processes: Trance Awakening and Ratification: Training in Posthypnotic Suggestion

E: I'm going to have you awaken shortly

for a lesson

in enjoying what your unconscious can do for you.

When I awaken you,

I want you to have a very profound feeling of comfort, as if you had been

sleeping for eight hours.

I want you to enjoy that.

[Pause]

Now you can start thinking

289

about counting backward from twenty to one,

waking up one-twentieth of the way at each count.

And you can begin counting backward from twenty to one, awakening at one.

And begin the counting *now*!

[Pause as Mrs. F silently counts to herself and opens her eyes and begins body reorientation in twenty seconds]

E: I emphasize that I am going to awaken her because I don't want her unconscious to awaken her. It's the job of her unconscious to turn up those memories. It's my job in association with her conscious mind to awaken her. I carefully separate the conscious and unconscious and keep them separate.

R: You begin the process of awakening her with a subtle posthypnotic suggestion that is very easy to accept. Her trance experience up to now has given every appearance of the deeply comfortable, receptive sort that is sometimes difficult to distinguish from sleep. You therefore *utilize* this to ratify her trance on awakening. Whatever behavior the patients manifest during trance (concentration, restlessness, emotions, etc.) can be used to ratify trance with a posthypnotic suggestion that allows them to respond with some expression about it upon awakening. This is your initial approach in training her to follow posthypnotic suggestions. You finally awaken her with that "now!" said in that bright and alert tone that will become an unconsciously conditioned stimulus for awakening.

Posthypnotic Suggestion Ratifying Trance: The Patient's Experience as the Focus of Attention

F: Hi! How was I? Oh, I felt like I went to sleep! You know? Like I went to sleep. That was strange.

E: A beautiful demonstration.

F: Did I go into a trance like I should have?

E: How do you feel?

F: It was sleep yet it wasn't sleep. It was like a borderline to sleep.

E: How do you feel physically now?

F: Much more relaxed. Much more at peace. I feel much more with it. I

290

heard your voice, and it became a little fainter, but it was there in the background.

M: But you ceased to hear individual words and sentences?

F: Yes, just a voice.

M: Did you hear my cassette recorder start and stop?

F: No, I did not hear any other thing.

R: Her first words on awakening are an obvious response to your posthypnotic suggestion to feel as if she's had eight hours of sleep. She is also ratifying trance at the same time. She describes the comfortable, quiet, and receptive type of trance where no conscious effort is being made in any direction. This is in sharp contrast with the deeply searching, concentrated, and furrowed brow that was characteristic of X's trance (sweating case). The dissociation wherein F could hear the therapist's voice in the background but not the individual words and sentences is very characteristic of trance.

E: My voice in the background is where I want it to be. It's in the background of *her* experience. Her own experience is in the focus of attention.

R: You evoke the patients' own inner experiences as the therapeutic factor so that they don't hear irrelevant things (such as the cassette recorder). This is the opposite of so many therapists who insist that the patients focus on the therapist's words and views.

E: I asked her, "How do you *feel*?" because I did not want her *thinking*.

R: It can be entirely valid to *feel* as if she had eight hours of sleep, but it would be a falsehood to ask her to really *think* she had had eight hours of sleep when you both know she has not. You are always careful to avoid anything that would cause disbelief and a loss of faith in the validity of whatever you say.

E: I always distinguish between thinking and feeling: Thinking can be valid but it's limited; a feeling can be anything even though it's an illusion from a rational point of view.

Somnambulistic Training: Indirect Posthypnotic Suggestion for Trance Induction by Catalepsy

E: Would you like a surprise?

F: OK what is it?

[The senior author silently reaches over and touches her right hand with a very slight guiding motion. Her hand lifts and remains cataleptic, suspended in midair.]

E: Close your eyes and go to sleep.

And you can really feel pleased,

and happy,

and rested.

> E: In her first trance I mentioned how she'd been taken by *surprise* many times in the past when her unconscious knew something before she did. That was an unrecognized posthypnotic suggestion that is now being used to induce this second trance with a surprise.
>
> R: This trance induction by catalepsy (Erickson, Rossi, and Rossi, 1976) is also a way of deepening her hypnotic involvement with a nonverbal approach. You then deepen the trance by utilizing the "sleep . . . happy . . . and rested" experience, which you now know she is very capable of experiencing. You are beginning somnambulistic training by giving her many experiences of entering and awakening from trance. What other means have you for facilitating the somnambulistic state?
>
> E: It's like learning anything else in life. The first time you read a textbook, you may not understand much; after you've read it two or three times, it begins to make sense. *Rehearsal of trance, posthypnotic suggestion, and further hypnotic training are all being given at the same time to develop somnambulistic behavior.*

Trance Awakening with Open-Ended Posthypnotic Suggestion

E: And if you wish,

you can leave your right arm where it is

after you awaken.

And you can begin counting backward from twenty to one, awakening at one.

And start the counting *now*!

(Mrs. F awakens with her arm remaining cataleptic in midair.)

> R: You now give a very open-ended posthypnotic suggestion to leave her hand there if she wishes. This open-ended approach is

fail-safe and tends to evoke an *acceptance set* by allowing the patient to express her own individuality. It is also a means of further assessing to what degree she is willing and ready to experience further hypnotic phenomena.

Trance Ratification via the Patient's Own Experience

F: Umm. What is my arm doing there? What is this? [She withdraws her arm from its cataleptic pose.]
Why was that up in the air?

E: Do you realize you've learned how to go into a trance?

F: I was thinking about that and just wondering if I have grasped enough to do this myself. I'll go home and try it unless you'd rather I not.

> E: I don't answer her question directly but ask her a question that would evoke her own experiential learning.
>
> R: Your question is an indirect hypnotic form that makes her search within and answer her own question about her hand in a manner that tends to ratify her experience of trance. Her hand does not usually act that way; therefore she must have been in trance. Her response of wanting to do it at home is now a direct acknowledgment of having experienced trance.

Third Trance: Induction and Posthypnotic Suggestion for Learning

E: You never waste a good skill on unimportant things. You use it only on important things. You would not use hypnotic anesthesia for a pin-prick, but you would use it for childbirth, surgery, for the pain of a broken leg.
Now do you want to see what you have learned?
[The senior author again induces an arm catalepsy by guiding her arm upward. Mrs. F blinks and closes her eyes and evidently goes into a trance.]
And you can leave your arm there and recognize what you have learned after you awaken.
And you can awaken by starting counting now.
[F awakens with her arm still cataleptic.]

F: That is . . . oh!
[F puts her arm down.]

R: You respond to her request for what amounts to autohypnotic training by first cautioning her to use trance only on important things. Why?

E: I'm forbidding any unimportant experimentation. The important thing is to get her memory back—not to see if she can levitate her hand.

R: Trivial experimentation tends to blur the distinction between the trance and awake state and lessen the dissociation between them, which in turn lessens the effectiveness of trance. After inducing the catalepsy, you give an important posthypnotic suggestion that she can leave her arm there and recognize what she learned after awakening. She does in fact awaken with the arm still cataleptic and then apparently has some inner realization and only then puts her arm down. Presumably she's learned an association between hand levitation and trance.

Fourth Trance: Autohypnotic Training via Training and Expectancy

E: Now suppose you raise your hand.

[F lifts her hand until it remains posed in balanced tonicity (catalepsy). She closes her eyes and evidently enters trance.]

R: In asking her to lift her own hand this time, are you placing trance induction more under her own control as a stage in autohypnotic training?

E: I did not tell her to go into trance. When you tell someone to raise or extend the hand, they are going to *expect* something. You're using that expectancy learned in everyday life.

R: And what else is there to expect in this situation except trance? You have built an association between hand levitation and trance so that she can expect and does, in fact, go into trance entirely on her own. This may look superficially like a process of conditioning (and it may be in part), but it's the element of *expectancy* as well as her own *motivation* for trance that leads her to experience it here.

E: I didn't define it as trance. I let her own experience define it.

Implied Directive to Ratify Trance: The Careful Study of Communication by the Therapist

E: And when you have recognized that you are in a good trance, you can tell yourself about awakening.

[After a few moments F awakens and reorients all on her own.]

F: Um! My word! I'm taken sort of by surprise by all of this.

E: A pleasant surprise.

F: The mind is an unbelievable organ, isn't it! This is wonderful.

E: All right. Now you know you can lift your hand and go into trance, and when you have been in a trance sufficiently, your unconscious mind can tell you to awaken.
Now you know you can do that. You have just had that experience.

F: Yes.

> R: You now use the implied directive as a means of having her recognize, explore, and validate her own trance experience. It is very important in autohypnotic training to give the patients an opportunity to recognize and ratify their own trance experiences.
>
> E: When she says, "I'm taken . . . by surprise," you know she's following my posthypnotic suggestion for a surprise. The validity of the experience is expressed in her own words, "The mind is an unbelievable organ . . . This is wonderful," not mine.
>
> R: Above all, hypnosis is experiential learning rather than intellectual or abstract knowing.
>
> E: I want you to notice how connected everything is even though it's all impromptu. *It is a language I've learned, a careful study. I know all the articles of speech and I know the meanings of all the words. Because I learned it carefully, I can speak it easily.*
>
> R: It seems casual but it's well-rehearsed in your mind.

Generalizing Successful Hypnotic Experience For Problem Solving

E: You can also know now that your unconscious can do what is necessary about that memory. And you can trust it to do it in the right way.

F: Yes. Is there ever a situation when you're in the trance and cannot come out of it? Like the door closes and you cannot get it open.
[Erickson gives examples illustrating that an individual in trance can awaken at will for any good reason.]

> R: You illustrate the potency of her unconscious in a concrete

way (via entering and coming out of trance) and then make this important generalization that her unconscious can also facilitate memory recall. That is, you immediately utilize her successful trance experience as a model of how the unconscious can contribute to her behavior and how it can facilitate a solution to her problem.

Unconscious Protecting the Individual

E: Your unconscious knows how to protect you.

F: There is some protection? I thought the unconscious was completely open?
[E gives examples of how the unconscious can protect the individual.]

E: Your unconscious mind knows what is right and what is good. When you need protection, it will protect you.

R: It is one of the most common misconceptions of hypnosis that you lose all your control and faculties. Hypnosis is actually a very selective form of attention.

> R: In one of your earliest research programs you demonstrated that it was not possible to force people into destructive behavior with hypnosis (Erickson, 1932). Do you still believe that is so? Does the unconscious *always* protect the person?
>
> E: Yes, but often in ways that the conscious mind does not understand.

Surprise and Indirect Suggestions for Caudal Anesthesia

[A general discussion about childbirth with hypnosis takes place. In a surprise move Erickson suddenly suggests the possibility of Mrs. F experiencing a caudal anesthesia as follows.]

E: By the way, did you know that you could produce your own caudal N . . . O . . . W.

F: Well, that would take a lot more time though, wouldn't it?

> R: The general discussion about childbirth seems innocent enough, but it's actually a means of structuring a new mental framework through indirect ideodynamic focusing; by discussing childbirth in the most general terms her unconscious will automatically initiate many ideodynamic processes she actually

experienced in her recent childbirth experience. These include, of course, a caudal anesthesia induced by chemical means. Her unconscious has a record of this experience, and when you ask her the *question,* "did you know that you could produce your own caudal N . . . O . . . W?" you are using two indirect hypnotic forms to induce trance and initiate an *unconscious search and process* that may help her reexperience her caudal anesthesia as a hypnotic response: 1) "N . . . O . . . W" spoken in the slow, low, insistent manner tends to reinduce trance as an unconsciously conditioned response; 2) the *question* initiates the *unconscious search and processes* for the ideodynamic memories of her chemical caudal anesthesia. This all happens automatically (hypnotically) even though her mind doubts, "that would take a lot more time though, wouldn't it?"

E: You did not recognize the element of surprise as a third factor.

Surprise and Vocal Cues for Reinforcing Anesthesia

E: **Now you listen to me because you are going to be very surprised** *because you can't stand up.*
[Mrs. F looks a bit startled, and her body remains perfectly still for about fifteen seconds as the senior author continues.]

E: **You don't know how to stand up, do you?**

F: **Well I did when I**
came in here.

E: *You've got a caudal!*

R: Since she did express some doubt, you then reinforce your suggestions with more emphasis on the *surprise* aspect of unconscious functioning (particularly since she earlier appeared to like this surprise aspect), and your slow, low, insistent vocal cues (in italics) which are by now well associated with hypnotic responsiveness.

Removal and Ratification of Hypnotic Response

[Pause as Mrs. F remains motionless for another fifteen seconds, then Erickson removes it as follows.]

E: **Now you can move!**

F: [She looks a bit incredulous and finally shifts her lower body a little.] Is this a joke or is this real? Because with the caudal the only thing I could move was my big toe.

E: That's right. You see, I know what a caudal is, and when I give a hypnotic suggestion that you cannot stand up, you lose the ability to use your leg muscles.

F: Oh, boy! What an education I've gotten today!

> R: You let her remain immobile for only eighteen seconds. Is that because you sensed she doubted her hypnotic response and may have broken out of it by testing it too much?

> E: You develop a sense for these things. I do know that I wanted to stay away from any dispute about her big toe.

Protecting and Further Ratifying Hypnotic Responsiveness: Unrecognized Posthypnotic Suggestion Via Generalization

E: Now don't try to explain your learnings to anybody. They belong to you and they are special, and when your child starts growing up and hurts his arm, you can remember how I told you gently, "You can't stand up." And you couldn't. You can tell your child he is going to feel all right now. You say it and you mean it. Your sincerity and your expectancy will cause that child to accept the suggestion, and his arm won't hurt.

[The senior author now tells a story about how he taught a physician to use the *surprise technique of anesthesia.*]

A farmer came into the emergency room with a serious wound, shouting over and over in a state of panic, "Doctor, you've got to help me! Doctor, you've got to help!" The nurse tried to get the farmer seated, but he just kept pacing back and forth and shouting. Finally the doctor said, "Shut up! Sit down! Stop hurting!" I had told the doctor he could do that, and he tried it out. Ordinarily you don't talk to a patient that way. The farmer was so surprised that he did sit down and stopped hurting. That is the surprise technique.

> R: You then protect her hypnotic learning by cautioning her about listening to any doubting views from others?

> E: Yes. When I associate her current hypnotic learning with *inevitable* things that will happen to her child, I'm extending

these learnings into her future as an unrecognized posthypnotic suggestion.

R: You're thereby generalizing her hypnotic learning to future life situations.

E: I now generalize it further with this other story of how I taught a physician the surprise technique of anesthesia.

R: The story also tends to further resolve any inner doubts she may have of her hypnotic response and thus ratifies it further.

Surprise to Initiate Another Unconscious Search

M: **Might I add one thing to her memory, as it is going to come in the picture. She is going to have one additional thing that will be a very delightful surprise when she recalls it. It will have something to do with the time of rotation (of the baby's head during the birth process). I'll just leave it at that. It will be the little flower on the icing of the cake.**

R: Dr. Moore's suggestion that the patient will have another "additional . . . very delightful surprise" is a further means of motivating her for a thorough *unconscious search* for the memories she wishes to recover. We will see the truth this suggestion brings forth in the next session.

Concluding Directives for the Unconscious Search: Focus on the Patient's Experience

E: **One thing more: Your returning memories will start. What time did you say the water bag broke?**

F: **About 6:40 A.M.**

E: **The memories will start by a sudden recovery of that memory, very intense, and then you can go on to the rest. You see, you weren't asking for the breaking of the water bag. You are asking for something hours later. Your unconscious will probably pick out the breaking of the water and then go on.**

F: **Because that was the start of the event?**

E: **Yes.**

F: **I remember that very clearly.**
[Mrs. F now recounts the circumstances of how her water bag broke and the unexpected suddenness of her child's birth.]

E: You've already outlined to me a memory you didn't know you had. And you are going to find it out.

F: The memory is going to come back in pieces?

E: I don't know how you are going to do it. You may get it back in one piece, you may get it back backward and not till it is all there will you straighten it out.

M: You might remember the nice things first.

R: Why did you give her these final very specific suggestions for recovering her memories?

E: I'm giving her a base within her own experience. She remembers 6:40 very well, and that can serve as a foundation for the recall of more memories. It's a marker around which she can organize her memories. When she lost her memories, she never really tried to restructure her recall as I'm now suggesting. When she now begins to recount the circumstances of how her water bag broke, she is following my implied suggestion where I've been telling her all along, "This is your experience. It belongs to you. I'm only a background. Your own experience is the foreground."

Part Two: Reorganizing Traumatic Life Experience and Memory Revivication

Two weeks after the preceding session Mrs. F returns to report as follows:

F: I had two items that came to me concerning the birth of my child. In that twilight state between being awake and asleep I recovered a vivid, detailed memory I had forgotten of being in the doctor's office. Why it came up I cannot tell you, but it did. The doctor came in the door and asked, "Have you felt life?" and I said, "Yes, since yesterday." The doctor said, "That's normal, that's when you should begin to feel life." I then woke up and thought, that's strange, I wonder why I remembered that? My mind seemed to pull it out of its memory bank.

[F reports that a few days after the above she had a more extensive recovery of memories while in another twilight state between being awake and asleep. She recalls being in the delivery room and her doctor being gowned in preparation for the delivery of her child. An edited version of her report continues as follows.]

300

F: All the details of that particular time frame came to me. Slowly—this has been a very slow process like you said it would be, it wasn't overnight. Very slowly the whole sequence of the delivery came more and more to the fore of my conscious mind. It was very slow over quite a few days. A little more sharper and a little more sharper. And it all seemed to hinge on two days when my mind decided to pull out certain memories or thoughts somehow. How, I don't know. I was surprised. Especially remembering sharply the part about the delivery. It was all related to the recovery of that earlier memory of the visit to the doctor's office, where he asked about feeling life. That's what was important to my mind.

I noticed also I'm more able to put into order the things that I can vividly recall. I can put them in order instead of a hodgepodge with nothing fitting as it should. That's what's transpired since the last time I saw you.

E: And was there any one or few moments during the delivery that became very vivid?

F: The most vivid memory was of those green leg coverings that the doctor wore. I know my mind exaggerated them. They were huge!
[E asks pointed questions, which elicit a train of associations suggesting that F's memory of "life" in the doctor's office was very important to her and associated with her memories in the delivery room because "life" was a strong reassurance against many negative and fearful stories she had been told about the dangers of childbirth. These negative expectations had been unfortunately reinforced just moments before the delivery of her child because she heard the painful cries of another woman who had just given birth to a stillborn child. She continues to recount with indignation a number of the hospital's "unnatural" procedures, such as tying her hands down during the delivery as if she were some kind of "wild animal without any sense," and not preparing her for the episiotomy. She was shocked to hear the "snip" of the doctor's instruments cutting her flesh during the episiotomy.]

Spontaneous Personality Maturation with Memory Recall

E: Do you want to find if you can remember better in the trance than in the waking state?

F: I think I would.

E: Have you noticed any change in yourself as a person since we last saw you?

F: Less anxiety in every way. The more uptight you become, the less well you remember, and it becomes a vicious circle.

E: How much older do you feel?

F: I feel my age. Sometimes I feel fifty, but usually I feel pretty good. That's a strange question, isn't it?

E: You appear slightly older now. Not in looks but in the sound of your speech and manner. The arrangement of your ideas is slightly older.

F: How come? How could I age in a week?

E: Because that memory was important to you, and you were so up-tight that you did not allow all the maturing possible to take place from childbirth. And that, I judge, constitutes some of the reason for your anxiety.

F: Oh, now I see.

R: Having that amnesia could retard a natural process of maturation. Someplace within her she understood that, and thus her concern to recover those memories in as clear a form as possible to facilitate her natural growth process.

E: Her unconscious knew something that she could not even dream and receive consciously. Now you see what I mean by unconscious wisdom?

F: Which is smarter, the conscious or the unconscious?

E: The unconscious is much smarter, wiser, and quicker. It understands better.

F: That's just fabulous isn't it!

R: You begin with a question about whether she would like to find out if she can remember better in trance, you obtain her assent, and then bounce onto this other question about her more mature manner. You evidently saw some behavioral resistance to trance at this point, so you delay trance induction till later.

E: [The senior author recounts clinical examples of how the natural process of personality maturation can be blocked by traumatic experiences that result in amnesias, since the life experience has not been integrated. The deeper meaning of her request to recover her lost memories is now evident: These memories are important for her current and future personality growth and maturation.]

Body Language in Trance Resistance

E: **What is your reluctance about going into a trance today?**
[E noticed that F had her legs crossed]

F: **Did I show that to you? I have no reluctance.**

E: **You have a minor reluctance.**

F: **Well, boy, you must be extremely perceptive. I don't, what is it that makes you feel this way?**

E: **I'm not going to prompt your conscious mind. I prefer what your unconscious tells me.**

F: **I did not notice any reluctance at all. Is it the manner of speech, mannerisms?**

E: **Don't try to guess it. Your unconscious is doing a beautiful job. It will let you know. DO   YOU   WANT   TO   GO   INTO   A
       TRANCE   TODAY?**

F: **Yes.**

E: **N . . . O . . . W?**

F: **Okay.**

E: **[To R] You've seen the answer, haven't you?**

R: **Yes, I think I do.**

E: **I didn't say. [To F] Uncross your legs please. [Pause as she uncrosses her legs and adopts the more typical posture for trance induction]**
N . . . O . . . W.
[Pause as F's eyes flutter and then close]
Go way deep into the trance.
[Pause]

E: At the end of the last session Dr. Moore suggested she would remember something that would be "the little flower on the icing of the cake," but she makes no reference to it in this initial

303

account. Since she has not tried to identify it, she may be reluctant to enter trance where she may be faced with it.

R: I notice she also had her legs crossed, which is the opposite of what you advise during trance induction. She keeps them crossed during your initial effort with the conditional "N . . . O . . . W" and doesn't enter trance until you ask her to uncross them. Then your "N . . . O . . . W" is effective.

Patient Deepening Trance with Hand Levitation

E: And entirely for yourself
in an objective fashion
review everything that you told me,
told us.
Review it slowly, carefully, objectively.
And if you notice any minor deficiencies,
it's all right to correct them.
It's also all right for you to correct them and not to know that you have corrected them.
[Pause as F's right hand begins to levitate upward very slowly in a barely perceptible manner]

E: She now deepens her trance by raising her own hand so that she can verbalize it without knowing it. She takes care of that by making certain that she goes deeper.

R: She is protecting her conscious mind by going deeper into trance. You offered some protection with your suggestion that she could correct "minor deficiences" without knowing it.

Self-Protective Mechanisms of the Unconscious

E: But I do want you to appreciate the ability of your unconscious mind.
[Pause]
The ability of your unconscious mind to perceive things.
And to release them to the conscious mind in
whatever detail
the unconscious considers
best.
[Pause]
And now there is a question I asked you.
And I'm going to try for an answer now.

Before the episiotomy,
perhaps subsequent to it.
But I wonder if before the episiotomy
you had some overlooked, forgotten feeling in your breasts.
You don't need to tell me.
[Long pause as her hand now levitates to about two inches above her thigh very, very slowly]
Your unconscious seems to be
telling me,
not letting you know.
[Long pause as hand continues levitating very slowly]

> E: As I get closer to anxiety-producing material dealing with the episiotomy her hand levitates more as a protective device by deepening trance.

> R: This appears to be a clear example of the self-protective aspect of the unconscious that you frequently talk about. The unconscious is deepening the trance to protect the conscious mind from knowledge it's not yet ready to receive.

> E: Yes.

A Cautious Open-ended Exploration of the Traumatic Aspects of Memory

E: Before you went into the trance,
your unconscious endeavored to tell me the same thing.
[Long pause]
And as far as I can judge,
your unconscious has not yet made up its mind
whether you should know or not.
[Pause]
As I told you last time,
records are made with the brain cells.
The only way to lose those records is to lose the brain cells.
And whether you find all the memories now
or later,
it is not important.
The only important thing is
for your unconscious to see to it that you really

feel comfortable
with all the memories you do have.
[Pause as her hand continues to lift, but her head and body slope downward]
I think it was a surprise to you
to find out
that you slowed up
maturation
in your need
for a more vivid memory.
Your unconscious has done a beautiful job
of giving you that maturity.
[Pause as her head and body slope further down]
Now slowly lift up your head.
Still higher.
And slowly tense the muscles of your back
until you're finally sitting up straight in the chair.
[Pause as she slowly realigns her body, with her hand levitating still higher]
It's perfectly all right not to know
that about your breasts.
It's also perfectly all right
to recover it later.
It's perfectly all right for me to be mistaken.
[Pause]
And you can look
with comfort
upon that
shock
connected with the episiotomy and the forceps.
You need have no regrets about that.
In fact, it is delightful to know
that you could have shock,
surprise,
and resentment
about your hands being tied down.

E: I'm taking all the resentment away from a particular thing (the episiotomy) and I'm focusing it on her hands being tied down.

R: You're giving her unconscious a series of cautious, open-ended suggestions to permit the memories and understanding of her situation to proceed in their own way and time. You also protect her from any misconceptions you may have with your remark about its being all right if you are mistaken. You're giving her own system the authority to declare what is valid for her own experience.

Facilitating new Frames of Reference

E: And you need know
that whatever interpretations were placed by others upon
your behavior,
you know what your behavior really was.
And that if they made an interpretation
you were fighting to get away,
you're psychologically altering
your psychosomatic position
to include forceps
and the altered view
of an episiotomy,
And you are so correct in saying
you heard the snip.
When using the word "snip,"
let's not dismiss it with that word.
You heard the cutting
like you hear the cutting of cloth,
and it's a very similar sound,
cutting of thick cloth with a large shears.

R: She was traumatized by not being told about the possibility of an episiotomy and thus not being prepared for it emotionally. You're here giving a series of suggestions about how she can now reorganize her perceptions and understanding of her experience. You don't tell her exactly how, but leave it fairly open-ended, to develop an "altered view of an episiotomy"; when she used the word "snip" earlier, it sounded very frightening. Your reassociation of the word to the fairly innocuous sound of cutting cloth, which is in the range of pleasant experience for most women, may help her reinterpret that "snip" into a more pleasant frame of reference. But it's only a most general example. Your basic suggestion is for her uncon-

307

scious to reorganize and reassociate that shocking experience into a more palatable frame of reference.

Dimming Irrelevancies and Traumatic Experience

E: Now your unconscious
can eliminate
the intrusion
of the other woman's sounds.
And let them become
the dim sounds,
the dimmed memories.
Your memories have that
pleasant and beautiful vividness
that belongs to you.
And you need to realize
in each first experience,
not knowing
prevents us from noticing
even though we do record.
[Pause]

R: You're here giving interesting suggestions for dimming the irrelevancy of the other woman's sounds and with them the traumatic aspect of her own fears of the dangers of childbirth, going back to the unhappy stories of her childhood. That is, you may be indirectly dimming those fearful images of her childhood so that her mind can now be free to deal with the realities of her current adult experience. You then make an interesting statement of what may be the essence of psychological trauma: The mind recording something it does not or cannot organize because it's a first experience that is overwhelming in some way.

E: Yes.

A Careful Awakening with Posthypnotic Suggestions of Comfort

E: Now straighten up still some more.
Still more. Still more.
Still more. Still more.
Even more. Even more.

308

Let your head be slowly upright fully.
And now,
as you slowly awaken,
I want you,
as you
awaken a bit at a time,
to increase
a bit at a time
your sense of comfort
and pleasure.
Enjoy life.
[Pause as her head lifts and she awakens, reorienting to her body]

> E: All this rather slow and elaborate awakening procedure is to
> get her away from any traumatic unconscious material that her
> conscious mind is not yet ready to handle.

> R: Yes, and you protect her further with your casual posthyp-
> notic suggestions for "comfort . . . pleasure . . . enjoy life."

The Reorganization of Traumatic Experiences

F: You said something that really hit home! The first experience! Because
you've never experienced it before, you don't know. It's unknown even
though your mind records things, it's still unknown to you. And it unfolds
to you. And that's how a certain mild shock—of a first unknown
experience. I don't know why. That really hit home. That really stood out
just like that! I don't know whether you intended this, but I saw a calendar
that has all the important dates flipping backward and backward.
It flipped through real fast all the items which I would consider a day at
home. There all of a sudden I was at my living room table. And there were
more details that had happened. You know, small things, conversations
came to me. More stuff (forgotten memories) came out.

E: That's fine.

F: That's weird, why did that happen?

E: I merely said the right words which you could understand, but
understand in your way.

F: Also, all this chaos—and that's exactly what it was, chaos. If you can
imagine it, there was only one nurse for that whole obstetrical floor. And

she had me to care for and my doctor and the hysteria going on next door (the stillbirth). Back and forth, I'm telling you! The phone ringing! Absolute chaos! Now that's dimmed, all that turmoil. That's what it was—turmoil and noises—and I don't know what-all was going on over next door. That's sort of dimmed. That's sort of taken second place.

R: Second place to your own experiences.

F: Right. And the awareness of what was happening to me is heightened.

E: [To R] Now you see it, don't you?

R: Wow, that's fantastic! Is that characteristic of this approach: The background fades into the background and the relevant matters take a sharper focus?

E: That's right. And psychotherapy would be much easier if everybody realized that.

R: A major function of psychotherapy is to let unimportant things fade into the background and only the relevant things come to the foreground. That's what hypnotherapy does *par excellence*.

E: That's right. And I didn't take hold of all these background things.

R: You let them be background.

E: I let *her* render them into the background. She didn't know why it happened, she just knew I said something that *really* hit the point.

R: There is a recording consciousness that is independent of a knowing and understanding.

E: Yes.

> R: She describes very well the "absolute chaos" that led to her traumatic experience and the effect of your suggestions in dimming that chaos so she can now focus on a heightened awareness of what was happening to her. This is an excellent example of your basic thesis that hypnotherapy can lead to a resynthesis and reorganization of unfortunate life experience.

The Person in the Physiological Process

F: I'm curious and tried to do some analyzing on my own. What relationship is there to your question about feeling in my breasts?

310

E: It's nice to know what you do understand.

F: [F again recites the traumatic aspect of being unprepared intellectually for the episiotomy and forceps, so that she felt herself shaking by the time it was over. The shaking actually continued for hours before it subsided completely.]

E: Dr. Moore mentioned that. Do you want me to tell you the rest of the meaning of that shaking?

F: Well, the doctor said it was normal. I don't know. You tell me, go ahead.

E: You said, "I don't know. You tell me."

F: Well, I just know what the doctor said—it was normal. He said it was a release of all the nervous system.

E: He doesn't even know! You are describing it well without even knowing what you are describing. I'm very glad you had the original shaking. I'm very glad you repeated it.

R: This is what Dr. Moore was referring to at the end of our last session as the "icing on the cake."

E: Yes.

F: There is a mind involved in all this!
[F outlines her experience of how her mind (thought, feelings, etc.) was very much involved with the birth experience. Even though the caudal anesthesia cut off certain sensations, there was much pressure and rhythmic contractions she could experience. She derides her young doctor's view that it was all just a physiological process.]

E: There is a person involved in it.

F: Right! A personality, so I think that all has something to do with it. It's the release of everything.

E: You want me to tell you how the person is involved?

F: Yes.

> R: She gives us an excellent statement of the importance of the person and the total personality that is so often ignored in modern medicine.

E: It's so difficult to get many physicians to understand this.

The Orgasm in the Birth Process: Individual Patterns of Knowing and the Resolution of Traumatic Experience

E: Think it over just a little bit. You got so close to it that Dr. Rossi here knows exactly what Dr. Moore meant.

F: [F now launches into another detailed set of recovered memories of the dynamics of the birth process: the way the doctor manipulated the baby's body, the fears and sensations she experienced, and so on. She describes how the baby finally came very suddenly as follows.] When the infant came out, it was like an explosion! I was never prepared for that. I just wasn't prepared! It was a weird feeling—like an explosion. I was dazed! I was absolutely dazed! Really, that explains it, I was dazed!

E: [E tells stories about the "joyful shaking" people have experienced when they have accomplished an important goal.] And the most beautiful *orgasm* a woman can have is when she gives birth to a baby.

F: That's what I was thinking! That's what I was thinking! It is really! The similarities, I'm not kidding you. The similarities between the two are quite the same and they go hand in hand. . . . The cry of the baby was like music . . . I was dazed, I couldn't believe it. [F now recalls many more memories of how she had to "educate" her young obstetrician about the process of carrying a baby, when it would be due, how much it would weigh, the sex of the child, and other factors in childbirth.] I was always one step ahead of that man.

E: The unconscious mind is very brilliant.

F: Was it my unconscious telling me those things?

E: That's right. There are a certain number of women who really do know those things, including what the sex of the child will be.

F: Why, my unconscious is more tuned in, or what?

E: Apparently you were trained in a *be-yourself way*. Your "education" never limited your behavior.

F: Well, it's a down-to-earth attitude.

R: That allows your natural self to be.

F: No pretentiousness that gets in the way of things.

312

E: Such women see no need for blocking out from themselves. So often you hear people say, "I wouldn't even think about that," and they don't.

R: Such people only learn to limit their perceptions and understandings.

F: [F again launches into a good-natured tirade of even more indignant memories about how she wanted to experience a more natural childbirth but was overwhelmed by the modern technology of the hospital delivery. This session finally ends with a general discussion of the interesting natural stages in an infant's growth that a mother can look forward to.]

R: The good-natured quality of her critical remarks is now very different from the fearful and tearful feelings she had when she first hinted at them in the beginning of her therapy. She has not only gained the complete set of memories she wanted in her original request for therapy, but she has also radically reorganized her perception and understanding of them. She has effectively dealt with a psychological trauma that was at the source of her memory problem, and has even resolved some of the early childhood experiences that gave her, in part, a predisposition to this trauma. Instead of being bitter at her young doctor, she can now understand him as a victim of his own limited education. She certainly has an enhanced sense of the worth of her own perceptions, feelings, and thoughts and a profound respect for her own unconscious processes.

CHAPTER 8

Emotional Coping

Case 11   Resolving Affect and Phobia with New Frames of Reference

Part One: Displacing a Phobic Symptom

Mrs. A was a highly intelligent, attractive computer programmer, recently married, who requested therapy for an "airplane phobia." She reported that she had been in a minor airplane accident involving a landing that shook her up a bit. The fright from this experience quickly generalized to any form of air turbulence or vibration when a plane was in the air. She was able to enter an airplane and even taxi along the runway with no fear. Her "phobia" actually began the moment the plane lifted off the runway. She was in great distress while airborne, but was comfortable again as soon as the plane touched ground.

She was eager to experience hypnosis and proved to be a very responsive subject. Because of this the senior author felt he could request a strong commitment from Mrs. A in her very first therapy session.

Commitment on a Conscious and Unconscious Level

E: I requested an absolute commitment from Mrs. A that she must agree to do anything I asked. I made her verbalize a promise to do anything I asked—"*good or bad, the worst or the best*. You are a woman and I am a man. Even though I'm confined to a wheelchair, we are of the opposite sex." If you only knew how grudgingly she gave that promise; she did not enjoy giving it, but she gave it. She thought about it for seven or eight minutes and finally said, "no matter what you do to me, it couldn't be worse than that awful fear." Then I put her in a trance and went through the whole thing again until I got the same promise when she was in a trance.

R: Why did you have to get the same commitment while awake and in trance?

E: Unconsciously you don't have to do what you consciously say you will. In everyday life, you may accept an invitation for dinner, and later your unconscious lets you forget it.

R: So this is an example of a mental mechanism in everyday life that can interfere with therapy unless you make provision for it as you do here. You aroused quite an emotional storm in her; she was really affected by your demand for an absolute obedience, which is rather unusual in modern psychotherapy.

E: Yes. It took an awful lot of courage on her part. Now why did I ask that kind of promise? She said she had an "airplane phobia," but I knew she didn't because it was only when the plane was in the air and she had no control over anything that she had fear. As long as the plane was on the ground, there existed a possibility of getting out. But up in the air she was in a state of absolute commitment.

R: So her problem was in giving a commitment?

E: Yes, and I made her give a commitment, a total commitment. The thing is, you couldn't do therapy with her except with the actual problem present. You can't remove a wart unless the patient brings the wart into the therapy room.

R: That's the dynamics of the situation; you had her reify her fears and bring them into the therapy session.

E: That's right, made her fears a reality I could work on, a reality I could then put in that chair she was sitting in and leave there.

R: By making her give you a total commitment, you brought her fear of total commitment into the therapy situation. By hinting about sex between you, the therapy situation became as fearful as her phobia.

E: That's right, there was a body threat in both. I had to make it so that it might all turn out terrible. I could not get a commitment by just asking her to imagine herself in a locked room. It had to be *this room*, something that would be truly horrible.

R: She might have been stuck with a dirty old man.

E: That's right.

R: You have guts to pull off these things.

E: She had to have her psychological problem with her at the time that I treated her. She then went into a trance quite easily. She was actually commited to do anything. She had no freedom of any kind. She was in a state of total commitment. Once in the trance state I had her board a plane and ride through a storm in her imagination. It was sickening to see; she actually went through a kind of convulsion. It was horrible to watch.

Concrete Displacement of a Symptom Outward

E: I let her go through that plane trip with great air turbulence, and then I told her that she would soon feel comfortable and at ease. She would then suddenly find that all her fears had slid off her onto the chair she was sitting on. She was then awakened. She immediately leaped out of that chair! I called in my wife and told her to sit in the chair. As she started to the patient yelled, "No, no, don't!" and physically prevented my wife from sitting.

R: You were testing the patient?

E: No, I gave her an opportunity to validate that the chair contained the fears.

R: I see! It was actually a way of helping her recognize and ratify her own therapeutic response of concretely displacing her fears onto the chair.

Posthypnotic Suggestion with Supportive Cues

E: I then gave her a direct posthypnotic suggestion that she was to actually take a plane trip in reality to Dallas. She had given me her absolute promise. I then told her it wouldn't be necessary to see her again until after she returned from Dallas. "You'll take a plane from the Phoenix airport. Of course, you'll have some question about it. When you get back to Phoenix from Dallas, you will have discovered how beautiful it is to ride a plane. You will really enjoy it. When you reach Phoenix airport on your return, call me up and tell me how you enjoyed it."

Before terminating that trance, I gave her other posthypnotic suggestions as follows: "You have lost your phobia for planes. In fact, all your fears and anxieties and horror are sitting in that chair where you are sitting. It's up to you to decide how long you want to sit there with those fears." You should have seen how she jumped out of that chair!

R: That's how you awakened her. You displaced all her fears onto the chair. That's why she suddenly jumped out of the chair. Such an immediate and vivid response was also the kind of feedback you needed, to know that she would follow your other posthypnotic suggestion to actually take a plane to Dallas.

E: I then wondered what I should do to be sure of the effectiveness of that single trance. I had my daughter take three pictures of that chair—one picture overexposed, one that was underexposed, and one that was normally exposed. I labeled the one that was underexposed, "Where your phobia and troubles rest and are dissipating into nothingness." The overexposed photo, where only the outline of the chair was darkly visible, I labeled, "Where your problems are sinking into the gloom of total doom." The normal exposure was labeled "The permanent resting place of your problem." I sent her those photos each in separate envelopes. They are her St. Christopher's medal.

R: You mean she carries them with her when she goes on a plane?

E: Yes. I don't care how educated people are, they still believe in good-luck pieces. Those photographs were her good-luck pieces; it's a part of everyday living.

R: Those photographs were supportive cues that she could take out of the therapy situation to reinforce the posthypnotic suggestion. Posthypnotic suggestion does not necessarily function because an idea is deeply imprinted in the mind during trance. Rather, posthypnotic suggestions are always in dynamic process and as such require outer and inner stimuli and cues to evoke and reinforce them. That's why it's so useful to associate posthypnotic suggestions with some inevitable patterned behavior the patient will experience after trance.

E: She followed those posthypnotic suggestions, and when she returned and called me, she said in an ebullient tone of voice, "It was utterly fantastic. The cloud bed below looked so beautiful I wished I had a camera." Months later, when she had occasion to return to the same room, it was ridiculous how she avoided that chair and prevented others from sitting in it.

Part Two: Resolving an Early-Life Trauma at the Source of a Phobia

The senior author developed a number of useful approaches to dealing with emotional trauma and facilitating an appropriate balance between intellectual and emotional experiencing. The most basic of these appears to be a separate experience of each before their final integration.

R: How and why do you separate the emotional and intellectual aspects of a life experience as a therapeutic approach?

E: You separate the emotional and intellectual content because so often people cannot face the meaningfulness of an experience. People cry and do not know why they cry, they feel suddenly elated and know not why. In using regression therapeutically you first recover the emotions in trance to help the patient recognize them. Then put the patient back in a trance; this time leave the emotions buried and let the intellectual content be recognized. Then put them back in a trance a third time and put the cognitive and emotional aspects together and then have them come out of trance with a complete memory.

R: You have them experience emotions and intellect separately and then put them together to integrate the now totally recovered memory.

Separating Emotion and Intellect

To illustrate this approach the authors decided to call upon Mrs. A, whose airplane phobia was discussed in Part One. While the senior author's unusual means of dissociating and displacing her fears had indeed apparently resolved her phobia (it was now two years after the therapy), it was felt that a more adequate resolution could be achieved by helping her develop greater understanding of herself. Mrs. A readily agreed to the idea of further hypnotic work because she was very interested in the experience and was willing to permit tape-recording and a number of observers. As the group assembled in Erickson's office a very friendly and positively optimistic mood was generated as we were all introduced and a few stories were told about how Erickson had helped one or another of us with hypnosis. *Rapport, response attentiveness*, and an interesting *therapeutic frame of reference* were thus facilitated in Mrs. A as she basked in the light of high therapeutic *expectation*. This was an illustration of how Erickson likes to use an audience to generate a therapeutic milieu. A hush gradually fell over the room as all of our attention was directed toward her. Erickson begins with the counting induction with which he had previously trained Mrs. A.

Trance Induction and Facilitating Posthypnotic Suggestion

E: One, five, ten, fifteen, twenty!
[Pause]
Very deeply in trance.
[Pause as Mrs. A closes her eyes and becomes quietly immobile with a relaxed face. She evidently has entered a deep trance very quickly.]

E: Now A, after you awaken I will ask you
casually,
"Are you awake?"
In a moment you will say "yes,"
and as you say "yes,"
there will come over you

318

all the horrible feeling that you experienced
sometime
before the age of ten,
feelings about something
that you can talk about
to strangers,
but
you'll have just the feelings.
You won't know what the thing is
that caused those feelings.
You will just feel feelings,
and you won't know what is making you
feel so miserable.
And you will tell us
how miserable you feel.
[Pause]
Get a firm grip on those horrible feelings.
You won't know about them until after
I ask if you are awake
and you say, "yes,"
and at that moment those feelings will hit you hard.
Do you understand now?

A: Um hum.

E: All right, twenty, fifteen, ten, nine, eight, seven, six, five, four, three,
two, one.

R: This is a basic approach for facilitating posthypnotic suggestion. You request a simple response like the answer "yes" that
is almost inevitable in response to your question, "Are you
awake?" You then associate that very easy response with
another, vastly more complex and difficult posthypnotic
suggestion to reexperience horrible feelings before the age of
ten without any awareness of the cause of the feelings. You are
facilitating the reliving of an old emotion by dissociating it from
an awareness of the cause of the emotion. The easy "yes"
response tends to initiate an acceptance set (Erickson, Rossi,
and Rossi 1976) for carrying out the more difficult posthypnotic
suggestion that is to follow. If you had noticed that a particular
patient tended to nod her head "yes" in everyday life, you
would *utilize* that head nodding as a vehicle to facilitate the more

difficult posthypnotic suggestion. By requesting responses that are already high in a patient's response hierarchy, it is more likely that you will be successful in facilitating an initial post-hypnotic response, and most importantly, you thereby initiate an acceptance set for the more difficult posthypnotic suggestions associated with it.

E: Yes, that's a beautiful wording. Notice I emphasize that she is to get a "firm grip" on those feelings. Then when I count down I skip from twenty to fifteen to ten, but then give an impressive countdown from ten to one by single digits as she gets a grip on the feelings that are to emerge.

Trance Reinduction When Carrying Out Posthypnotic Suggestions

A: Oh, I like it. It is so restful. I didn't want you to count.

E: Are you awake now?

A: Yes.

[Mrs. A looks a bit startled and becomes quietly self-preoccupied for a moment or two. Her face frowns, and she obviously begins to experience some internal stress.]

R: Her slight startle and quiet self-preoccupation are actually indications of the momentary development of another trance as she begins to carry out the posthypnotic suggestion (Erickson and Erickson, 1941). Although talking and acting as if she were awake, she is probably in what you define as a somnambulistic state as she experiences the fearful emotions recorded in the next section.

Emotional Experience Without Intellectual Insight

E: What's the matter, A?

A: I don't know, I don't want to look. There is something I don't want to see.
I don't know what, but I don't know what to tell you.

E: Talk about your feeling. Tell me what you are feeling.

A: No, I'm afraid. There is something there that I don't want to see, and I don't want to look. I'm afraid of what it is, and if I look . . I don't want to look.

E: You don't need to look. Just talk to me about it.

A: It is just fear. I, I want to forget. It will go away if I don't look, OK?

E: I don't think the feelings will go away.

A: Yeah, because . . . because I'm just afraid. There is something I . . . I don't know what to tell you about it, but I am afraid, I'm afraid.

> R: Mrs. A is genuinely frightened and only apparently awake following your posthypnotic suggestion to experience a horrible feeling without knowing why she is experiencing it. You have thus accomplished the initial part of this hypnotherapeutic approach by having her first experience these feelings separate from their source and intellectual content. You now release her by counting to twenty again to reestablish a comfortable state of trance.

Reinducing Trance Comfort With Posthypnotic Suggestion for Intellectual Insight: Protecting Patients in Trance: A Feeling Approach

E: One, five, ten, fifteen, twenty.

Now you feel comfortable.

[Pause]

And you will again,

now,

can't you?

A: I'm beginning to.

E: That's right.

[Pause]

Now the next time I awaken you, A, I have a different kind of task for you.

When next I ask you casually if you are awake,

you will say 'yes,'

and then

there will come to your mind

something that could have scared you

years ago.

But you won't feel any emotions at all,

is that all right?

It won't scare you,
is that all right?

A: I will remember, but I won't be afraid?

E: You'll just remember, "Yes, when I was a little kid I was scared."
That's the way you'll remember it.
You will be able to laugh about it
and take an adult person's view.
I'll be cautious,
A,
to make certain
whether or not you should
identify it,
OK?

A: All right.

E: I ask for her approval to view the past when I ask, "Is that all right?" I describe what she is to do and get her agreement. Each pause in my final sentence is an independent message saying that I will protect her. Each part is a separate reassurance.

R: Each phrase is a reassuring suggestion in itself within the overall sentence about being cautious for her sake.

R: After her previous experience of an uncomfortable emotion Mrs. A is rather hesitant about going on. It's therefore important that you reassure her by letting her know she will be able to laugh at it from an adult person's point of view. Most patients are vulnerable in trance; they need the therapist's protection. Therefore you let her know that you will be "cautious" and make certain it will be OK for her to identify her experience. If it was about to become traumatic, or not the sort of material she could share with strangers, for example, you could easily shut it off by distracting her, telling her to stop, or giving her the counting signal to reenter trance.

E: My approach is very casual even with this difficult material, and that makes it easier for her. It's hard to say "no" to a casual easygoing approach.

R: This illustrates how you often work on a feeling level: Intellectually a person might want to say "no," but that seems ridiculous on a feeling level where you are so casual, warm, and permissive. It feels wrong to say "no!"

Trance Awakening with Intellectual Insight: The Transformation of Painful Affect: A Genuine Age Regression with Adult Perspective

E: Twenty, fifteen, ten, five, four, three, two, one.
Not a restful trance.

A: Not as restful as before.

E: No?

A: No. I, I feel an apprehension. I don't know why, and I don't know what is causing it, but I feel apprehensive.

E: Want to ask Dr. Rossi? Are you awake yet?

A: Yes.
[Pause as Mrs. A looks a bit puzzled. She is again apparently experiencing a momentary trance as she begins to carry out the posthypnotic suggestion for recall without emotions]

E: Would it be all right to tell us?

A: What is in my mind is a void. It is, um, a void, I don't know how to describe it, but it is like looking at, un . . .
Oh . . . yes! Fantastic! I know what it is! Shall I describe the scene to you?

E: Oh, yes!

A: Oh, yes, it is a bridge. Do you remember when I told you before I was afraid of bridges? The scene is coming up a bridge . . .
as you come up you see nothing of reference, but a void. The car or whatever I am in, and it must be a car, I'm sitting in it in such a way that I see nothing. I don't see the superstructure of a bridge if there is any, or the hood of a car. I am looking out and see nothing all of a sudden. Where I was looking at before and seeing—trees or grass or something, pasture, that I can relate to. All of a sudden there is a void and I see nothing to give reference. And it is a bridge. I know where the bridge is. I am aware of where this bridge is. I can't relate to how old I am or whom I am with or anything like that.
But, yeah, OK.

E: Tell me something about the bridge.

A: Where is it? Well, it is on the way to my grandparents in northern California. And it is a bridge that has a very steep incline so that as you are

323

driving up, you then reach the top and you break over so that as you are going up, you are not aware of anything, there isn't anything. You can't see anything to relate to unless you are looking out at the side, but if you are looking straight ahead, there is nothing until you break over onto the top of the bridge.

E: How soon do you think you will discover your age?

A: I don't know because I have gone on that bridge many, many times as a child.
Eight comes into my mind, but I don't know why eight. Because I could have been any age, going over the bridge so many times, not just one time.

E: Is that sufficient, Ernie [R]?

R: Yes, I think so.

> R: Whereas before she was greatly distressed with the emotional component of the experience, she now appears to be fascinated and even a bit elated ("Fantastic!") when she recalls the scene with intellectual insight. Affect is thus not completely eliminated in this second phase, when you supposedly have the patient discover the intellectual component of the experience alone. All negative affect has certainly been dissociated from the memory, however, and she does indeed experience it with an "adult person's view," as you suggested. The fear and anxiety she experienced as a child have been replaced by the curiosity and fascination she can feel about the experience as an adult.
>
> E: In my previous session with her I said the view from a plane would be "fantastic," and she uses that word here.
>
> R: This suggests that there is a transformative aspect in her hypnotic work that is restructuring a previously painful affect into a new frame of reference where it can be experienced as "fantastic!"
>
> E: When she speaks of "car . . . I am in . . . I'm sitting in it in such a way that I see nothing . . ." it is in the present tense, which indicates she is really there.
>
> R: That aspect was a genuine age regression in which she was acutally reliving an early life experience rather than simply remembering it.
>
> E: Then I ask her to tell me about the birdge, and she experi-

324

ences a transformation of the trauma into a more adult recollection. First she was an adult being a child reliving a past experience, then she is an adult and understands it. She is in two identities simultaneously; child and adult are working together, becoming integrated.

Trance Reinduction and Comfort

E: One, five, ten, fifteen, twenty.
Now you have done beautiful work so far today, A. Very good work. Now this time
I am going to awaken you, and I want you to feel really comfortable, very rested, very relaxed,
feeling as if you had eight hours of rest.
You will be surprised when you look at the clock and notice the time.
And again I'll ask if you are awake.
Immediately after
You will say "yes."

R: You now prepare her for the final task of integrating the emotional and intellectual aspects of the experience by suggesting that she will first feel comfortable and relaxed as if she's had eight hours of rest. This is another example of giving an easy and much desired posthypnotic suggestion to initiate an acceptance set for the more difficult posthypnotic suggestion you will associate with it. It's also a way of rewarding and reinforcing her for the work she's already done when you tell her she's "done beautiful work so far today, A. Very good work."

E: Suggesting eight hours of rest also utilizes what we experience in everyday life: You frequently sleep on something in order to deal with it.

Posthypnotic Suggestion for Integrating Emotions and Intellect, Child and Adult

E: The entire episode will flash in your mind
with utter . . .
with utter and complete vividness.
Now did you understand my words, A?
[Pause]

A: Um?

E: Your first look at the clock.
You'll probably be astonished that it is not later,
a lot later,
than this.
You can feel so rested. Tell how rested and comfortable you feel, how much
you enjoyed this trance state.
And then I ask you
if you are awake,
and you will say "yes,"
then immediately
this entire episode
will flash
into your mind very vividly.
Is that all right?
[Pause]

A: Um. Last time
you said "complete."
You said "complete and vividly."

E: That's right.
Completely,
intellectually and emotionally
complete.
So that you will know what your feelings *were then*
and
everything about how you felt *then,*
even knowing yourself then.

A: I'm confused.

E: It is perfectly all right, A.

A: I will know my feelings, or I will feel my feelings?

E: You will *recall* your feelings.
[Pause]

E: Just as long ago and barefoot on the first day of spring, I felt so good to
be barefoot, I jumped and landed on some broken glass. I can recall my
agonized shriek of pain and my bitter feeling of disappointment that it
would be a week before I could go barefoot again. But I can be amused by

326

that now. It did hurt and I recall how it hurt. I can feel it in my heel right now, my right heel.

I can laugh about it, and that bitter feeling disappears. I can go barefoot tomorrow and I just persuaded my mother to let me go barefoot that evening.

I can be amused by it now. You will recall your episode, you can describe it fully and describe the feelings you had then. Now do you understand?

A: Um hum.

> R: You're now making an effort to help her integrate emotions and intellect, child and adult. Why do you resort to giving her a personal example of what you mean?
>
> E: I can always *show* you what I mean rather than explain it. Can you describe a fishy handshake?
>
> R: I wonder, too, if such concrete, imagistic illustrations make better contact with the right hemisphere, where such personality integrations may be taking place (Rossi, 1977). Such concrete illustrations also evoke ideodynamic processes much more readily than abstract and intellectual formulations. From this point of view it can be regarded as multiple-level communication.

Integrating Emotional and Intellectual Experience from an Adult's Perspective: Reassociating and Reorganizing Inner Experience

E: All right.
Twenty, fifteen, ten, five, four, three, two, one.
Feeling comfortable?

A: Um?

E: Feeling comfortable?

A: I feel like I am waking up.

E: How much do you feel you have slept?

A: I feel like I have been asleep for a long time. Like it is time to get up. Oh, dear!

E: Are you awake now?

327

A: Yes. Um. Um.

[Pause as Mrs. A appears lost in thought. She is again apparently experiencing a momentary trance as she begins to carry out the posthypnotic suggestion.]

E: What are those um's about?
Tell it fast.

A: Oh, there are so many things to tell! It is a cloudy day and I am in a car with my parents and my sister. I don't know where my brother is. I'm wearing, I can't think of what I am wearing. I'm wearing a cotton pinaforelike dress, but I don't understand why I am wearing that dress when it is so cloudy outside. We were going to my grandmother's and my grandfather's and it is, how did I know it was Sunday?
It's Sunday, how could I tell?

I guess because my father is not working, but he does work on Saturdays, but it is Sunday. It is Sunday afternoon. We are going over to my grandmother's and grandfather's and my grandmother has promised me chicken noodle soup for lunch. And we are in a blue car. I wonder if my parents had a blue car? They must have. This is like a newsreel in my mind. Events are happening in my mind.

We are driving down the road, and it's the Sacramento River Bridge. My mother is unhappy about something, and she asked me to sit back in the seat. I don't know why, maybe Diane and I were playing. I'm sitting back in the seat and I'm looking out straight ahead. No, I had gotten up again and am holding onto the back of the seat, looking out the front window, and we are driving and there is nothing.

And I close my eyes because I couldn't see anything, I wasn't aware of anything to relate to. I was aware of bouncing over and knowing that if we made the next bump I'd see something. And that's all.

It's like a newsreel in my mind. If I just wait long enough, some more will happen. I opened my eyes when we went over the second bump.

E: How old are you?

A: I seem to be eight. For some reason eight comes into my mind. I feel eight but I can't be eight, but the dress that I am wearing would be a dress that I would wear at that age, I think. But I don't see my brother. I don't know where my brother is. If I am eight, my brother should be five, but I don't know where my brother is, but my sister is there.

Eight comes to my mind, but I can't tell you why. Maybe because I said it

328

earlier, that I felt eight, but I don't know why. There is no fear, though. I am not afraid of anything.

E: How was it?

R: It seems very fine.

A: How was what?

R: Your work in dealing with these experiences.

A: It's not frightening anymore.
There isn't the fear.

E: Now it will be all right for you to remember the fear.
You just showed it to us a few minutes ago.

A: Oh, it seems very innocent now. There is nothing that I am afraid of.

E: A few minutes ago, how did you feel?

A: Why was I afraid? Now I'm not, it doesn't frighten me in the least. It was just an incident as a child.
I was afraid, though, I remember, and that's why I was very afraid.

E: What happened to her fear?

R: I wish I knew.

> R: Integrating the emotional and intellectual aspects of the experience from an adult's perspective now enables her to relive the experience without the child's fear. This is an emotionally corrective approach that helps the patient reassociate and reorganize her inner experience in a therapeutic manner. Once a certain amount of catharsis of the traumatic aspects of the experience takes place (in the first phase of the reexperiencing the emotions without the intellectual component), the entire experience can be integrated and worked through from a new adult perspective in another relatively brief trance. It's interesting that under this third trance condition, where she is to reexperience both the emotional and intellectual aspects of the experience, she recalls much more detail than with either alone. That this is something more than a simple recall of a lost memory is indicated by the fact that she reports it as a "newsreel in my mind," wherein it seemed to come to her autonomously as an unconscious process unfolding itself spontaneously, rather than a labored effort of the conscious mind to remember.

329

E: She was able to restructure her early life experience to remove the pain associated with it. Even though she did restructure this early life experience, you can always, again, separate that life experience into its emotional and intellectual components and have her reexperience the child's painful emotion.

R: What do you feel is actually involved when you speak of restructuring a life experience? Do we simply give it new associative connections so it is not isolated in a pathogenic manner? What is restructured?

E: [The senior author gives the example of a patient overcoming his fear of swimming. The patient reported that if he just wades halfway into the water, as he used to, he can feel the old fear somewhat within. When he takes his new position and swims, however, the old fear disappears. A potential for the old fear remains, but new activities can generate emotions that can replace or restructure it in modifications of the old situation.]

R: In restructuring an old life experience we are developing new associative pathways, facilitating new responses to the old fear-provoking life situation. The old memories and pathways are still there. They will always be there.

E: We are giving the patient new possibilities and we are taking away the undersirable qualities. Usually it's best to have patients experience the emotion first and later the intellectual, because after they have experienced the emotions so strongly, they have a need to get the intellectual side of it.

R: I see, this dissociative approach enables emotion to surface more easily and then strongly motivates them to get the intellectual. Do you have any other means of dissociating experience other than this separation of emotions and intellect?

E: Yes. You can have the patient recall one single facet of the emotional experience—then an unrelated intellectual facet, like a jigsaw puzzle. The entire experience can be recovered, the whole meaning can be put together, only when the last piece is put into place.

Part Three: Facilitating Learning: Developing New Frames of Reference

After a leisurely discussion of the foregoing events by the group Mrs. A described some of her current problems with a course of academic study that made great demands upon her time. The senior author now decides to utilize her motivation for more efficient study habits to facilitate her learning processes. He induces hypnosis in his usual fashion with her and continues.

The Utilization Approach

E: The alterations I'm going to suggest, the first is this:
homework is tedious, tiring, exhausting. I think
homework
carries with it
a sense of something
well done, well accomplished,
and the feeling
it is going to be done,
is being done,
and has been completed will carry with it
a very partial feeling
that will enable you to
concentrate better,
learn more rapidly,
and enjoy the entire process.
[Mrs. A nods her head "yes" in the rapid, abbreviated manner that is characteristic of a conscious intentional process]
You think it over,
don't nod or shake your head yet,
think it over.

E: You don't want the patient to agree with you too soon. It's nice to think it over before you buy a house.

R: As is highly characteristic of your style, you begin by first accepting her own frame of reference, "homework is tedious." This opens an acceptance set. You then add your initial suggestion, "homework carries with it a sense of something well done." Your suggestion is a truism—anyone would have to agree with it—and that further establishes the acceptance set. To this you finally add the easy-to-accept suggestion, "a very *partial* feeling that will enable you to concentrate better, learn more rapidly, and enjoy the entire process." You don't directly command her, you simply state truisms about better learning and associate them with her own inner experience in such a way that she cannot deny them. She accepts them as valid for her own experience and thus she receives and accepts your

331

suggestions. You do not add anything new with these suggestions. Rather you evoke and utilize her own real-life experience; anyone who has ever, at any time, done their homework (or any other kind of learning) usually has had a feeling of accomplishment, and this is invariably associated with "a very partial feeling" that they can learn even better some time or other. Your suggestions about better concentration and more rapid learning thus reinforce aspects of her own experience which you have evoked. You (1) establish an *acceptance set* and then (2) *evoke* aspects of her life experience that you can then (3) *utilize* to help resolve her current problem. This is a typical example of your utilization approach to therapeutic suggestion. She accepts this so quickly with a nodding of her head that you must tell her to think it over. You want to let her unconscious have enough time for a thorough search of the relevant inner processes that can implement these suggestions.

E: I let her have a little taste of a good thing with "a very *partial* feeling," so she will soon tell herself that she wants the whole thing. It's a common life experience to take a taste and then want the whole thing. A mother says, "Just take a little bite." But our patient didn't even hear me say, "Just take a little bite."

Generalizing a Learning Frame of Reference to Restructure a Phobic Problem

E: The other alteration is
this question of flying.
The initial apprehension
that can be
transformed possibly
into
a sense
of the task,
the responsibility
of doing the task.
One can always be apprehensive
about a task.
You always know that you can fail,
then you are hooked
and realize
you've done this sort of thing before. You have enjoyed it before and you

can actually **enjoy starting out on new assignments. Instead of boredom**
there is a time
when you enjoy being within your body,
a feeling of resting,
feeling of comfort,
while your mind's eye
is exploring
the things that really give you pleasure.
[Pause]

R: You now generalize the learning frame of reference you've just developed to help restructure her understanding of her fear of flying which you helped her with some time ago. This is something of a surprise; she could not have known you were going to bring up this old problem again for a new and more adequate resolution.

E: Yes, I'm now transforming the phobia problem by placing it into a frame of reference of dealing with intellectual tasks, where she is really an expert.

R: Although she's asking for help as a student, she is, relatively speaking, an expert in solving intellectual tasks.

E: She has a very strong desire to do good work. She is strong there, so I'm using that motivation to deal with the place where she is weak—her airplane phobia.

Illustrating Open and Flexible Frames of Reference

E: I know flying to France
at night,
the plane was crowded
I was physically rather uncomfortable at the time.
I knew we'd arrive in France at breakfasttime,
and we'd barely get our dinner eaten
before we were handed our breakfast.
But throughout that flight
I kept thinking about
my boyhood concepts
of what the ocean was.
Its unlimited span,

**and how that contrasts
with my current understanding.
I thought about all of my daydreams as a boy
and how they had evolved.
[Pause]**

> R: You now introduce a pair of illustrations about how one can maintain open and flexible frames of reference to become more adaptable to unusual life contingencies. The second illustration from your boyhood has particular relevance for her because your conception of an "unlimited span" of the ocean corresponds with her early fear of the void over the bridge. You are attempting to help her restructure some of her early fearful childhood associations to "void" with a more adult perspective.

Associating Therapeutic Themes

**E: In going back to the first change,
a sense of accomplishing something,
of knowing that you have a good job to do,
that you are doing a good job,
that you are reaching in,
that you have concluded with a joyful sense of accomplishment.**

> R: You now return to the problem of academic learning. By associating this academic problem with the phobia problem you are implying that they can both be resolved by the same process of learning to adopt and maintain more open and adaptable frames of reference.

Restructuring Sensory Experience: Translating Therapist's Words into the Patient's

**E: A farmer knows he has done a good day's work because his back is comfortably very tired.
And so you can accomplish homework
with profound feeling of accomplishment
and the knowledge that you can go to sleep and sleep soundly,
your homework is done,
and that the overall picture
of your homework is
a good thing and also a good thing to have in the past,**

334

and the nice feeling comes during the process.
So that
the whole is worthwhile and
is not going to distress you.
Is that all right?
And now the transformation,
the alteration that I have suggested
in regard to flying I have suggested one
way.
But I expect you to translate everything I have said,
both connections,
into your words,
your phrases,
so that the alterations
are set in your terms,
not mine.
And I don't need to know those.
You do.
[Pause]

E: What does "comfortably very tired" mean?

R: The farmer's tired back is his cue that he can be comfortable knowing he's done a good day's work.

E: The mind restructures the tired feeling into a comfortable feeling. You don't have to have a Ph.D to do it!

R: You end this section with an important suggestion wherein you encourage your patient to translate your words into her own. Your suggestions are therefore received in an open-ended manner that allows the patient's own individuality to utilize them in an optimal and personal way.

Patient Feedback and Further Therapeutic Illustrations

E: I have a
former alcoholic as a patient.
Last time
he saw me
he said, "Let's go out and have a good drink."
The wife and I went with him to have a good drink.
We had daiquiris and he had a glass of milk.

Now all three of us had a good drink.
Now I was suggesting
a very nice feeling
for you
in your definition
of a nice feeling
in two regards:
homework
and travel
Relaxed? All right.

A: Um hum. In the case of homework the end result is what you say, it becomes a sense of accomplishment and pleasure. It is the process of after a hard day of concentrating on a lecture, that it takes a lot of concentration and discipline to sit and then study another three or four hours at night. After being tired all day, the only thing that pushes me to do that is the fact that I know that I will be happy when it is done and will feel better. And when it's done I will sleep better. So those are the reasons for doing it. The problem is not realizing the end result. I do realize what I want the end result to be, which it is. The problem is the concentration and the discipline necessary to do that.

E: All right, now I'll explain further.
I worked out this plan.
I borrowed six novels from the library.
I grew up in a home where there weren't many books and I knew
my knowledge of literature was very poor,
and so I would sit down and read fifty pages of one novel,
study hard in chemistry
for twenty minutes,
shift into another set of gears and study
physics for twenty minutes,
and another fifteen minutes on my English assignment,
read part of the next novel,
and keep going around
from novel to textbook,
perhaps another novel,
another textbook, all shifting gears.
Because every time you shift from one pattern of physical activity, you rest from the previous activity.

336

On the farm I learned to pitch hay right-handedly and left-handedly.
When my right arm got tired, I rested it by using my left hand.
In chopping wood—right- and left-handed. Always resting first one arm
and then the other.
Alternating in hoeing in the garden, I did the same thing.
In studying
chemistry,
it is so different than reading a novel.
Reading a novel is one kind of an exercise, and a chapter from a psychology
book is another kind of exercise,
so I was always working at top speed at each of the things that I was doing
and resting from all the other things.
Now working all day tires you. Studying your homework at night is also
tiring.
But
to untense that part of your body fatigued by the day's work
and work with the rest of you on homework.
Listening to lectures is one thing,
doing paid work is another thing,
and studying is a third type
of exercise.
You alternate them and understand that you can rest
the lecture-receiving apparatus
while you're doing homework,
and rest from homework activity when you are doing office work.
Because it all requires different sets of patterns of functioning.
Do you understand?

A: Um hum.

E: Now you can elaborate that in your own understanding?
When a friend entered medical school,
she heard lectures from eight in the morning until five at night. And then
from six to eleven she was in the laboratory.
It took her a while to discover that she could use different parts of herself
for the lectures in the day and different parts of herself in the laboratory at
night. When she got back to her room
she rested all of herself.
She has been rather startled to see how neatly and precisely she can divide
herself up in accordance with her needs. And she has added to that

crocheting shawls and baby blankets and afghans. It is so restful when she is starting to crochet an afghan. And the joy of crocheting an afghan for her sister in Ethiopia really soaks up the fatigue of studying.
In a very delightful way of doing it,
in a careful
unconscious thinking it out,
you can devise
a mastery of your own functions
so that you can
work out patterns
of function.
Do you think you understand me now?

A: Yes.

E: You can think about those things at your own convenience. You can decide whether or not to accept these alterations.
I think they are good,
perhaps you can find them good.
But it's your advantage,
your comfort
in your ease in studying
and hearing lectures,
in understanding homework
that I really
want to promote.
And I want
your work
while you're overseas mentally
to carry with it something enjoyable,
overtones and undertones.
Over hills to grandmother's place
is very nice,
appealing,
to everybody.
Then jingle bells
all the way,
overtones and undertones.
I don't know what your acquaintance is with
sleighs and jingle bells,

338

you undoubtedly know the song,
There are so many things that have
overtones, undertones of enjoyment.
I can think of how much easier it was to churn butter
for my grandmother than it was to do it at home.
Same job
but in a different setting.
Any question, A?

A: Not really, I'm fine.

E: Now
because what you can do can be your own
in some future time, you might like to talk about it.

> R: In this section Mrs. A gives you some valuable feedback on
> how she is receiving your suggestions, so you are able to adjust
> your orientation to fit her needs more exactly. You give her
> more illustrations of how to facilitate her own learning proces-
> ses and continually offer your suggestions in an open-ended
> manner so that she has to do continual inner work in organizing
> your words into her own terms. This is a state of very active
> trance learning. She is not at all passive. There is an intense
> rapport between you; it's almost as if there was a kind of direct
> mind transfer between you.

Confusion and New Learning

A: I'm having trouble.
I understand about studying and homework, and that makes sense to me,
but I'm confused about flying
and about what you said earlier about doing the tasks that I face.

E: It's okay, A.
Recognizing that the task ahead of you
has sufficient proportions
to mean a great deal.
You look at your work the way a surgeon looks at an operation.
It is a simple appendectomy, but if you are a good surgeon,
you know
that in the United States,
quite unexpectedly,

a certain number of simple appendectomies die
from surgery.
Therefore,
you know there isn't such a thing as a simple appendectomy.
So you set about
making it
a simple appendectomy.
Taking care to omit
nothing that is important.
And have the good feeling this
is going to be a simple appendectomy because you are doing it.
A very good surgeon feels
just a simple operation and it is going to turn out right because
he is not goint to omit anything and he is going to enjoy doing it
and the patient is going to enjoy having had it done.
You give the proper amount of respect
to the task in hand,
realizing
that there are hazards in any human performance,
which have to be met
by each functioning human being,
and then
the enjoyment
of looking forward to doing it, a simple act of appendectomy tomorrow,
looking forward to enjoying that flight tomorrow,
looking forward to the enjoyment of preparing
whatever it is.
And letting that take over boredom.
Boredom narrows your vision
and restircts the freedom of your mind to think.

A: How about enjoying anticipation of bad weather?

E: There is nothing more pleasant
than the sound of raindrops on the roof
when you are lying on the hay in the barn,
knowing at least you won't be out in the hot sun pitching hay.
And knowing that you have a few good meals under your belt
before you get out in the field,
and then the rain.

Most bad weather for the farmer is
in regard to cutting hay.
Well, it certainly isn't a blizzard.
If it were a blizzard,
a blizzard is terrible
in so many different ways.
And bad weather,
30,000, 35,000 feet up is
a different kind of weather than at
zero feet.
I often wonder,
when I was at 30,000 feet above sea level,
what would it be like if
I could sense
how a plane was dealing with that air
at that speed.

A: I do, I do that. I do two things that you suggested. I try to think of and enjoy the clear air turbulence that wasn't expected. I try to think of all the feelings of whether it was a roller coaster feeling or a bumpy car feeling. What kind of feeling it was.

> R: In this section Mrs. A clearly illustrates the utilization of trance as a state of active learning. She is confused about how to generalize her acceptance of a more adequate approach to academic learning to her phobia for flying. Her confusion, of course, is itself proof that she is in the process of giving up an old, less adequate frame of reference for a new one that she does not yet understand. You now take advantage of this situation to facilitate more openness in her frames of reference in the following sections.

Depotentiating Habitual Mental Sets: Facilitating Flexible Frames of Reference

E: But you had no frame of reference.

A: Then I try to think about what was happening to the aircraft in terms of structural stress and knowing that the structural specifications allowed for stress of this magnitude.
But I was uncomfortable and quite relieved when it was all over.

E: All right, I will give you an example

that shows what I have done for you before.

Could you plant ten trees in five straight rows with four trees in each row?

A: Ten trees in five straight rows, four trees in each row?
[Pause]
[After a number of futile attempts, the senior author shows her the following star-shaped diagram as a solution to the problem.]

A: Oh, I didn't think that. I was trying to relate it to air turbulence.

E: You can't understand air turbulence, can you?
You can't understand it in terms of air turbulence on the ground.

A: I can understand it intellectually in terms of what happens atmospherically. How it forms and how it affects bodies and that sort of thing. I can't understand my response emotionally.

E: All right, and how can you understand
you have two responses; intellectual and emotional?

A: Oh, yes, that's for sure.

E: Now sometimes you can have intellectual knowledge of it,
and you may be emotionally behind it.

A: I can't separate the emotional in this case. Intellectually I can understand a lot of things that I fear—in this case air turbulence.
But a lot of fear as it was before,
is an uncomfortableness.

E: Now that puzzle there,
five straight rows,
four trees in each row,
only ten trees. What you did was you dragged into my presentation the definition of a row,
and a straight line, a second row.

A: Yes, I did.

E: It would be nice if this puzzle could be a way of treating air turbulence

because you can only understand it
in certain frames of reference.

A: I'm not relating this to air turbulence. I understand intellectually air turbulence.

[Here Erickson distracts her by ostentatiously tearing up the sheet of paper on which he had shown her the tree problem. He then shows her another of his set-breaking problems. He writes the number 710 and asks Mrs. A to read it in all possible ways. Most people are not able to break the number set sufficiently to read it as OIL when they turn it upside down. Erickson typically reveals the answer by first asking the patients to make an "S" near the upside-down 710. If they still don't get it, he has them make the "S" right in front of the upside-down 710 so it reads "SOIL." At that point most people succeed in shifting from the number to the letter set.]

R: This was a typical example of another of your approaches for depotentiating a patient's habitual mental sets to introduce the possibility of experiencing more flexible frames of reference. With the trees and 710 problems, you have patients experience the rigidity of their own mental sets and you give them a bit of training in developing more flexible frames of reference.

E: You always have patients experience as much of themselves and their limiting mental sets as possible within therapy. *The most important thing in therapy is to break up the patients' rigid and limiting mental sets* (Rossi, 1973).

Phobia as a Limited Frame of Reference

E: You can have a numerical frame of reference.

A: Which I definitely do.

E: I know, you work on a computer. Now, what is the proper frame of reference for air turbulence at 30,000 feet up? Is it words or numbers?

A: It's feelings, really.

E: The feelings that you learned on the ground?

A: No. I'm not aware of feelings, having that feeling on the ground.

E: You learned certain feelings of fear on the ground, and you carried them aloft with you. Know what right feelings you should have up there.

A: So are you saying that when I fear an air turbulence, I think only in a fear frame of reference instead of a logical frame of reference?

E: Neither logical nor fear. There is a new frame of reference for you to discover.

A: You mean how I should think of it?

E: Yes. A frame of reference that is really a totally new and different feeling unrelated to any feelings you have had.
Stop to consider, what did the astronauts encounter in space?

A: Total unknowns.

E: Total unknowns! Now what I'm telling you is that air turbulence can't be understood in terms of ground experience, just as the astronauts found out they couldn't understand the absence of gravity. They could pour water up, they could pour water down, or pour it sideways, and I don't know how they could spit.

A: So how do I do that?

E: I don't know how the astronauts learned about no gravity, but they did.

> E: She learned fear of heights on the ground and she carried it aloft on a plane where ground fears are inappropriate. In a plane you can hit an air pocket and fall hundreds of feet and it can be a delightful experience. What feelings should you have when you're in the air? Not ground feelings!
>
> R: On the ground it could be a disaster to fall only a few feet.
>
> E: I'm asking her to adopt a frame of reference that is totally new and different.
>
> R: You genuinely don't know how she will experience the new frame of reference. Her conscious mind does not know either. Your job as a therapist is to point out and possibly depotentiate some of the limiting and biasing sets of her conscious mind so her unconscious may have a better opportunity for becoming manifest with the new. This case illustrates the essence of a theory of phobia. Phobic behavior comes about from the problem of using an old frame of reference inappropriately in a new situation. The old frame of reference really doesn't fit, and this lack of fit gives rise to the anxiety, negative affect, and avoidance behavior so characteristic of phobia. The anxiety and avoidance behavior is actually an accurate signal indicating that

the patient's old frames of reference need to change. When the patient does not recognize the signal aspect of the anxiety, it is experienced as a negative affect without any appropriate intellectual component: The patient experiences anxiety and fear without knowing why; she has a phobia. We can infer that when a phobia develops in a apparently familiar situation (such as school phobia, agoraphobia, etc.), it means something has changed in the patient's relation to that situation, but this change is not recognized and the appropriate inner adjustments (modifying old frames of reference or creating new ones) have not been made. Phobia is due to a too-limited frame of reference. Its permanent resolution requires insight and expanded frames of reference. This is essentially a new theory of phobia that is inherent in your work, and you didn't know it, did you?

E: There are a lot of things that I know I don't know.

Further Illustrations of Growth via New Frames of Reference

E: You know the measurements show that the astronauts grew one inch in space, and they lost that inch very promptly after reaching the earth. When children experience a sudden spurt of growth, when a child measures himself against his mother,
you know what happens:
"How tall I am!"
Everybody in the house knows it.

A: He bumped into things.

E: He was bumping into things!
Striking things with his hands.
The awkward stage is the growing stage.
And he had
to figure out how long his arms were,
how far he stepped.
He had to build a new set of measurements for himself.
Now what set of measurements will you form for turbulence?
[Pause]
You have an oppurtunity there to find out.
[The senior author now gives other examples of new life experiences requiring the formation of new frames of reference, not merely the use of an old frame inappropriately in a new situation.]

E: The growing age is the awkward age; growing pains.

R: Yes, awkwardness should be applauded as a sign of growth and new learning.

E: You give many examples so that patients are more likely to find one that's personally convincing and actually helps alter their behavior. The only things that I say to you that cling are those that touch upon your experience in some way. You always study your patients for evidence that they are accepting what you say.

Autohypnosis to Facilitate Therapeutic Change: Flexibility in Mental Functioning

A: I am satisfied with not being terrified of flying. To find it enjoyable, that is asking a lot, I think. You think I will?

E: The astronauts didn't know what on earth it was like to be in space.

A: There is a difference. I can be apprehensive about something unknown, knowing that it is going to turn out OK at the end. That kind of apprehension. But there is no way that I can logically relate to being afraid. I just am. Logically I know I shouldn't be and I know that there is nothing to worry about and I can recite all these statistics and——

E: And you know how very easily I can put you in a state of terror.

A: Yeah.

E: And wipe it out just as quickly, right?

A: Yeah, the terror.

E: And wipe out your happy feeling, too.

A: Yeah.

E: That is, your fear or your pleasure can' be removed and reassumed.

A: Can I do it in advance? I tried hypnotizing myself in a situation and I can't concentrate. Like when we hit turbulence.

E: Try to count from one to twenty.

A: Right now?
From one to twenty? [Mrs. A closes her eyes and evidently goes into trance momentarily. She then opens her eyes, shifts her body, and is obviously awake again.]

346

E: You didn't get all the way to twenty did you?

A: No.

E: That's right.
[Pause]
And now future accomplishments are future accomplishments.
[Pause]
And they can be enjoyed. [Pause]

A: I was just thinking. I can't wait to get out of here and fly.

E: Well you are at liberty to leave at any time you want to, or stay.

A: That's fantastic. I can't wait to get on an airplane!

E: I facilitate a certain flexibility in mental functioning when I remind her how easily her pleasure and fear can be "removed and reassumed."

R: Her residual fears about flying are apparently resolved when you give her the tool of autohypnosis with which to help herself. If trance is conceptualized as an altered state or shift in frames of reference, we can understand how autohypnosis can be particularly useful for phobia or any situation where the patient needs to cope with difficult emotions. Her momentary autohypnotic experience here was enough to let her know that from within she is experiencing a high degree of therapeutic expectancy—so much so that she can't wait to get on a plane!

Selected Shorter Cases: Exercises for Analysis

Uncovering Techniques: Dissociating Intellect and Emotions to Uncover Traumatic Memories

E: In this matter of uncovering techniques I think one of the most important things is to recognize that if your patient has something covered up, she's got it covered up for a very good reason, and you'd better respect that fact. You ask the patients to respect the fact that you personally do not think it needs to be covered up but that you are going to abide by their needs, *their actual needs*. Now you've told them you will abide by their needs, but they don't hear you qualify it to their "actual needs."

R: This is an example of indirect suggestion through two-level communication. The first portion of your statement about abiding by their needs is readily accepted by a patient's conscious mind and tends to open a yes or acceptance set for the qualification that follows regarding their "actual needs," which may be very different from what they think they are. The unconscious does pick up this qualification (which may be subtly emphasized with a slight vocal intonation or gesture), however, and uses it to initiate an inner process of search for "actual needs." This search on an unconscious level may finally result in new insights that will depotentiate the patient's previously limited frames of reference and thus facilitate therapy.

E: Yes. You actually have two issues here: Does it need to be covered up? Can it be uncovered? You then point out to a patient that there are various ways of remembering things. Undoubtedly, when we cover up a memory, we usually cover up a lot more than the memory itself. That is, trauma of a shaved head might be covered up as an uncomfortable memory, but along with that would be covered up the room in which it was done, perhaps the address of that particular place, and other things that happened that year. Does the year need to be covered up? All the other things that happened that year? You thus emphasize that the patient undoubtedly covered up many things that didn't need to be covered up. So why not uncover every one of those things that are not safe to uncover and be sure to keep covered up the things that are not safe to uncover? You then define the situation as one from which the patient can withdraw at any time. You point out, "Suppose you did accidentally uncover something you didn't want uncovered. How long do you think it would take you to cover it up again?" That is the little bit of assurance that you always give your patient.

You then point out to a patient that it is perfectly possible to remember the intellectual facts of something but not the emotional content, and vice versa. You point out that once, when you felt downhearted and blue, you couldn't for the life of you figure out why, but there must have been a reason in the back of your mind. You experienced the emotions but you didn't have intellectual content. In recovering a traumatic memory you can uncover deep emotions and not intellectual content. If you want to, you can remember the actual intellectual content; you need not remember whether you felt sad, mad, or glad. It will be just a memory, as if it happened to somebody else.

An example of this was with one of my medical students who was going to flunk out of medical school, he absolutely and irrationally refused to attend the lectures and the clinics on dermatology. He wouldn't open his book on dermatology. He was warned and called up before the dean and told, "You're either going to attend dermatology lectures and clinics and study it or you'll flunk out of medical school. We can't pass anybody who arbitrarily refuses to take one of the courses." Bob said, "I can't." The dean said, "What do you mean, you can't, you're going to!" Bob meant it, however, he couldn't.

Bob came to me very worried about it. I knew Bob was a very good hypnotic subject and I asked him if I could use him as a demonstration subject to the medical class. He said, "Yes." I told him that there had to be some explanation for his peculiar behavior about dermatology. I asked him to spend the next week trying to remember what it was he had forgotten.

Bob spent a week trying to remember and then came to the class. In class I asked, "Bob, did you remember what you had forgotten a long time ago?" Bob said, "How on earth do you go about remembering something you forgot a long time ago? You don't even know where to look! You've forgotten it! It's unavailable, it's unreachable, it's untouchable! It's forgotten—it's gone!" I agreed and sent him out of the room so I could raise the question with the class. They all agreed it would be an awfully blind sort of thing to try to find such a memory. Then I called Bob back and induced a deep trance. I told him, "You know why you are here. You've been thinking for a whole week about remembering something that you'd forgotten. Have you remembered it?" Bob said, "No." I said, "All right, you are in a deep trance. I would like to explain a few things to you. You know what a jigsaw puzzle is? You can put a jigsaw puzzle together in two ways: You put it together right side up, and then you will know what the picture is; you can put it together reverse side up, and there you have just the back of the jigsaw puzzle. No picture on it—just blankness and no meaning, but the puzzle would be together. The picture of the jigsaw puzzle is the intellectual content—the meaningful content of the repressed memory. The back of it is the emotional foundation, and that will be without any picture. It is going to be just the foundation. Now you can put that jigsaw puzzle together by putting two pieces on one corner together, two pieces in the middle together, two pieces in another corner together, two pieces in a third corner, two pieces in a fourth corner, and then, here and there, you can put two or three pieces together. You can put some of the pieces together face up, some pieces together face down. You can put them all together face down, put them all together face up, but you do what you want to do."

What did he want to do? I didn't know, but that question left the burden of the responsibility upon Bob—namely, that he had a jigsaw puzzle of a repressed memory that he needed to recover and put together meaningfully. I asked Bob, "Well, you don't really know what to do. Suppose you haul out from your unconscious just a few little pieces of that unpleasant memory." Bob thought a minute and then perspiration began to form on his forehead. I asked, "What is it Bob?" He said, "I'm feeling sick in a funny sort of way. I don't know what kind of a way." I said, "That's fine, so you're feeling sick in a funny sort of way; you don't know in what kind of a way. All right, forget about it." With that Bob developed an anmesia for the material that was making him feel funny. I then continued, "Suppose you reach down into your repressions and bring up a few pieces of the picture." Bob did essentially that and said, "Well, there is water and there is something green. I suppose that is grass, but that green isn't grass." I said, "That is fine, now you shove that down. Now bring up some more pieces of emotion." Bob brought up some more emotion and then said, "I'm scared, I'm scared. I want to run," and he was really perspiring and trembling. I said, "Shove it down again. Let's bring up a few other picture pieces."

We alternated in that fashion for a while; getting a few associations and then repressing them when the emotion became too threatening. As we got more and more material, Bob began digging up bigger and bigger pieces of emotion so that I would have to bring him out of the trance and let him rest. Bob would take a deep breath and say, "I'm all worn out. I don't know what is happening to me. I'm awake, my shirt is all wet, my trousers are wet with perspiration. What has been going on here?" I assured him that the medical students in the class were just about as sick as he was of seeing that perspiration spurt out on Bob's forehead each time he'd experience an emotion.

Finally I suggested, "Let's put all the blank sides together again and do a complete overhaul." So he put it together again, and you should have seen him trembling and perspiring. He was actually shivering, so periodically I gave him a suggestion to blank it out and rest: "Take another deep breath and look at that blank reverse side of the jigsaw puzzle with the amnesic traumatic experience." He said, "Whatever is on the other side of that is something awful—it's just awful." I then told him to forget the entire emotional side. We'd turn the jigsaw puzzle over and see it intellectually only, without emotions. He described, "Two little boys, about eight or nine years old, they looked like cousins— they're playing in a barn, they are wrestling. Oh! Oh! One is getting mad with the other. Now they are hitting at each other. Now they grabbed some forks, they start stabbing at each other. Oh! Oh! One of them stabbed the other in the leg. That one is running into the house to tell. The one that stabbed him is a little bit afraid. He runs along, too. The boy's father isn't mad; the mother isn't mad; they are calling the doctor. The boy's father makes him sit on a chair to wait. There is the doctor driving in. The doctor is going to stick something in the boy. Oh, my goodness, what a funny thing. Look at that boy's face. He is lying there.

His face is swelling up, his eyes are swelling shut, his skin is turning a funny color, his tongue is so thick, and the doctor is scared. He is getting something else. He's got—it looks like a needle or a pump of some kind, and he is pumping something into the boy, and now that swelling in the boy's face is getting less, his tongue is getting smaller, he is opening his eyes, and everybody is breathing deeply. The father grabs the other boy and takes him down to the horse trough. The father sits on the horse trough, hauls the boy over his lap, and starts spanking him, and he is really spanking him hard. The boy is looking down into the horse trough and he sees that green slime on the water and he is crying. There is something awful bad about this, and I don't know what it is. There is something awful bad." I said, "Well let one corner of the back of it soak through, and then another corner, let the back of it soak through, soak through, soak through." You should have seen poor Bob as he began uniting the ideational content with the affect. Shuddering, trembling, crying out, horrified, he said "I can't stand it."

I again told him to develop a complete amnesia. "Take a rest Bob. You have a little more work to do. Maybe if you rest five minutes, we'll have enough strength to do a little more of the work." Then about five minutes later I asked him to continue. He dropped the amnesia until he couldn't stand it any longer, and then another amnesia, a rest, and then again another recovery, until finally he said, "That little boy that stabbed the other one is me. That's my cousin, and that was the fork we used for cleaning out the barn, and the doctor comes and gives him an antitetanus shot. He gets an anaphylactic reaction with all that edema, and everybody expects him to die including me. Then the doctor gave him adrenalin and he recovered, and then my father took me down to the horse trough and spanked me. I couldn't even stand the way my cousin looked, and there was my father spanking me and that nasty green slime on the water in the trough—that horrible green slime and that horrible color of my cousin's face. No wonder I couldn't study my dermatology." That was the end of that. No wonder he didn't like dermatology.

Too many therapists try to recover the total experience all at once. In everyday life we frequently notice people with an attitude of indifference. They may have an intellectual appreciation of their position but an emotional indifference. Well, I think that in hypnotherapy we need to recognize the tremendous importance of indifference, detachment, and the possibility of extracting only one fragment here and another fragment there. It was sufficient that Bob recover something and then develop an amnesia, because when he developed an amnesia for any part of it, that was at my request. That was not his own spontaneous involuntary amnesia under pressure. This was something where he was being responsive to suggestion, and therefore the amnesic behavior was under his control. It was just as effective as a repression, but it allowed that traumatic material to be available for examination—and available in varying degrees, in small portions in relation to emotional healing and the ideational content.

The class began at six P.M., and I think it was somewhere around midnight when I finished with him. I cautioned the class to say absolutely nothing to Bob because I knew there was a dermatology class the next afternoon. Everybody cooperated, and when they went to dermatology class, Bob came in casually, matter-of-fact as could be. I told them just to greet him casually and ask him where he is going next but say nothing at all about it. You know it was almost a week before Bob recalled that he was attending dermatology. He just simply took it so-matter-of-factly that he didn't realize he had missed previous lectures and clinics. Now that is an approach I have used with a lot of different patients.

R: Is it necessary to develop a deep trance state for this particular type of thing?

E: It was with Bob, but it's not necessary if you get that state of indifference and ask the person to think of himself more or less as being in the next room undergoing a certain experience. "Of course you can't see it, you can't hear it, but think of yourself as undergoing a certain experience—the experience of recovering a lost traumatic memory, and as you sit here you are not really in a deep trance, you're not really in a medium trance, you are in a light trance. You don't feel like moving, you don't really feel like doing anything, but your mind seems to be rather far away and you are thinking about yourself in the other room—remembering something, and I wonder what part of that memory you're remembering?" There you are getting associations, and the patient can start remembering.

R: Your request that the patient simply imagine himself in another room recovering a lost memory is itself an indirect approach to hypnotic induction. You (1) *fixate attention* with that request, and if the patient takes you seriously, you certainly have temporarily (2) *depotentiated his habitual conscious framework.* The patient is thereby engaged in a (3) *search on the unconscious level,* since the conscious mind certainly doesn't know how to do it. The trance induction is further emphasized with your suggestions, "You don't feel like moving, you don't really feel like doing anything, but your mind seems to be rather far away." You are utilizing indirect suggestions in the form of not doing, and a dissociation between the personality sitting with you and the mind "thinking about yourself in the other room." The patient's own associations and (4) *unconscious processes* then take over and mediate the (5) *hypnotic response* of recovering the lost memory.

352

Hypnotherapy in Extreme, Sudden, Acute Emotional Disturbances*

Much has been said and written about the need for intensive searching into the remote past of patients to discover the "psychodynamics" underlying personality and behavioral disturbances. Alarmist statements have been made about the damage that might result from employing hypnosis in situations of acute emotional distress and disturbances without an adequate knowledge of the patient's past experiences and personality structure. To this author such alarmist statements suggest only lack of knowledge and a sense of personal insecurity when facing problems of stress in others.

The adaptability of hypnosis in meeting critical situations, the ease with which it can be used without altering natural physiological and psychological processes (as contrasted with pharmacological assaults and electric shock), suggest the desirability of its more frequent and ready use in sudden emergency situations. Following are two illustrative accounts, one given in greater detail than the other because of their essential similarity. For the reader's orientation certain general information will be given that was obtained by the author only subsequent to the handling of the acute emergencies.

The patients' presenting problems were handled in the same emergency fashion as one would handle an accident case with acute injuries and a broken leg (that is, first splint the leg and then undertake complete local treatment before taking a detailed history.)

Both of these patients were in their early thirties and both manifested essentially the same behavior, the development of which had, in each instance, been an intense quarrel between husband and wife. Both women were definitely insecure, dependent persons, unstable emotionally and easily rendered tearful. Neither was ever regarded as even latently psychotic, but both were considered to be passively dependent, emotionally insecure, mildly psychoneurotic persons making reasonably good adjustments in the childless and protected environments in which they lived.

Decondition a Hysterical Catalepsy: Case Report One

This patient was a thirty-three-year old wife of an internist who, with the aid of his partner, practically carried the patient into the senior author's office and placed her in a chair. She sat there rigidly, staring

---

*Previously unpublished paper written by the senior author and edited for publication here by the junior author.

vacantly into space, with fully dilated pupils, in a state of complete unresponsiveness to all stimuli.

The husband explained that she had become hysterical during a quarrel at the office and that she had begun to scream uncontrollably. This had resulted in the husband's partner coming into the office to ascertain what difficulty had arisen. Both had frantically tried to reassure her but could not secure her attention. In desperation they had agreed that perhaps it would be possible to "bring her out of it" by a sharp slap on the face. This has served to "freeze her completely" in the state she now presented. They had tried all manner of stimuli to attract her attention, but to no avail. They were alarmed about the bilateral fixed dilation of her pupils because of uneasy feelings about intracranial injury, but felt a bit reassured because the pupils were equally dilated. They had attempted to reduce the pupils by the use of an extremely bright light, but she had stared unblinkingly into the light with no change in her pupils.

Because of the husband's state of emotional distress, he and his partner were excluded from the office, and the husband's request for some suitable intravenous medication to allow her "to sleep it off," and his statement that "if necessary, I suppose electric shock could be used," were disregarded. The senior author preferred a psychological approach to the patient's psychological reaction in a period of emotional distress. A psychological approach should certainly be regarded as a method of first choice, to be attempted before resorting to drastic assaults upon the patient's body.

Since the two physicians had, at the scene of the inception of the emotional disturbance, tried flashing a powerful light into the patient's eyes, the author decided to capitalize upon this fact. Securing a small blinking light (a child's toy), the senior author placed it at the opposite side of the office so that it would be within her field of vision. Seating himself beside her, he softly repeated a long series of brief, gentle suggestions, synchronizing them with the blinking of the light. (Past experience in research had taught the senior author that conditioned responses can be effectively established even when the subject is not consciously aware of the stimuli.) These suggestions were, "Off in the distance, see a light. Now it comes, now it goes. Off in the distance, see a little light. Now it comes, now it goes." With monotonous regularity these suggestions were repeated for about twenty minutes. A slight quivering of her eyelids led to a change in the suggestions to the tripartite suggestion of "as it comes—and goes—try harder to see," synchronizing the first and third part to the appearance of the light.

After about five minutes of this triple suggestion, her eyelids began quivering and her pupils started to contract. Further synchronized suggestions were given slightly more urgently: "As the light comes, your lids will close; as it goes, they will close more. As it comes, your lids will close; as it goes, they will close more." Within two minutes the suggestions were changed to, "As the light comes, so tired; as it comes, so sleepy; as it comes, eyes close, so tired; as it comes, eyes close, so tired; as it comes, soon asleep; as it comes, soon sound asleep; and sound asleep and sounder asleep, and sound asleep and now sound asleep." There followed, since she responded well, "Staying asleep, resting comfortably," repeated a number of times. She was then instructed to "rest comfortably," to "sleep deeply," to "relax so comfortably and completely," to "feel so good, so much at rest, so ready to tell" the senior author anything he wished to know about, but "too tired to be worried, too sleepy to be scared, just softly to tell" the senior author whatever he asked, and "doing so, just understand everything."

Within forty-five minutes this patient related an informative account of her early youth, when she had seen a neighbor's wife develop an apparently causeless screaming episode that had terminated suddenly in a mute, catatonic, schizophrenic stupor with resulting commitment to a state hospital. She related this as a past unhappy memory that she had "forgotten years ago." When she was asked to continue, she showed mild emotional distress and somewhat hesitantly related the circumstances of a quarrel with her husband about a vacation trip. This had caused increasing anger on her part. The trip, as she wished it, would have taken her to her childhood home, but her husband wished to go elsewhere. Realizing that he would have his way, she screamed in futile rage, and then the memory of that neighbor's wife screaming came to her mind. She "wondered if I could stop screaming, and that scared me terribly and I kept screaming. Then someone—my husband, I guess—slapped me, and that paralyzed me. I just couldn't see and I couldn't hear. I was just looking helplessly at nothingness, getting more scared all the time. Just thinking about it makes my skin crawl. It won't happen again, will it?" She was reassured and asked to continue.

"Well, nothing happened forever and ever it seemed, and then I thought I saw a little bright light and I began hearing a voice. At first I couldn't tell what the voice said, but it seemed that I began listening better, and soon I could hear better, and pretty soon I heard you talking to me. I know I didn't know you, but I was tired and sleepy, and some way I knew you would take care of me. You will, won't you?"

Again she was reassured and she was asked what next she wanted. "Tell my husband." She was asked if she did not think she ought to remember the entire episode when she awakened. Her reply was the inquiry, "Will I get scared again?" She was answered with, "Not unless you want to be." "I don't," was her earnest assertion. Accordingly, she was aroused and, with no further instruction, consciously retold the whole story with embarrassment and some slight distress about the extremes of her behavior. She was then asked if it would not be well for her to relate the entire story to her husband. Her reply was, "Oh yes, or he will worry about me." She also agreed that her husband's partner could be present when she learned that he had participated in the situation.

Her husband asked, "Were you thinking about that neighbor when you insisted on the vacation trip, including going to your old home?" "Oh, no! I haven't thought of her for years. It's just that I got a letter from Ann [a girlhood friend], that girl I used to know that you didn't like, and I wanted to go back and see her." Further conversation and discussions were not significantly informative. Suffice it to state that the vacation trip did include her desired visit and that her adjustments have improved during the years that have elapsed. Her husband's comment on the correction of his wife's problem was, "Well, I suppose it helps people to get things out of their system, but I'm not sure I would recommend starting it that way."

The entire therapeutic process for this patient required not over two hours, and the passage of about a half dozen years indicates that it was adequate.

Conditioned response; Compound suggestions securing attention and initiating inner searches and responses.

Deconditioning Hysterical Catalepsy: Case Report Two

In the case of the second woman, aged thirty-one, with a personality structure very similar to that of the first patient, and also childless, the immediate emotional difficulty had arisen at the breakfast table. She had timidly told her husband that, on returning from a trip the previous evening, the car had collided with the side of the garage. She had bent the fender slightly and broken the headlight; because of the lateness of the hour, she had not told him because of possible unpleasantness. Her anticipatory fears were justified, as the husband explained in accounting for her condition. "I just ranted and raved like a prize idiot, and she got madder and madder, and so did I. She finally grabbed her purse and threw it at me, and it fell open and things spilled out. Her pocket mirror slid along the floor and stopped right where the sun was shining on the floor, and I could see how it reflected the sunlight so that it hit her right in the face. She froze instantly, just froze right like she was, with her face all mad, her eyes glaring, but she just seemed as blind as a bat and as deaf as a stone.

"I yelled at her, asking what was the matter, but she didn't make a move. So I shook her and finally she limbered up a little and I brought her in. Did I make her lose her mind, and can you help her?"

The man was reassured briefly and dismissed from the office. The woman, who had entered the office with her husband anxiously propelling her like an automaton, now sat listlessly, with her eyes open but apparently unseeing.

After studying her appearance for a few minutes thoughtfully, the senior author touched her gently on the shoulder to attract her attention. The effect was electrifying. Her body jerked to rigidity, and her mouth opened widely as if to scream. Her eyes were wide open, the pupils fully dilated.

The senior author, recalling that she had become "frozen stiff" when the sunlight had flashed into her eyes, decided to try a technique essentially comparable to the one used above.

Placing the toy blinking light within her field of vision, but keeping it obscured until the suggestions had been phrased, the author began the use of a technique of suggestions similar to the one used with the first patient. A bipartite suggestion was used, synchronizing the first part with the appearance of the light and the second part with the disappearance of the light. Also the two parts were said with distinct but different emphasis, the first part being emphasized as a fact, the second part as a reassurance.

For about fifteen minutes, in repetitious monotony, the senior author carefully stated over and over, "You are frightened, but feeling better." As the minutes passed, the second part was more firmly emphasized, until finally she began to relax physically. Then the suggestions were progressively changed in the following fashion: "You are less frightened, you are feeling better; you are less frightened, you are feeling better and relaxed; you are feeling still less frightened and more relaxed and better; less and less fright, more and more relaxed, better; just a light fright, so much better; fright going, going, gone, relaxed, comfortable; all better, ready to relax; to sleep, to relax, to sleep; and deeper, deeper and deeper and deeper asleep."

About ten minutes of this graduated change in suggestions resulted in a comfortable, relaxed state of deep hypnosis.

A new suggestion was offered: "And now you can look back on last night as if it were last week or even last month—who really cares now? Just feel comfortable and just as if you were another person. Tell me what happened to that young woman in her kitchen that scared her."

With very light urging and only slight emotional display she answered, "Light in her eyes, scared, she thought automobile going hit her. Scared, couldn't move." She was told, "Now I want you to understand all I say. That young woman was you, and you were scared, but that's all over now. You are here, talking to me about it. Just tell me everything. Just remember I don't know a single *little* thing about it, so be sure to tell me all even if you think parts are *not important* (the italicized words were intended to minimize the whole event without doing so noticeably)."

357

She told a story of a bitter quarrel with her brother and of striking him and turning to run, of how she ran into the street, of how her brother yelled, and then she started to look toward him. It was evening, and a car with glowing headlights was bearing down upon her. She was too paralyzed to move, and she stood staring helplessly even after the car swerved by her. She was forcibly hauled out of the street by her irate father, who soundly spanked both her and her brother. This incident had, to the best of her knowledge, been long forgotten, but the quarrel with her husband over a car, the associated headlight, her assault by throwing her handbag at her husband, and the mirror flashing sunlight in her face had all combined to revivify, in a violently emotional situation, a comparable emotional situation of long-past experience.

The course of handling was similar to that of the other patient. She and her husband were seen for an additional three hours, primarily to meet their current needs. The beneficial results of the therapy, brief as it was, are still persistent.

Fixation of attention, compound suggestions with vocal cues; Pun (light fright); Dissociation initiating inner searches and responses; Two-level communication.

A little needs to be said about the underlying experiential factors and conditionings that long afterward were manifested in the highly disturbed states that developed in these two women. In the limited meanings ascribed to the term by various schools of thought these two problems were clearly "psychodynamic" in character. But that the handling of the problem therapeutically must necessarily be based on a ritualistic, orthodox, or classical method of approach is, to the senior author, neither reasonable nor profitable. The patients presented a problem that needed to be handled at once. The problems were remote in origin, recent only in manifestation. To search for those remote origins would have been impossible until the traumatic course of stressful emotional events rendered the patients more accessible and probably more permanently damaged. Past experience with many similar patients suggests the importance of a ready approach to the immediate problem by dealing with it directly.

One can speculate on what would have happened had a pharmacological approach, electric shock, or extensive psychoanalysis been employed. The senior author has seen patients he believed were similar to these so treated with adverse consequences.

In the treatment given these patients it is apparent that hypnosis is a modality that offers possible methods of approach to patients difficult to reach by ordinary interpersonal methods. *Hypnosis also offers the opportunity of dealing with the patient at two levels of awareness,* so that the patient can safely approach a complete understanding of a traumatic experience that was previously repressed as intolerably painful—that is, at an unconscious level of mentation and then at a level of conscious awareness.

An Instance of Aggression Tranformation*

From almost the first day in medical school Anne had made herself unpopular with both students and professors. She was always in sight at the classroom door well ahead of time, but she nevertheless entered the classroom from five to twenty minutes late. Each time she would walk across the front of the room, down the far side, and find a seat in the rear of the room. If she had to enter the room from the rear, she walked down the side aisle, crossed the front of the room, and then sought a seat in the rear of the room.

Repeatedly she had been privately and publicly rebuked by her teachers, some patiently, some irately. She always listened courteously, would apologize to them, and then in subsequent classes she would penalize them for the rebuke by being later and more ostentatious. Her classmates came to resent her, some of them intensely and rudely. Nothing availed, and everybody continued to resent this constant irritation by Anne.

A new professor was added to the faculty, and when his student management methods became known, Anne's reformation was gleefully predicted.

The professor's first lecture of that semester of Anne's attendance of his classes was at 8:00 A.M. He arrived at 7:40 A.M. and was greeted cordially by a large number of students, including Anne. One by one the students filed into the classroom and took their seats expectantly. Anne was not among them. The professor closed the classroom door which was at the front of the room, took his place on the podium, and began his lecture. At fifteen minutes past the hour Anne entered. Instantly the professor paused in his lecture, extended his hands palm up to the expectant students, and silently motioned for them to stand. Then he turned toward Anne and silently salaamed, and so did the students, until she had taken her seat. The lecture was then continued as if there had been no interruption.

At the close of the hour the students rushed out to spread the news. Everybody who met Anne—student, secretary, professor, even the dean—salaamed silently, and her entry into any classroom that day was an orgy of silent, respectful salaaming.

Anne was on time for all classes the next day—in fact, she tended to be the first to arrive.

---

*Previously unpublished paper written by the senior author and edited for publication here by the junior author.

Several months later she sought out the professor to ask for intensive psychotherapy and established excellent rapport with him.

The rationale for this treatment of Anne is rather simple. Her tardiness, whatever its remote origin, had become an aggression, was received as such, continued as such, and was universally regarded by her colleagues and instructors as an intolerable but continuing affront. The entire situation called for an effective aggression against Anne that would eliminate, and thus abolish, her aggression.

By the simple process of a silent salaaming, Anne's aggression was instantly transformed into a totally different kind of thing that offered not an opportunity for aggressive retaliative attack but a joyous participation by all others in the transformation of the aggression. Yet Anne was, in essence, left unscathed as a person, since there still remained with her the control of the aggression. This she promptly manifested the next day by her own abolition of her aggression.

Don't Think of the Baby

This report concerns a problem of brief duration, decidedly acute in character and marked by terrified, obsessional, insistent demands.

The patients were a young couple in their early twenties. Both were attending college, and they had been engaging in sexual relations regularly for nearly a year. They had just discovered that there existed a pregnancy of about two months' duration. Both sets of parents were furious and unforgiving and asserted emphatically that "It better be gotten rid of, or no more college" (one more year of college for each remained). Extreme and unreasoning emphasis had been placed upon the shame entailed for all relatives and friends. The young couple had planned to marry but not until after graduation from college.

The couple was seriously distressed by their situation and by the parental attitudes that had developed to include "no college and no marriage unless you spare us this shame." The father of the young man furnished him sufficient money and advice on where to secure the abortion. A friend of the young man, knowing about the situation and aware of the highly disturbed emotional state of the couple, suggested that they see the senior author and get "tranquilized" before undertaking the risks of an illegal abortion.

Their distress was greatly augmented when the senior author uncompromisingly discountenanced an abortion. Nor would they listen to the senior author's suggestions of other more reasonable possibilities. For two long hours they insistently repeated demands that the senior author approve the abortion and that he undertake the task himself by using hypnosis to induce physiological activity, thereby making it "legal," and that he prescribe tranquilizing drugs to "calm" both of them. They expressed fear that their overwrought emotional state, in view of the senior author's lack of cooperation, might cause an abortionist to reject them as too much of a risk, since neither could keep from bursting into hysterical sobs at frequent intervals.

Brief, scattered bits of information disclosed that each was an only child, highly protected by rigid, domineering parents, and that each was completely dependent on their parents for everything including even their opinions in general. They were genuinely in love and were expecting to be married with parental blessings upon being graduated from college. Among the planned wedding presents were a secure position in the firm of the father-in-law-to-be for the young man and a beautiful home from the young man's parents. Now all of this, their entire planned and desired future, was at stake unless they abided by parental commands and secured the abortion.

Two full hours of desperate endeavor failed to make the slightest impression upon their insistent, hysterical, highly obsessional, repetitional demands.

Finally the senior author decided to capitalize upon the obsessional fearful behavior they were both constantly manifesting by using that very behavior itself. As everybody knows, it is impossible to hold a stop watch to time oneself and to avoid thinking about an elephant for one whole minute. This simple, childish challenge seemed to present a method of dealing affectively with the problem they presented.

Accordingly, the author emphatically demanded, "All right, all right, quiet now, quiet—if you want the help you ask. Quiet, and let me tell you how to ensure getting the abortion you are desperately trying to prove to me that you want. You have told me you want the abortion. You have told me that there is no other choice. You have told me that, regardless of everything, you are going to go ahead with the abortion. You declare most emphatically and resolutely that nothing can stop you. *Now let me warn you about one thing that can stop you, that will surely stop you, against which you will be totally helpless if you are not warned about it in advance. Quiet now! Listen attentively because you need to know this if you really want the abortion, if you really intend to get the abortion.* Now listen quietly and attentively. Are you listening?"

Both nodded their heads silently, expectantly. The senior author continued, "You do not know an important thing, a vitally important thing. That essential information is this: You do not know whether that baby is a boy or a girl. You do not see, cannot see, the vital connection between that question and the abortion you have told me that you want. *Yet that question will prevent you from getting the abortion since you don't know the answer.* Your personalities, your psychological makeups make that question important. You do not know why, but who expects you to know? Let me explain! If that baby were going to be kept by you,

you, not knowing if it were a boy or a girl, would have to think of a name for it that would fit either sex, such as Pat, which could be either Patrick or Patricia, or Frances for a girl or Francis for a boy. *Now that is the very thing you must avoid at all costs.* Under no circumstances, not even once, *after you leave this office,* are you to think of a possible name for that baby, a name that would fit either sex. *To do so and to keep on doing so would compel you psychologically to keep the baby,* not to get an abortion. Hence, under no circumstances are you to dare to think of a name for that baby. Please, please don't, because then you won't get an abortion. Every time you think of a name, that thinking will definitely deter you from getting an abortion. You will be forced into taking the money you have and seeing a justice of the peace and getting married. You want an abortion, and you can't have it if you think of a name, so don't, just don't, don't don't think of a name, any name for the baby *after you leave this office, because if you do you will keep it, so don't don't don't think of a name, any name.* Now without another word, *not one word, not a single word, especially not a baby's name,* leave this office at once.'' Thereupon the senior author took them by hand and led them quickly to the door to hasten their departure.

Several days later they returned smiling in an abashed fashion, stating, ''After we got married—*because we just couldn't help thinking of dozens of names, and every name made the baby more precious to us*—we realized that all you did was bring us to our senses before we did something awful foolish and awful wrong. We had just lost our heads, and our parents didn't help either—that's why we acted like such awful fools in your office.''

Inquiry disclosed that both sets of parents accepted the elopement instead of an abortion with a profound sense of relief. The original plans for setting up the young couple were carried out when the husband was graduated.

The young mother had to delay her graduation for some time. Then the grandmothers alternately babysat so that the young mother could complete her college work. At the present time little Leslie has several young siblings.

From the very beginning of the interview with this distraught couple the extreme obsessional character of their behavior, thought, and emotions was most marked. They seemed, as persons, to be sound, yet caught in a situation they could not handle. Hypnosis was obviously not a suitable procedure, but it was realized, as observation of them continued, that hypnotic technique of suggestion, seemingly worded to favor undesirable results, could effect positive results and that a specious psychological contingency could be so emphatically suggested to them that their own hysterical, obsessional behavior would make it effective in securing a desirable end result. The presentation of the problem so emphatically of not thinking of a name befitting either sex *outside of the office* and only incidentally mentioning marriage by a justice of the peace, without actually suggesting that they resort to it, precluded any tendency for them to rebel because they had been "told what to do." This created a favorable climate for their voluntary marriage by a justice of the peace, since they were not recognizably so instructed. Fundamental to this evolution of results was their own sense of guilt, their own desire for marriage, their need to do something, the unexpressed, unrecognized anger at their hitherto loving, permissive parents, their outraged feelings at the rage and demands that they obey their parents' commands, and the suggestion of the friend that they seek "tranquilization." All this resulted in a disturbed emotional state that left them in an essentially irrational state. The author then simply, deliberately, *utilized* their own state of irrational thinking to effect a favorable outcome by the use of a hypnotic technique of the presentation of ideas in a fashion conducive to acceptance despite their overwrought emotional state. Additionally, that technique of suggestion subtly transformed the problem from "we must get an abortion" to "we must not think of a name for the baby." This could only be a losing battle, and the very desperateness of their efforts not to think of a suitable name could only serve to bring them closer and closer to marriage, as indeed it did.

The use of *negativity* (they must *not* think of a baby's name) is of decisive significance in this case. Since their whole situation was permeated with negativity (their parents would *not* help them, they could *not* finish college, *not* have a baby, *not* get married, etc.), the senior author was utilizing a dominant mental set by phrasing his suggestion in a negative form. Since negativity was the dominant mental set, it was the most effective one to achieve the desired results.

Utilizing the patient's own patterns of obsessional thinking and affect; Questions initiating unconscious searches and processes; Negative suggestion; Posthypnotic suggestion tied to behavioral inevitabilities.

CHAPTER 9

Facilitating Potentials: Transforming Identity

Case 12   Utilizing Spontaneous Trance: An Exploration Integrating Left and Right Hemispheric Activity

SESSION 1: Spontaneous Trance and Its Utilization: Symbolic Healing

Jill was an attractive thirty-year-old mother who was college educated and highly talented as an artist. She visited the senior author to learn if her spontaneous states of reverie were actually a form of hypnosis. She reported that she would sometimes lapse into spontaneous periods of reverie when she was painting such that her body suddenly became completely immobile in the middle of a brush stroke and she experienced herself as being deeply absorbed in fantasies and visions that would cross her mind like a vivid dream. These periods might last anywhere from a few minutes to hours. She reported that she often experienced deeply meaningful insights during these periods, and at the present time many of her inner experiences served as inspirations for her art.

Immediately upon entering the office for the first time, before a word was spoken, Jill focused on a wooden dolphin that was one of many unusual carvings on top of a bookcase. As she sat with her attention still fixated on the dolphin, she began to speak in a soft, "faraway" voice about the "dolphin who swam away to sea, the dolphin is lost." It was immediately obvious to both authors that Jill had lapsed into one of her spontaneous periods of reverie; from a clinical point of view she appeared delusional. After a few minutes of talk about the dolphin, Jill seemingly blinked and came back to the reality of the office situation with E watching her intently and R fumbling to get the tape recorder operating. Dr. X, a psychologist with academic training in experimental hypnosis, was also present. E first questioned Jill politely to determine if she had been taking any drugs, but she blushed smilingly and assured him that she had never taken any psychedelic drugs. Such behavior was "normal" for her.

Individual Differences in Trance Behavior

E: How far away were you?

J: As far away as the ocean.

E: All right. Was I there?

J: No.

E: You were alone, I thought so. [To R] She showed a lack of movement that we all show in the absence of others. The dissociation of her right arm was acute. The left arm somewhat. There was a failure of head movements. Her eyelids sank to a one-half level. As she is behaving right now, she is much more in contact.

R: So that was classical trance behavior.

> E: She is evidencing here her own pattern of trance behavior. There is no such thing as pure trance behavior.
>
> R: There is no such thing as "pure" or "classical" trance behavior: Everyone manifests their own individual pattern. Certain behaviors like body immobility and altered eyeball behavior are typical, however.

Spontaneous Trance Equivalent to REM Sleep?

J: Would a person in such a state—call it "leaving" or whatever you want to call it—can that take the place of sleep sometimes? Sometimes I'll be very tired and I'll want to go and paint something. I'm tired, but I'll make the decision to paint anyway. But what happens a lot is, that I'll be painting and I'll still think I'm painting but it's like, I'm not asleep exactly, but it's like I'm somewhere else. Totally. It's not just a thought, like thinking of something else.

Just the other night I realized I did this. I did not realize I did this until, oh, four days ago, when I saw my hand holding a brush in the same position for about at least twenty minutes or a half-hour. And I thought I was somewhere else in this kind of imaginative conversation. And I thought I had not slept for a long time and I had woken up from a dream. But I realized it wasn't [a dream], since the brush was there. And I did not feel tired anymore. I painted for a few hours longer, and then I was surprised to see it was even getting to be morning. I'm a little shy about talking about it since it is essentially such a private kind of thing that I do.

E: It is a very nice kind of thing. [Pause]

E: It is a state similar to the hypnotic, and you can rest, you can be comfortable. You can paint. You can trust your unconscious mind.

> E: She does a remarkable job of explaining. How on earth do you get across to a person that you have experienced a totally different feeling? She knows that she has different feelings in trance, but she really doesn't know how to describe them, and neither do I.

> R: The feelings are so private that she has no external references to develop a communication bridge. Her description of these spontaneous trances suggests that for her, at least, there is an equivalence between trance and the REM stage of dream sleep, since she comes out of trance refreshed as if she had been asleep.

Negative Hallucination in Sequential Stages

[J now evidences minimal cues of entering a trance as she listens to E. Her eyes are in a fixed stare at him, and her body remains completely immobile.]

E: Now you have forgotten the presence of the others.
[Pause]
How completely have you forgotten the presence of others?
[Pause]
How much?

J: I don't know how to measure it.

E: But they were awful vague to you just now, right?

J: Yes, yes. Although I think I was just on the surface.

> E: You lose a knowledge of the presence of others first by losing the number present, then losing which sex, and only then the positive identity of the person. When you lose your identity or recognition of who is present, then you finally can lose the totality of their presence. I don't know why that is, but it always follows that progression. Her remark about not knowing how to

measure it is very revealing: Consciousness does not have available all the knowledge that is in the unconscious, which actually governs our perceptions and behavior.

R: Losing first the number present makes sense, since number is probably the most abstract left-hemispheric function. The loss then progresses by degrees until you finally lose "recognition," or the most concrete perceptual right-hemispheric aspect of the situation.

Trance in Everyday Life: Right and Left Hemispheric Dissociation in Trance?

X: When you asked about her attending to the rest of us, she came out of it, her state.

E: And you saw her come out of it.

X: Immediately.

E: And you saw her recognize it. She came from somewhere to here. Now you can use that for very constructive purposes. Emotionally constructive, artistically constructive, and constructive as far as thought is concerned.

J: Can it be done on purpose? I mean can I will it? Can I use it that way? Because I know that I feel better when I am doing some painting and I, I don't know what words to use to label it, when I go into that, when that happens, when I experience that.

E: Yes, you can do it intentionally.

J: Is that the same as when you are listening to music and you have the feeling of actually entering the music? Or being inside of colors instead of just using them on the outside? It is very funny to talk about, because it is not just something to talk about, exactly. I feel a little shy.

R: This slight falling into trance or reverie is a normal aspect of everyday behavior. You and Dr. X are trained observers and can pick it up immediately. You can use this awareness of the spontaneous beginnings of trance to choose the most appropriate moment for inducing or encouraging further trance. Do you wait for such moments to induce trance?

E: They are going to be *interested* in what makes me think they can be put into a trance. So I merely make use of their interest and keep away from formal trance induction.

R: How do you make use of their interest? You direct it to the inner parts of their own world?

E: Yes. And there I stay with them.

R: Her continued emphasis on not knowing what ''words to use to label it, when I go into that . . .'' strongly suggests there is a dissociation between the verbal aspects of left-hemispheric functioning and the right-hemispheric experience of trance, wherein one has the feeling of ''entering the music'' and ''being inside of colors.''

Indirect Induction of Trance by Focusing on Inner Experience

E: Don't be shy. A woman who thinks as an artist attended one of my lectures and told me she could not be hypnotized. I told her that was all right and asked her what type of music she liked. She said she liked orchestral music. I asked her if she could pick out the second violinist over there. And she picked him out. She described his clothes, she found a redheaded musician. Do you know that orchestra then played all her favorite pieces of music? I knew from the way she talked that she could do it, but she didn't know it. She went into that dissociated state and heard the music and could see the people very nicely. And that is a very excellent thing to do. Sarah Bernhardt in her acting was having a quarrel with her husband in a play. She unintentionally took off her wedding ring, and she *really* took it off.

You do get inside things, and there is nothing wrong or abnormal about it. Every person who has a lot of feeling has hangups about how other people feel about it. Now what pleasures do you like? Do you like swimming?

J: Yes, all the pleasures! All the pleasures! That's it! [She now begins to cry.] I try not to, I don't want to be that way, but I do feel guilty about enjoying all the things I enjoy. Whether it is doing my thing in art and really going into it. That's why I cry.

R: You can induce trance most subtly and easily by simply letting a person focus on what is of most interest to them. Trance is initiated when they become absorbed in something they are really interested in. This is the basis of all indirect induction of trance.

E: Yes. I did not ask that woman if she wanted to enter trance. I simply asked her if she could pick out the second violinist.

R: You find an interest area of the person. An area where there are strong programs built into the person, and you just focus on that to induce trance.

E: That's all!

R: But why do your subjects become so absorbed in their interest areas that trance behavior is evident? We all talk about what's intensely interesting to us in normal conversations every day without falling into trance.

E: *Because I stick to that one thing!*

R: The conversation does not jump to something else. You focus on one thing, you intensify that absorption, and that's what trance is.

E: I don't let the conversation jump to anything else. Yes, trance is a focusing on one thing. Watkins has written a paper describing a trance as dropping all the peripheral foci and narrowing it down to one focus. I agree with that.

A Rapid Age Regression and Therapeutic Reorientation

E: I think that is a very nice thing that you enjoy.

J: I do too. It is not the me now, it is probably the childhood thing. As a child it was always put down. That's it! That's where it comes from. It's as though the tears I feel coming now are not me here now crying. It is the child-feeling from long, long ago. It is an old, old feeling that is coming out now.

[E now questions Jill about her family background, number of siblings, and other details of her early life.]

E: How would you like to go for a swim in the ocean now?
[Pause]

J: [In a very soft, faraway voice] Immediately when you said that I was there.

E: Close your eyes and go for a long pleasant swim in the ocean all alone. Swim a long way
from three years.
[Pause]

A long way
from three years old
to your present age.
And enjoy every stroke of it.
[Long pause as Jill closes her eyes and very evidently follows internal
imagery as her eyes shift rapidly under her closed eyelids.]
And my voice will be meaningful sounds in the water.
[Long pause]
And you'll see that little girl,
[Pause]
a bigger girl
[Pause]
a young lady.
Look at her carefully,
[Long pause]
and you'll learn a surprising number of nice things about her you didn't
know.

R: She describes so well how it's the child side of her who is
crying now. Did you choose this method of induction because
she had already demonstrated that the theme of swimming in the
ocean had spontaneously induced a trance in the beginning of
this session in her association to the dolphin? In other words,
you were again simply *utilizing* a subject's own inner programs
to induce trance?

E: No. I was primarily interested here in getting her as far away
from her family as possible, since it was becoming too emotionally involving for this situation. I wanted to help her with her
tears by distracting her from her emotional distress. I was
creating a situation where she would be free from stress and free
to enjoy. A patient has to be talented to be able to make such
quick jumps as she, but the therapist has to be able to recognize
the situation and know where the patient should jump.

I picked three years because it's reasonable to assume that
she had siblings by the age of three—problems with them. Since
she is showing early-childhood emotions, and early memories
usually begin around three years, I assume that is the age from
which her emotions are actually coming. I ask her to swim away
from them to get the relief she needs at this point. She was
regressing too much in her emotions, and I wanted to yank her
back to her present age. I ask her to become a bigger girl and
finally a young lady.

R: You use a very short period of age regression to simply touch the source of emotional distress and then have her quickly leave it. You permit a momentary catharsis and a very rapid resolution of the problem for the time being. You then introduce a therapeutic reevaluation of her early childhood by suggesting she learn the nice things about herself, since she earlier told you about her deprivations and guilts. You are thus *utilizing* her need for positive self-affirmation to deepen trance and at the same time effect therapy.

Validating Inner Trance Work

[Long pause after which J spontaneously smiles, stretches, and awakens]

E: Hi!

J: Hi. My dolphins are swimming also.

E: Now share only the things you can share with total strangers. Tell us the nice thing you were able to discover, something you had forgotten.

E: The "Hi" is informal. This is tremendously important in therapy, that you keep things informal so you give the patient the privilege of concealing just how important some of these things are.

R: Because if the material becomes too important, the conscious mind will start blocking it out. She apparently came out of trance spontaneously, but actually she was probably following the implications of your remarks to awaken before doing a certain amount of learning.

E: By implication I'm asking her to work at all the things and to communicate only what she can share. That now by implication *confirms* all the others! She has to select only one bit of trance behavior out of many. When she does that, she is also confirming or validating the others, and that's what you want your patient to do. It also is implying that there may be bad things.

Symbolic Language: Linguistic Cues of a Shift in Hemispheric Experience?

J: The beautiful way the light was showing through these bushes that need to be trimmed but shouldn't be trimmed at all. I saw them this morning, the way the light shimmered through the leaves, and these shoots were making designs. It was so beautiful, and I hoped that the gardener wouldn't trim them. It was very pretty. I wish I could have gotten through to people to tell them how beautiful these bushes were in their natural state.

E: How old were you then?

J: It's now. This morning.

E: Now!? How many shades of green were on the leaves of the bushes?

J: At first I saw so many shades, but I didn't want to see all of the different shades. I just wanted to go into one. When I finally stared at it long enough, it turned into more like chartreuse.

E: But you can see different shades.

J: Yes, I see them. It's a good feeling, too.

E: Society says, "Trim those bushes."

R: Trim down your behavior; get in line. But she is saying here that she does not want to be trimmed, she wants to be free to grow in her own natural way.

E: That's right! And she does not know on a conscious level what she is saying. She is not talking about bushes, she just thinks she is. I then get away from that in a hurry and distract her with talk about shades of color because I don't want to put any emotional pressure on her. That was a therapeutic opening, but she did not come here for therapy.

R: In saying "I just wanted to get into one [shade of color]" she is repeating her earlier theme" of actually *entering* the music . . . or being *inside* the colors." I wonder if such language implies that her ego identity (associated with left-hemispheric functioning) is allowing itself to be surrounded by, or under the dominance of, the more artistic experience of the right hemisphere?

E: Yes, I think that could well be. You frequently find that patients say being in trance is being in a different part of themselves: "You know you are you, but you are in a different you."

R: That "different you" is the more intense, experiential functioning of the right hemisphere. Sperry (1964) has said we all exist in at least two worlds of experience (the right and left hemisphere). Hypnosis can be a way of more clearly differentiating these worlds of existence. When she speaks of "going into" trance, she actually means going into the world of right-hemispheric experience. According to this view artistic talent consists in the ability to give in to right-hemispheric experience (Rossi, 1977). Artistic development would involve the discipline of the left hemisphere's learning to submit itself to right-hemispheric experience and then forging some expression of it in a consensually valid art form.

Life Review in Trance: Time Distortion

E: **What about the swimming? Anything you can share with strangers?**

J: **Yes, I was swimming. At first I was alone, and then the dolphins came. But I did not feel awkward at all because they have no destination anymore. And when I started swimming back, I came into a net of dolls and old toys, childhood things. And my immediate thing was to swim through it. But I knew I could not do it because my fist got stuck in the net. So I put my fist out and I could still swim and I felt my legs being very strong kicking the water. And I gently moved the net of childhood things over and pushed it out to sea, so it was free again, and I swam some more. Whatever obstacles there were, different things from my family, etc., I just swam gently through them after that.**

As I was swimming, my body changed; it became older. I was swimming in a plaid dress from when I was ten, and then I was swimming in this long cape I bought when I was an adolescent, and then the suit I got when I was married. It's really weird! And then when I had my children, I remember the things I wore and I was also swimming in that. And the various things I had on until now. Until suddenly I was in a lovely form watching the ocean.

> E: Here again by emphasizing that she should reveal only what she can share with strangers, I'm keeping her on the surface. I'm protecting her. She then outlines the course of therapy she wants to discuss.
>
> R: How to cope with these childhood things. She actually goes through a life review with so many details in so short a time that she probably experienced considerable time distortion (Cooper and Erickson, 1959).
>
> E: She comes up to the present and is ready to deal with the present situation.

Facilitating Creativity

E: **All right. Close your eyes.**
[Pause]

And go for another swim in something
you've never worn before. Something very happy.

> R: Is this an example of facilitating creativity? You may be asking her to synthesize some new psychic structures when you ask her to wear something she has never worn before.

> E: Yes. It's a break from the past when she becomes aware that there are other things she can wear, that she has never seen or experienced before. You're also giving her permission to do something she has never done before. Also, symbolically, something you've never worn before can be an experience! It isn't necessarily clothes that we are talking about.

Validating Trance Behavior

E: And have a long and tiring swim,
but enjoyable.
At the end you will feel rested.
[Long pause]

> E: Why tiring? You're tired when you really have done a good day's work, a fruitful day's work.

> R: So by suggesting she be tired, you are introducing an element that is associated with doing work and thereby validating that she is to do or has done important work in trance.

> E: Yes. "Today's tool has earned tonight's repose." Longfellow. But enjoy it and feel rested.

Utilizing Time Distortion

E: A lot of time will pass.
But pass very rapidly.
[Pause]
It will be a delightful surprise
to find out how rested you are after being so tired.
[Long pause]
And only tell the part that you can share with strangers.
[Long pause]
And just a bit more fatigue before you go into that nice restful state.
[Long pause]

And there is a surprise for you
at the end.
[Pause]
The destination becomes clearer.
[Pause]
Almost there.
[Pause]
And you may continue to enjoy
the rested feeling
after you arouse.
[Pause]

E: First you let the patients know they have a wealth of time so they will do all their work. Then you distort the time so it can all be done in a short time.

R: That's your approach to utilizing time distortion: Give a lot of time, then let it pass quickly so the work is quickly done.

E: Implying there was a lot, of which she should share only a bit. You then validate further by confirming her fatigue. You keep validating your suggestions as you go along.

R: You're validating that she has done important work. When you imply she has done important work, that reinforces any tentative steps she has made in that direction. And however little she may have done, that is immediately reinforced so she is more likely to work even better in the next trance.

Surprise and the Creative Moment: Secrets in Facilitative Psychological Development

E: **And be greatly surprised by the new and pleasant understanding you have reached.**
[Long pause until J begins to awaken, to reorient her body, and open her eyes]
Only tell us what you wish to share with strangers.

R: Is this emphasis on *surprise* a way of facilitating the development of the new? Since surprise is usually associated with *new insight,* suggesting surprise would tend to facilitate an ambience where creativity and new mental structure could be synthesized.

E: Yes, that's right. What pleases a little child? A surprise and a secret. All children like them! [Here E tells a charming story of how he cured one of his daughters of bed-wetting before it became a real problem. The daughter began bed-wetting when her younger brother was born. After a week of this bed-wetting, E told his wife to tell his daughter that after she had a dry bed for a week, she could go to E's office and say he had to give her a quarter but he could not know why. It was a secret. Daddy could not know why he had to pay her a quarter because it was her secret. After a week of dry beds she came in and demanded her quarter. She got it with no questions asked, so her secret remained intact. She came in the next week for another quarter. The third week she forgot to ask, and she has had a dry bed ever since. She had accomplished her own secret wishes since she didn't like a wet bed either.]

R: So secrets and surprises motivate children!

E: A secret for the child so they can surprise the adult.

R: When you are surprised, I would speculate that a creative moment is taking place wherein new protein structures are being synthesized in the brain that then serve as the organic substrate of new phenomenological experience. The experience of surprise is the reaction of consciousness, the old frame of reference or set that has been governing consciousness, reacting with a startle to the new that has just been synthesized and now appears on a phenomenological level for the first time. The surprise implies that the old frame of reference must now be expanded or changed to accommodate the new (Rossi, 1972, a, b & c; 1973a & b).

E: Yes, every time you surprise a small child, you widen its range of responses.

R: Every time adults do a "double-take," you widen their range of responses. So we are always trying to facilitate surprise as creative moments in therapy.

E: Yes. And when you keep a secret, you widen your understanding of how things work.

R: Wait a minute! How does that work?

E: One must widen a whole lot of receptors to uncover a secret. Every time you try to keep a secret, you have to find ways of hiding it. That is an important learning process, too! Just keeping a secret makes you learn how to erect guards, defenses. It broadens all of your understanding to keep a secret.

R: When you increase your defenses, you also increase your understanding?! That's the opposite of the classical psychoanalytic view! Of course there is a difference between the use of unconscious defenses, which would limit your understanding, and conscious defenses, of which you speak, that actually can increase understanding. You could actually, under certain circumstances, facilitate a person's psychological development by asking them to keep a secret. By telling a child to keep a secret, for example, you are telling that child to put certain defenses under conscious ego control, to develop creative tact, etc.

Symbolic Language: Fantasy to Work Through Traumatic Material

J: All of it! I was swimming alone this time. No animals, nothing, just me in the water. The water was very intensely colored. I did not want to swim on the surface, so I went almost the whole way underwater. And when I got under there, the colors were like nothing the sun could make on top. I was so happy. The whole way I felt happy! And I could really swim underwater. It is hard for me to keep that up in a real pool. As I went deeper and deeper and deeper, there were shells like you've never seen. And then I even found some that looked like stones and gems and could even breathe underwater. And I took them and I just threw them up so hard they went on top of the water and they changed colors outside because I could see through the water. And I did this all the time. I'd just swim underwater and find these beautiful shells and even these discarded, uh, like dishes, I don't know what they were, but they were beautiful and when I tossed them, they changed. And I did that all the way to shore.

As I got to shore I could sense that, I could see it underwater—you know—you can sense how the shore is building up when you are way down there and the rocks change after so many feet. Like geographical.

E: When she says it's "just me" in the water, she is saying she is nude. She is not covering up anything. There is no need to cover up. "I did not want to swim just on the surface" means she is going deeply. The shells are the empty things of the past, shells that once had something, problems, agonies in them. She

377

can see them as empty, but she doesn't know she is looking at her past and its problems here.

R: She sees this symbolically without consciousness understanding its significance, as we are now.

E: She is detoxifying the situation.

R: She is detoxifying the situation for her conscious mind right now because it would be too traumatic to burst out in tears and depression, looking back again at these old problems. When you say the shells are empty now, you mean that she has already dealt successfully with the problems they once contained? If the shells were full, that would mean she was still carrying all those old problems.

E: Yes. There is a willingness to let the bitterness, frustrations, and disappointments of the past remain in the past. She's taking the first step toward the recognition that she is no longer carrying them.

R: So this was a good psychotherapeutic movement that she took in this fantasy. Fantasy can be a way of detoxifying or working through emotionally traumatic material.

E: She is describing therapy here with these gems and stones that she throws up to the surface of the water! She is describing therapy in symbolic terms, but she is only recognizing the words and not the meaning behind them.

R: Therapy is like taking the gems from underneath the surface and throwing them up to consciousness. The gems would be the valid insights.

E: And the stones would be the not-so-good things. In successful living you can always afford to throw away a lot of gems because there are always a lot more available to you. Those gemlike friendships of childhood can be given up because there are other things for the adult. Now the beating a playmate gave you—that is a stone you toss aside.

R: So she is describing a good therapeutic movement.

E: Her unconscious is doing it in symbolic terms. Her conscious mind does not yet understand it fully. But there is an understanding present that allows her to say these things that way.

E: The shore is society. The closer you get to it, the more complicated it is.

Psychological Healing Through Symbols: Right- Versus Left-Hemispheric Healing?

J: I knew I was coming to shore and it was OK. But I wanted to take some of them with me. I did not want to leave them all there. So, I wasn't wearing anything but paint. That's what I wanted to wear. It wasn't ordinary clothes. I was painted from toe to my earlobes. My face was just plain. All kinds of designs, and I realized the designs on my body mirrored the designs underwater. It was like one.

And so I got out of the water, and the designs were still there. But I took off the designs; it sounds weird, but all the designs kind of came off, and I wrapped all the shells in them and I pulled them to shore like in a net. And they made a round circle, and when I saw that, I did take one of these gems with me. I hadn't meant to but I did anyway. And when I noticed it, it got very bright! And the more I looked at it, the brighter it got! Until it seemed to burst into flames, but it wasn't a hot flame, it was just a flame flame. And I lay down in it and it was so bright! So light! It was beautiful, you really should have been there. And I lay down in it, and it wrapped me over, and I didn't need any paint, I didn't need any clothes. I didn't need any makeup, I didn't need anything. I just lay down in it, and it wrapped me up and closed me in. And it sort of elongated and filled out the shore, and I just looked at it. It was very beautiful and very bright!

I don't think you could look at it if you saw it out here. I feel very intensely good, like in every cell in my body!

E: "From toe to my earlobes," a rather peculiar way of speaking. Toes are very physical, and earlobes are where you hear: Touch and hearing are involved, and paint says vision.

R: So you are saying she has many of the senses in there close together: She is a sensual person.

E: Yes. When she takes off the designs and pulls them to shore like a net, she is describing what she is doing with a past trauma.

R: The designs are symbols of a trauma of the past that she is successfully coping with.

E: It could be the loss of a childhood friendship, a childhood injury, anything.

R: It could be anything, but this design and gem image is the way her mind is dealing with it on an unconscious level.

E: Yes, on an unconscious level. She is dealing with it very intelligently and very comprehensibly. She's putting everything down for the conscious mind to understand later.

R: Would you say then this was a healing on a symbolic level?

E: It is a healing on a symbolic level.

R: So while she was going through this symbolic experience, a process of healing was taking place. She tells you about this symbolic experience, but her conscious mind still does not know that a healing has taken place.

E: She shared it with me, a stranger. She told me, and she can't take away any more what she has told me. There is no longer any way for her to deny it.

R: She has validated the healing process by telling it to you even in these symbolic terms. She has confirmed it, she has stamped it in. So she can heal herself on a deeply symbolic level, and once she tells it, she can't undo it. You feel a healing process took place while she was in trance, and this is one of the ways hypnotherapy can heal people.

E: Yes.

R: She is walking out of your office after this experience healed in some way. You do not know in what way or to what degree, but you do know some trauma has been dealt with. The whole problem may not be resolved, but some increment of resolution has occurred in this fantasy that has a successful tone to it and is associated with such happy feelings at its conclusion: the symbolism of light and good body feelings.

E: With a sudden burst of light comes "Oh, that is what it is!" The light of day dawns.

R: Light is associated with new insight and learning. She is saying that the light, the insight was so beautiful.

E: Yes.

R: That is exciting to think that that is the actual moment when a curative process is taking place. I'd hypothesize that this was the creative moment when new proteins were being synthesized in the brain and new phenomenological structures could come into consciousness.

E: Yes, therapy is like reading. First you read the alphabet, then different combinations of letters. First short ones and then longer ones—words. Then combinations that are connected—

sentences. Then a theme and a plot. She's recognizing and describing the essential steps in therapy in this section.

R: She is symbolically describing increments in the therapy process: Her experience here was but one step, one letter, word, or sentence in the total process of a redevelopment of her life.

E: You let the patients use their own words to describe the process.

R: You let them utilize the structures that are already present to express the new. For Jill, *flames* and *gems* and *stones* and *shells* were the currency of her mind for expressing the therapeutic process of change and growth. Therapy on a symbolic level uses the language of the patient. A growth process can be talked about in any terms. Whatever terms you use can facilitate its progress merely by being experienced and expressed. Since these are all highly imagistic terms, it's tempting to speculate that this form of symbolic healing is characteristic of the right hemisphere, whereas the more classical type of Freudian therapy that analyzes problems back to real-life events is more characteristic of left-hemispheric healing. Patients who are strongly dominated by left-hemispheric functioning would do well in the classical forms of insight therapy, but those dominated by their right hemisphere could do better with symbolic therapy. This could also account for the undercurrent of antagonism that has always been present between the classical forms of insight therapy and people with artistic temperaments. Artists have always been suspicious of Freudian analysis with good reason! The Freudian tends to translate everything into terms understandable by the reality-oriented, ego consciousness of the left hemisphere, while the artists' natural proclivities incline them to the symbolic approaches of the right hemisphere. Religiously inclined people who find healing through evangelical or miraculous experience would also be utilizing their right-hemispheric capacities for symbolic healing.

E: A good author can outline a story or plot line but then finds that his characters run away with him. The characters seem to have a will of their own, and the story turns out differently than the author had planned. There again you may have the right hemisphere intruding upon the plans of the left. In the introspective accounts of such authors they will say, "I never intended so-and-so to be married, but he did. Then I thought he should have two children, but more turned up."

R: What fascinates me is that whatever the language of the

patient is, when you talk in that language you can effect a therapeutic change. When she has a hypnotic experience utilizing that language in a positive and constructive fantasy that leaves her feeling good, then an increment of healing or growth has taken place. Whenever something "good" happens in a fantasy, on whatever symbolic level, then healing has taken place. Would you agree with that?

E: Yes. We can reinforce the value of that experience by speaking well of it to the patient even though we do not know exactly what it is referring to. You don't know how long the patient will need to digest the new material. It could be a day or a week or whatever. So you need not see patients on a rigid schedule. It is best to let them call when they need to. A therapist should have flexibility in his schedule to accommodate the patients' needs.

R: So they should come to therapy when their particular healing process needs to be reinforced or extended.

Facilitating Self-Healing: Integrating Left- and Right-Hemispheric Functioning

E: And you can feel good anytime you want.

R: You can utilize these states.

J: I'd really like to learn how to do it.

E: I'm going to let you discover that you can. In the other room is an Indian portrait painted by a young woman who had absolutely no art training at all. You go out and look at it and pick out all the good things in it and come back.
[J goes out to examine the portrait and returns in a few minutes.]

E: Did you like it?

J: Yes. I like the mouth, the eyes, the muscle right here. It was beautiful.
[E now tells something about the background of the picture. A casual conversation takes place for about five minutes about one of E's successful cases.]

E: Here I'm putting the good feeling, the healing process, under her own control. She is an artist, so I want her to pass judgment on another artist and thus reinforce the artist in her.

R: You are helping her validate herself. You elevated her by giving her this task without her knowing that you were giving her a boost. By having her judge an artistic production, you are utilizing and facilitating or reinforcing her natural right-hemispheric tendencies and integrating them with the left. Judgment is probably a left-hemispheric function, which you are joining to her right-hemispheric sensitivity to art.

E: By discussing and giving reality to the other artist, I'm giving more reality to her judgment.

R: You are probably fostering a whole new phenomenological world here in which she can integrate left- and right-hemispheric functioning.

Rhetorical Questions Engineering Responses

E: **Now I'm going to ask you what I've not yet asked you: What do you have to do?**

J: **There is nothing to do. Nothing. I've just fully enjoyed talking to you. Your eyes are incredible!**
   May I look at them more closely?
[**J bends closer to E and studies his eyes.**]

E: You don't want your patients to feel as if they are under a great burden, so I carefully gave her a chance to give this answer.

R: How did you set her up to give that answer?

E: The question I asked seems so damn precise, and yet it is not the least bit precise. It is just vague. What can you do with a question that is so vague it has no meaning? I thus engineered that "I've got nothing to do" answer.

R: You engineered her into saying in effect, "I've got nothing to do; I'm satisfied now, doctor." I can hardly believe you really did that with premeditation! That is fantastic!

E: I've been practicing this sort of engineering for some time!

Self-Hypnosis Training: Further Symbolic Healing
E: **I'm going to tell you to go in the other room and return in five minutes and tell me where you have been.**

[Jill leaves for five minutes after E explains that he wants her to have some practice in developing her altered state by herself. Up to the present her altered state came upon her spontaneously and unwilled. Now she is to learn to bring it on when she wants to and thereby learn to control and constructively utilize her gift for achieving altered states. When she returns, she continues as follows.]

J: I'm interested in my attitudes toward people and things. I suppose it is basically a conflict between attitudes I have and those I should have. When I was in there, I sat down and went someplace. I was on a desert, and all of a sudden I noticed a peacock come from this cactus. Suddenly it got very big, and I jumped on its back and pulled out a feather, and suddenly it became night. I got the feeling somehow that on the peacock, it raises its tail feathers—that is where its beauty is. I know it is weird, but somehow I would here discover my attitudes to things.

As we rode through the night, I pushed the feathers apart, I wanted to see what was underneath. And there were other colors—every color, even more than you could imagine, so I knew this was my peacock, so to speak.

Then, as we arrived, suddenly these fingers began pointing, and I laughed because I knew they were old, wrong attitudes in me. And all of a sudden we had to stop because the mailman was there with a letter.

E: So you've made a few trips. Now you've got to go out there and make your own.

J: I am! I am! But as you make it out there, there is a lot that changes inside, too. On my last trip in there I was lighting a few lanterns. I think that's my attitude toward things now. I felt good about that.

> R: She obviously succeeds in going into a self-induced hypnotic state where she experiences this visionary state with the peacock, her body getting big, and so on.
>
> E: Two words—"night" and "tail." Slang terms for sexual ideation. She is saying that sex is beautiful. She is exploring her attitudes toward sexual things. The colors are facets of emotions.
>
> R: Is this another process of symbolic right-hemispheric healing taking place, when she laughs at the pointing fingers? She has solved the guilt problem implied by all the pointing fingers and can now laugh at them. She might have been overcome with guilt with all these sexual feelings coming out, but here she has gained an increment of therapeutic change by not falling into

guilt. These symbolic fantasy trips are actually solving inner problems on an unconscious level. As long as a person is going on these fantasy trips with a good outcome, they are solving little increments of an inner problem.

E: Yes, they are solving them for the purpose of reaching a consciously recognizable goal.

SESSION 2:

Part One: Facilitating Self-Exploration

This session begins the next day with a casual conversation about hypnosis. E then gives an extensive example of one of his wife's hypnotic experiences of recalling early memories. J gradually grows quiet, closes her eyes, and apparently goes into a trance in response to the gentle cadence of E's voice.

Hypnotic Induction by Indirect Associative Focusing

E: Now my daughter investigated through hypnosis a great many things, seeing them as she actually saw them at the time and later seeing them for their significances. In other words an infant has a fragmentary memory: A hand lifting is only a hand that is lifting. There is no arm involved. It takes some time to connect the hand to the forearm, the upper arm, the shoulder, the self. And to discover that the hipbone is connected to the kneebone and so on. Some time to discover it. Adults seldom realize the learning process that is involved. As an artist you should be interested in those memories.

You've got to be creative.

Colors for a child are bright and stimulating. Just what does a brightness stimulus mean?

[Pause]

And the thrill of lifting something heavy. That counts.

[E tells a story to illustrate individual and cultural difference for about five minutes—how his son-in-law brought a Vietnamese child home to the U.S. and the trials of teaching the child to eat solid food like an American.]

And you've got so many memories and so many understandings you don't realize you have that can enrich your understanding in so many ways.

[E now tells a brief story about a heroin addict who was an artist and his patient. E asked him to sit on the lawn and discover something. The patient discovered new ways of seeing the sheen on the grass, the direction of the trees, and so on.]

E: I use personal examples frequently because they are best known and carry a greater sense of conviction.

R: You're beginning this session with many examples of self-exploration and early learning. All these examples are together indicating a direction for her own inner efforts. You do not tell her specifically what to do; you simply lay down a suggestive network and allow her own unconscious to respond by picking up and elaborating this or that aspect of your network. In Chapter Two we called this the process of indirect associative focusing.

E: You depend upon the patient's natural associative process to put things together. If I want you to talk about your family, the easiest approach and the one least likely to arouse your resistance is for me to first talk about my family.

R: If you have a target area, X, you want a patient to talk about, you first talk of the associated topics A, B, C, D, etc. that all converge upon X. Gradually the area X is stimulated to the point where it is expressed by the patient. You're beginning this session by giving her associative process many possibilities of response by talking about many things. Your target area does seem to be associations about *childhood, individual differences*, and *creativity*. We will soon see how effective you've been when we learn what her responses to your introduction are.

E: It is desirable to do it indirectly, so that the patient does not feel under attack. It is a way of obviating defenses.

Spontaneous Movements Funneled into a Therapeutic Framework: Contingent Suggestions

[J begins to make small movements with her hand, and then her entire arm begins to move gracefully and easily, as if floating. Her entire body gradually takes on a rhythm as if it were swimming or flying. Even her legs lift in slow motion, with delicate flowing motions in coordination with the rest of her body. She remains seated, but flows easily around in her seat.]

E: Now of course I don't know what you are doing. There is a possibility that you are exploring—

infantile learnings

subsequent learnings

and reaching understandings. You are making realignments of understanding, realignments of words.

[Pause]

One of the things my daughter put to me was: "Daddy, how old was I when I first had tears? Because I know I did not have tears when I cried when I was very young?''

I told her that's right. The month at which one gets tears varies from one individual to another.

[Pause]

Her discovery that she had not had tears till a certain age, but not when, gave her a new understanding of tears.

[E now outlines for a few minutes the stages in the development and expression of anger from infancy to adulthood.]

What I want you to do
is to begin
being yourself.

[Pause]

Accepting yourself.

And knowing that you can control yourself.

[E tells one of his favorite stories about one of his baby daughters, who screamed for days because people walked and she knew she was a "people." She finally got up and walked her first hundred steps with no hesitation.]

You want to do something.

You control yourself.

You focus your efforts.

[Another story about one of his daughter's persistent and finally successful efforts to enter medical school.]

> R: She is obviously in a state of deep inner involvement with all these apparently spontaneous movements. It's nice to know that even you, with all your fifty years of experience, really don't know just what she is doing. You do, however, utilize these moments to suggest that she is making therapeutic progress by realigning her understanding. Whatever the original significance of her movements, you are funneling them into a therapeutic framework. This is a form of contingent suggestion in which you tie your therapeutic suggestion to her ongoing behavior.

Facilitating Self-Exploration

And it is a wonderful thing
to explore,

to discover,
the self.
[Pause]
Now there are discoveries you make.
Some are personal
and belong only to you,
and some can be shared with certain others,
and some can be shared with others in general.
And one of the nice things about it is this:
You don't know what you are going to discover,
but you are going to have a delightful time discovering it.
[J's motions are now fuller and more luxuriant. She is smiling broadly at times. There is a happy atmosphere in the room.]
Just like the small child who says,
"I'm building something,
and when I get it done
I know what I really began."
The same things applies to the infant in a crib.
[Long pause]
And for anybody to watch you
and interpret your behavior
can be looked upon as futile
as that
of looking at an infant in a crib
who really doesn't know what
she is doing.
But she is doing something.
[Pause]
You can find out what
you are doing.
Because you have the background of understanding,
and it has to be your background
to understand it.
[Long pause]
[E describes how an infant can repeatedly reach for its own hand and each time not understand what is happening as the hand moves. The adult watching the infant is puzzled that the infant is making this continuous reaching movement.]
Now I have talked,

388

trying to give you
a general
background
from which
you can start
your own self-exploration.

[E gives many clinical examples of the source of psychopathology in the inhibition of self-exploration due to parental and societal structures.]

R: So, in general, one of your first steps with a new patient is to initiate some self-exploratory programs. When you introduce trance with these self-exploratory programs, you are actually laying down a foundation for future deep absorption in trance.

E: Yes. You encourage patients to do all those simple little things that are their own right as growing creatures. You see, we don't know what our goals are. We learn our goals only in the process of getting there. "I don't know what I'm building, but I'm going to enjoy building it, and when I get through building it, I'll know what it is". In doing psychotherapy you impress this upon patients. You don't know what a baby is going to become. Therefore, you wait and take good care of it until it becomes what it will.

R: The very fact that you don't know makes you take extra good care.

E: Life isn't something you can give an answer to today. You should enjoy the process of waiting, the process of becoming what you are. There is nothing more delightful than planting flower seeds and not knowing what kind of flowers are going to come up.

R: So you were setting Jill on a self-discovery program without knowing what she was going to discover. That is very characteristic of you and your work. You can carefully engineer things, but you also enjoy blind exploration.

E: That's right.

Facilitating Individuality: Indirect Ideodynamic Focusing for Hallucinatory Experience

I'm suggesting
a comfortable examination.

An examination
which will show you
how your understanding grew and changed.
[Long pause]
Now I'm going to add one new
dimension
to what you are doing.
And that is this:
[E describes how once when he demonstrated hand levitation, all the observers thought the subject failed until he proved that the subject hallucinated his hand levitating.]
That hallucination was just as effective as a real hand movement because it was the inner experience that was important.
You can at any time you
wish
make use
of the engrams.
I think you know that word.
Imprints for various learnings and experiences.
But you don't need muscles
and bone and flesh.
[Pause as J moves gracefully as ever]
And you can see colors
with your eyes closed.
[Pause]
And you can feel heat and cold
while your body remains comfortable.
[E gives further examples of hallucinated feelings and sensations under hypnosis. At one point he has J open her eyes and, finding that she knows nothing about a tapestry hanging on his office wall, E proceeds to give her a little lecture about the pre-Columbian origin of its symbols, etc.]

E: This also gets the person into their own individuality. In psychotherapy we are looking for the individualities. A patient, all too often, does not have much.

R: This is a way of facilitating their individuality with self-exploration leading to more self-recognition. As you then talk about the hallucinated hand movement, you are touching indirectly upon whatever her own hand movements may mean while also indirectly facilitating the possibility of hallucinatory experience by ideodynamic focusing.

E: Yes, but I'm especially focusing on "the inner experience that was important." What are her really important inner experiences?

R: Yes, the common denominator of most of your suggestions finally comes through very clearly here when you say she can "make use of the engrams . . . imprints for various learnings and experiences." This is very characteristic of your approach. You first tell stories and give many interesting examples of what you later more directly suggest the patient can now do. Your initial patterns of indirect associative and ideodynamic focusing initiate many autonomous search processes within the patient, so that when the more direct suggestion comes, the unconscious is ready in terms of its own mechanisms and the conscious mind is eager to receive whatever it can.

Criteria for Genuine Creativity: Psychosynthesis

E: Now I'm going to speak to Dr. Rossi.
There is no way whatsoever to interpret any of these movements correctly.
Any meaning we give them is our meaning.
They may be completely infantile movements manifested by adult muscles.

R: And a different time orientation, perhaps.

E: And a different mental orientation. A different emotional orientation.

R: This is a general exploration program you've put her on.

E: And she can remember at any level that she wishes.
I know that I can remember what happened at three weeks old.
If I can so can others.
[J continues her movement, seemingly oblivious to the conversation between E and R.]

R: What is of interest to me is that she may be going through an emotionally corrective experience. Is there any way we can find out? Is her mind actually synthesizing new psychic structures? Is she at this moment synthesizing new proteins as the organic substrate of new phenomenological experiences? How could we ever find that out? As Dr. X said the other day, he liked the hand-levitation induction because it gave him continuous feedback as to what was happening in a subject. I'd like to get more feedback and yet not disturb her experience.

E: You permit the patients to find out that they can solve a problem that previously was insolvable. So you do know there was something added.

R: Yes, something is synthesized. Something is being put together.
[E tells a detailed example of how an apparently "spontaneous" naming of a street by an adult was actually a response coming from the adult's childhood. What may appear "spontaneous" or newly synthesized may thus simply have roots in past experience that we are unaware of.]

R: There is no way of knowing exactly what is going on, but you sense something good is happening, so you just let it continue.

E: I don't know if it is important or not. She is obviously having a good time.

R: Yes, I expect a very creative time. It must be pleasing for her to know she can do this on her own for any constructive purpose.

E: You never know, her slow motion could be subjectively perceived as rapid motion.
[E gives a clinical example of this.]

> E: You know there is something "synthesized," to use your favorite word, because when patients find something new, never again can they function in the old incomplete way. Their world is permanently changed.
>
> R: The most self-evident criterion for genuine creativity or psychosynthesis is that the patient's world view, attitudes, and behavior do change. Anything less than this simply means the patient is only paying lip service to the therapist for whatever insights are purportedly developed.
>
> E: When do patients have a good time? When something has been cured!
>
> R: So having a good time, positive affect in a patient under these circumstances, means something is being healed.
>
> E: That something desirable is occurring no matter how unpleasant it may be.

392

R: So positive affect is another important criterion of satisfactory work.

Three Types of Trance: Self-Absorption, Rapport, and Somnambulism

R: Would you say J is in a somnambulistic state now? How would you describe her trance?

E: Call it "deep"; it is self-oriented. Somnambulistic means you have a certain relationship outside. She may be achieving certain purposes, but they are all inside herself.

R: There seem to be at least three basic types of therapeutically useful trance: (1) *The self-absorption type* like this, where the patients are so absorbed in self-exploration that they are seemingly oblivious to the therapist; (2) the more popular conception of trance, when the patients are very much in *rapport* with therapists and responding to suggestions and (3) *somnambulism*, where the patients' eyes may be open and they may talk and act as if awake, yet respond hypnotically to the therapist's suggestions.

E: In practice you have all kinds of admixtures between them, but those would be the extremes between which useful trance work can be done.

Spontaneous Awakening and an Unexpected Reinduction

[With a slight startle J. awakens, apparently spontaneously at this point.]

R: How would you compare your spontaneous trance experiences with your hypnotic work with Dr. Erickson today?

J: This is longer, for one thing. But also . . .
[At this point J's eyes close and her arms again take on their spontaneous trance movements.]

R: During the first few moments after awakening one is still in a light trance state (Erickson and Erickson, 1941). This together with my question about trance was apparently enough to reinduce her into another deep trance.

SESSION 2:

Part Two: Automatic Handwriting and Dissociation

Utilizing Spontaneous Trance for New Learning

[While J is in trance the senior author continues.]

E: Now there is something else I'd like to have you learn.

[Pause]

I'd like to give you the opportunity to learn a totally new thing.

[Pause]

And are you willing to learn something totally new?

Without much effort?

[Pause; J finally nods her head very slowly. The senior author arranges four sheets of paper and a pencil on the desk between them, so both he and J could have easy access to them.]

> E: Notice my pauses in this section. To ask someone to learn something new is a threat, so I pause and then I slowly say "without much effort" to make it less threatening.

Converting Self-Absorption to Rapport

E: Now whatever you are doing

can be discontinued temporarily.

And you can come back to the office and join me.

And can move your chair closer?

J: Umm?

E: Move your chair closer to the desk and writing materials.

[J's eyes remain open after she adjusts her chair, but the staring quality of her eyes and slow body motions indicate she is still in trance.]

> R: Here you are asking her to come back into close rapport with you. In the first part of this session you let her indulge in the *self-absorption type trance*. Now your remarks are beginning to convert her over to the type of trance were she is in close rapport with you so she can experience new hypnotic learnings by following your directions closely and exactly.

Automatic Writing, Age Regression, and Dissociation

E: Now I'm going to treat you like a child.

Is that all right?

J: Sure.

E: There is paper there and pencils.

J: Can I act like a child? And treat me like one?

E: No, you are going to stop acting like—
I'm going to stop treating like a child.
[Pause]
But you can lean forward.
Now while looking at me, what do you suppose your hand might do?

J: Clap! [With a happy childlike laugh]
I don't know what it would do.

E: Touch the pencil to the paper.

J: It's hard to control [as she picks up the pencil awkwardly].

E: You can control, you can write.
[Pause]
And you could write something you didn't know you were writing.

J: Not know I was writing?

E: And you could write a question to which you do not know the answer
consciously.
And only know it unconsciously.
[Pause]

> R: You introduce the possibility of automatic writing by first
> establishing a childhood or early learning set. Just as she first
> learned to write as a child, you hope a more childlike set will
> help her automatic writing. But she seized too eagerly onto the
> child role, so you had to correct it. Actually she was responding
> too literally to your earlier statement that you were going to
> treat her as a child.

> E: Yes. She is responding as a child out of desire. I had to get
> her away from that because children can be pretty irresponsible.

> R: The awkwardness she experienced in holding the pencil is a
> revealing cue about her state of age regression. You then give
> your first direct suggestion regarding automatic handwriting:
> She can write without knowing what she is writing. This not
> knowing, of course, facilitates further dissociation from her
> adult consciousness.

Indirect Ideodynamic Focusing to Facilitate Automatic Writing

I'll give you an example of that.

[The senior author here describes an example of automatic handwriting. A patient who felt "troubled about something" requested that she be allowed to write a question and then an answer. Erickson distracted her with conversation as she spontaneously wrote her question and answer on different parts of a sheet of paper. He folded up the paper and put it in her purse. Three months later she reported that she found the answer to her question and requested permission to look at the paper that was still folded. She now unfolded the paper and saw she had actually written two questions. The first was, "Will I marry Bill?" The answer was, "No." The second question was, "Am I in love with Howard?" The answer was, "Yes." She was now actually engaged to Howard. Thus the automatic writing three months earlier had reflected her major conflict at the time and indicated feelings about Bill and Howard that would later become manifest in breaking up with the former and getting engaged to the latter.]

E: Now all of us have such questions.

That patient knew from my behavior that I would not read the question she wrote or the answer she wrote.

Let your hand wander as it takes hold of that pencil.

[Pause. J picks up the pencil.]

Now suppose you talk to me about something other than what your hand will write.

R: This is very typical of your approach when a subject seems to need help in trance. When a new hypnotic learning is still in the process of being formulated or expressed for the first time, you begin quietly and casually to give many examples of the desired hypnotic behavior. This seems to motivate subjects and give them unconscious clues as to how to proceed. It also gives time to make the necessary inner connections that will make the behavior possible; time for the subjects to realize that you really mean it, and you are willing to wait for them. It's the basic process of indirect ideodynamic focusing again. Your mentioning "Now all of us have such questions" tends to facilitate unconscious processes of search within her for some meaningful material to express itself in the writing. You attempt another dissociative approach by asking her to talk to you about something other than what she is writing.

Amnesia and Protecting the Patient in Trance

[Pause. J stares unblinkingly into Erickson's eyes, and as he stares back into her eyes, her hand with surprising quickness and firmness writes a clear sentence. When her hand finishes the sentence and it is apparent no more writing is forthcoming immediately, he quickly and subtly turns the four sheets of paper over so the writing is now covered and a blank sheet is on top. J continues to stare into his eyes and apparently does not notice his paper shuffling.]

J: Was it a question?

E: Humm?

J: Was it a question? I wrote some questions?

E: Where?

[J now sees the blank sheet of paper, and a look of puzzlement comes to her face.]

You wrote a question?

J: Did I write a question?

E: Where?

J: Down here. [Much obvious puzzlement]

[Pause]

I thought the pencil moved somewhere, I think.

[Pause]

I guess I didn't. I'm holding a pencil. Why am I holding a pencil?

[Pause]

Did I dream something? Did I fall asleep? No, I didn't fall asleep because I have vivid memories of things.

R: Why do you cover up the writing she has just done?

E: You cover it up so she will feel safer: You are not trying to pry. You are also teaching her a sustained amnesia.

R: Even while in trance you are protecting her from seeing too much of that material.

E: Yes. That gives her an opportunity to write more. She knows then that you are not going to take advantage of her. I don't pry, I don't read it at that point myself.

R: All this puzzlement and doubtful self-questioning are indications of her developing amnesia as well as dissociation. So precarious is her ego consciousness that she's not sure if she's been dreaming or asleep.

Classical Description of Dissociation

E: Vivid memories you can share?

J: Yes, I had a very important one for me. You really want to hear it all?

E: Was the presumed question important?

J: I don't know. I just had a feeling of importance, of something important. I was holding a pencil, my hand felt as if it didn't move. I felt very stiff. When you hold a pencil and you are writing, you pinch your fingers together. But the pencil wasn't pinched in my fingers.
That's why I felt like something was odd.
I was holding a pencil, and the only reason I can think of that I'd be holding a pencil is to write.
But I didn't feel like I was holding a pencil. It doesn't make sense. I don't feel like I was actually holding a pencil. But I see the pencil in my hand so I assume I'm holding it, right? But my hand still feels kind of stiff. Not stiff like a board. But it is not—I don't know how to describe it—it's kind of numb almost. It has a different kind of feeling in there, right now.

E: Does this question seem to make sense? Does your hand want to write again?

J: Again? It feels like it wants to write but it can't because it doesn't want to hold the pencil to write. Do you know what I'm talking about?

E: I do.

J: You hold a pencil, you have to hold the pencil with the tips of your fingers so that you can control it and let it go the way you want it to.

> E: What she is describing is the dissociation of her writing and that part of her conscious awareness. This is a classical description of dissociation from a subjective point of view. Her unconscious wants to hold the pencil differently than she holds it in the normal state.
>
> R: Why?
>
> E: Because its unconscious material! Just like when you are on vacation you dress differently. How different? Just different!

R: The fact that the pencil is held differently is a sign of the genuineness of the phenomenon of automatic writing.

E: Yes.

Body Dissociation and Depersonalized Language

J: My hand holds the pencil and *it* feels as if *it is* going to write, but it is not, it doesn't hold the pencil to write. It doesn't hold the pencil in the accepted manner to write.

E: Maybe it's automatic writing.
[Pause]

J: That's possible. I never thought about that before.
But how can it be? Your hand still has to—all right, wait a minute. The muscles still have to hold the object to make it work.
Don't they? I don't feel like I'm even holding the pencil!
[She has in fact been holding the pencil throughout this discussion.]
But I *see* I'm holding a pencil! I don't feel the pressure.

E: Ordinarily a person knows he is holding a pencil, he doesn't have to see he's holding a pencil.

J: Right, that's how I feel, but I don't feel I'm like really holding a pencil, but I see that I'm holding a pencil.

E: Yes, that's right. Maybe it's because your hand wants to do some more automatic writing.
[Pause]
It is possible to put your hand in a position where *it* has an opportunity.
[Pause]
Maybe you'd like to watch it and see what it is writing, only, of course, you won't *know* what it is writing.
[Long pause. J's hand finally begins to move with decisive firmness and quickly writes a few sentences.]

J: Could I read it? There is writing there, is that my handwriting?
My hand feels very strange, like it's my hand but it didn't write anything.

E: Notice her language when referring to her own hand: "*it* feels as if *it* is going to write . . ." *It* is no longer herself.

R: Her dissociation is leading to a depersonalization of the dissociated body part and its activity.

E: She has to actually see the pencil to know it's being held. This again is evidence for a separation of conscious and unconscious.

E: Notice how I accept and reinforce the depersonalization by using "it" and contrasting it with the part of her that I address as "you." She can *see* what she is writing, but this in itself implies she will not *know* what she is writing. You can see without knowing. I can just see those books, for example. Her questions and the strange feeling are all characteristic of the dissociative process.

A Dissociation Between Thinking and Feeling

E: **Look in this place.**
[The senior author thus distracts her vision for a moment and then deftly turns the paper over so J is again confronted with a blank sheet of paper.]
You look puzzled by something. Now do you want to read it?
[Pause as J looks in vain for her writing on the blank sheet of paper.]

J: **Did I dream it? (In a very soft, faraway voice)**
[Pause]
Did I dream it?
[The senior author now reveals one of the sheets of J's writing to her.]

E: **Is this the writing?**

J: **What about this writing? It doesn't look quite like my handwriting, does it? Is that my own? First of all you have to tell me, did I write that? I** *think* **I must have, but I don't** *feel* **I did.**
I found myself holding a pencil and therefore I put it back together: I must have written something because usually I don't hold pencils unless I do something with them. But I don't feel as if I wrote anything. This hand is my hand. [Referring to her left hand that did not write] This hand [her right that did the writing] feels more separate than this one [her left]. But they don't know, they don't feel as if they actually wrote.

E: **Now just express here your intellectual impression: Did you write the writing on the other sheet?**

J: **I don't feel like I did.**

> R: Her remark, "I *think* I must have, but I don't *feel* I did," indicates a clear dissociation between *thinking* and *feeling*. It's

interesting to note that her ego consciousness associated with the *thinking* of her left hemisphere is retained as a part of her identity, while *feeling* that may be more associated with right-hemispheric experience is dissociated off.

E: All these questions and attempts at logic and rationalizing are highly characteristic of a genuine dissociative state.

R: It is as if her left hemisphere with its logic is trying to rationalize an act that may be outside its range of experience, just as patients with right-hemisphere lesions and deficits use their intact left-hemispheric logic to rationalize their behavior without ever recognizing its incongruities (Luria, 1973).

Furthering Dissociation: A Conflict Between Thinking and Feeling

E: **All right, let's see what your hand thinks. Let your hand point to the writing that you did. Now just watch your hand start pointing.**
[J's hand lifts.]
It might pick up the pencil and write, "yes."
[J's hand does write "yes."]

J: **How can it know if I don't know? I feel that it can know, but my mind thinks I feel that, I feel that it knows that it wrote something. Something, somewhere! But I**
[Pause]
I wrote something, but it's very
[Pause as J seems to fall deep into thought]

E: **Very what?**

J: **My thinking isn't very clear right now [faraway voice].**

E: **Why?**

J: **I'm very relaxed. My thinking—it's like my feelings don't want my mind to think, particularly.**

E: **Let your hand point . . . to automatic handwriting.**

J: **But it's going to point to nothing.**

E: **Perhaps it will write "yes" or "no."**
[J's hand lifts the pencil.]

E: I thrust upon her a "yes" when I said the hand might write "yes." This furthers the dissociation because it shows her she can write automatically, but she can also do responsive writing (response to Erickson's suggestion to write "yes"). At this point she does not want to think that she obediently wrote "yes," so her feelings do not want her "mind to think, particularly."

R: You have precipitated a conflict between her thinking and feeling.

The Subjective Experience of Dissociation

E: That's what we mean by "automatic." Would you like to try to guess what it is going to write?

J: No. I don't want to try anything. I just want to let it go by itself.

E: Yet you can guess. The hand will write the correct answer.

J: I would think yes and no—because it doesn't feel like I wrote when I thought about how it felt when I was holding the pencil.

E: My question is: Did it write?
[Her hand begins to write.]

J: It's moving by itself. It's moving by itself. Strange, I'm so aware of it. [Whispered very softly] It is going.
[Pause]
It's holding a pencil. It feels, I don't know, it feels like my hand is a cosmic hand. I see it as a part of my body, but it's like a cosmic hand coming out of the clouds.

E: Do you think you might like to try more?

J: Not my forehead, but the rest of my being feels as if it's going to write more. But just not my forehead. It's like my forehead is pulling against the rest of my body right now.

E: Let your hand pull over on top of the paper.

J: Humm? [Faraway voice]

E: Write.

J: Should I start it writing or just wait? I don't know how to do it. I mean I don't know how to.

E: Is it enough? Is there any writing undone that you would like to do?

J: Yeah, I think so.

E: Let your hand start writing.
[Her hand begins to write several sentences as she looks at Erickson's face. As usual with automatic writing, the hand picks up speed till it's writing at a furious speed, seemingly much faster than normal. When she has finished, she shuffles the papers without any apparent awareness on her part so a blank sheet is again on top.]

> E: By asking her the first question of trying "to guess what it is going to write," I facilitate the dissociation and I let her affirm that she herself wants to do the automatic writing. She then gives many beautiful subjective expressions of the dissociation between mind and body by a person relatively naïve about hypnosis.

A Question Structuring an Amnesia

E: Now we can ask: Do you think you can do automatic handwriting? [As if no writing had taken place]

J: Pardon?

E: Tell me honestly: Do you think you can do automatic handwriting.

J: I think I can. Anything is possible in the world. I think anything is possible.

E: I'm just talking about you.

J: I don't know too much about it. How *do* you begin? I mean my hand feels like—it's just a little bit mine, you know. Because it looks like it's mine but it doesn't—and the only way I've written is to hold the pencil between the pads of my fingers. I tried it with my toes once. Also my mouth and teeth. [Her automatic writing was sometimes done holding the pencil awkwardly between her second and third fingers with a closed fist, like a child's first efforts.] But right now, to be perfectly honest, my hand does not feel like it is holding the pencil to write with. You know what I'm talking about? I feel like I'm babbling.

E: You're talking and making sense only you don't know it. And Dr. Rossi's finding that out. Would this paper be all right to try automatic handwriting on?

J: Well, sure, I'll try it, but I mean, still tell me how to begin, exactly. I let my hand feel it, right? It feels like I'm not using my hands. So how do I know if it felt that it wrote, exactly? It felt like a hand coming out of a cloud that I could watch and see move maybe if I looked at it.

R: This question at this point tends to give her an amnesia for the writing she has just done. You are actually reorienting the conversation to a point in time before the handwriting was done so the writing activity tends to fall into an amnesic lacuna. This is what we have called a structured amnesia (Erickson, Rossi, and Rossi, 1976).

E: Yes, it sets the act of writing in its own cubicle of time. She then gives many classical expressions of the dissociative process: "It looks like it's mine but it doesn't."

R: Her feeling that she is only babbling is another sign of the dissociation within her. Her words make perfect sense to us because we understand both sides—conscious and unconscious. But she cannot put the picture together with understanding even though she is trying, and thus her own efforts sound like "babbling" to her.

The Economy of Automatic Handwriting: The Variable Language of Yes and No

E: All right, now I'm going to do something. I would like to have you be interested and pleased.

[The senior author now reveals the first sheet of her automatic handwriting—Figure 1.]

J: I did that? Oh, my God!

E: You're amazed that you did automatic handwriting?

J: I wrote that? Can I read it?

E: You don't know what is written, you haven't read it, to my knowledge. You may want to read it or you may not want to read it, that's up to you.

J: I want to!

E: This is the second part. [Reveals the second sheet as well—Figure 2]

J: I don't know how to spell too well, do I?

E: Automatic writing is characterized by misspellings.

404

J: Oh, really.

R: You've done very well!

> R: She writes her words with unusual clarity for automatic writing.
>
> E: Yes, usually there is more economy of effort. A "yes" answer can be condensed into a vertical line and a "no" into a horizontal line.
>
> R: So a vertical line is actually an abstraction of "yes" and a horizontal line is an abstraction of "no."
>
> E: That's right. And an "I don't know" can be a horizontal with varying degrees of angle to mean it is more like "yes" (toward the vertical) or more like "no" (toward the horizontal). Thus:

yes | no —

I don't know   //

> A "yes" line written on the opposite side of the paper could mean a "no." A "yes" line on top of the paper is "yes," but if it is written on the bottom of the paper, that could signify the reverse, a "no."

Multiple Meanings in Automatic Writing: Caution in Interpretation

J: Can I read it out loud? [She reads.]
"To rest and be at one with the sun is okay.
To get down again just slide down on a moon beam."
Gee, that means you have to wait till night time and the sun cools down to get down.
[The senior author now reveals the third sheet of her automatic writing—Figure 3.]
I wrote?
Gee, what strange writing!
It doesn't look like mine, that I know! [She reads.]
"The sun is not too hot to splash in.
I love the sun and I am at one with the sun's center.
We are the same and I leave the fire whole again, not burnt.
And love is like the sun."

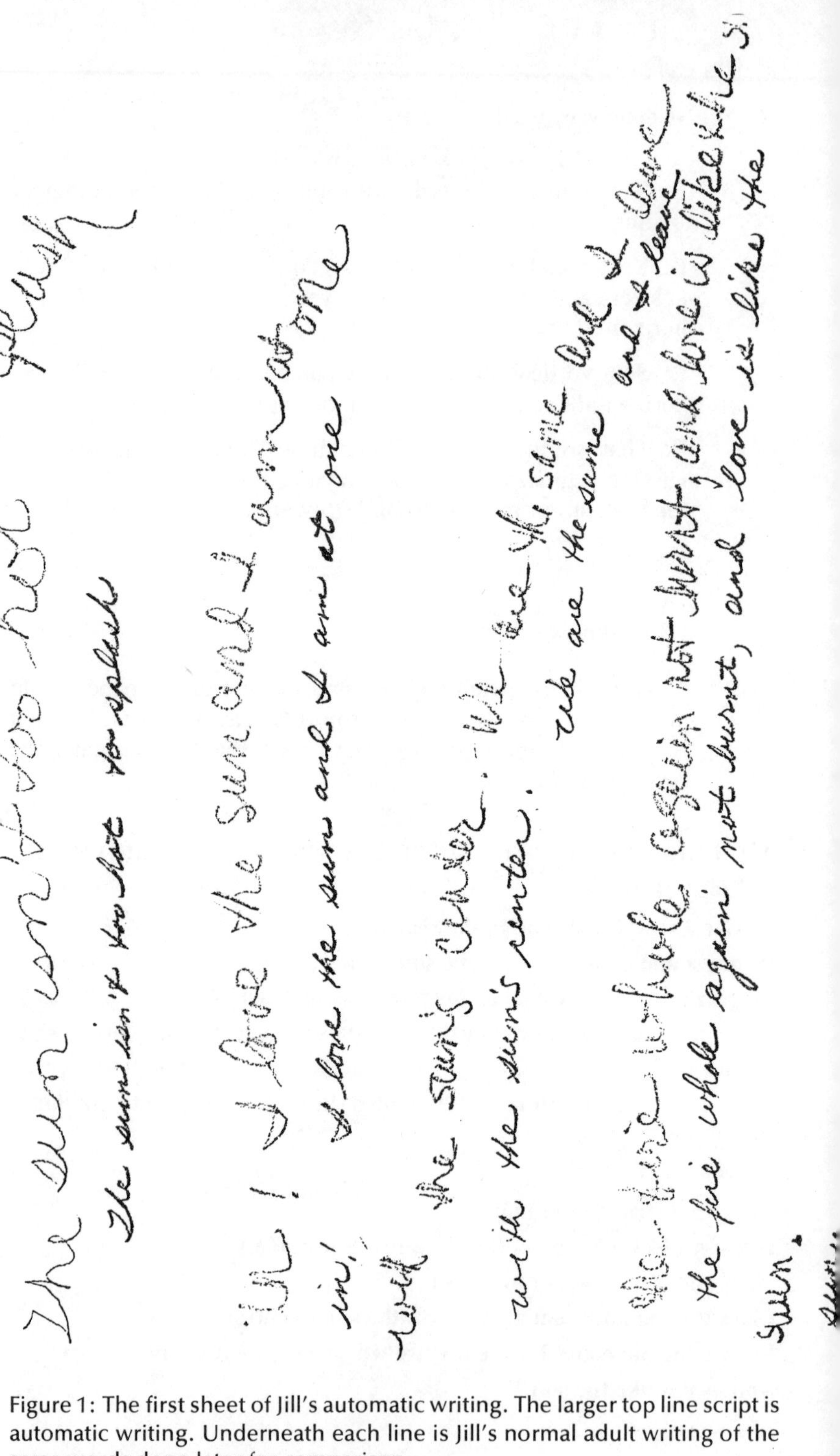

Figure 1: The first sheet of Jill's automatic writing. The larger top line script is automatic writing. Underneath each line is Jill's normal adult writing of the same words done later for comparison.

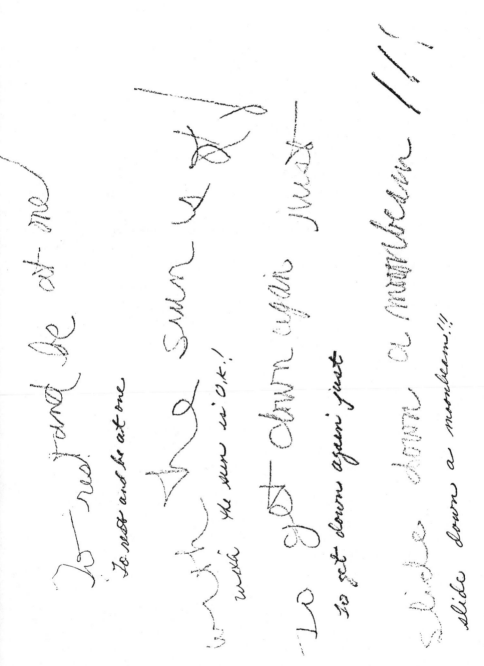

Figure 2: The second sheet of Jill's automatic writing. The large script is the automatic writing, and beneath each line is Jill's normal adult writing of each word done later for comparison.

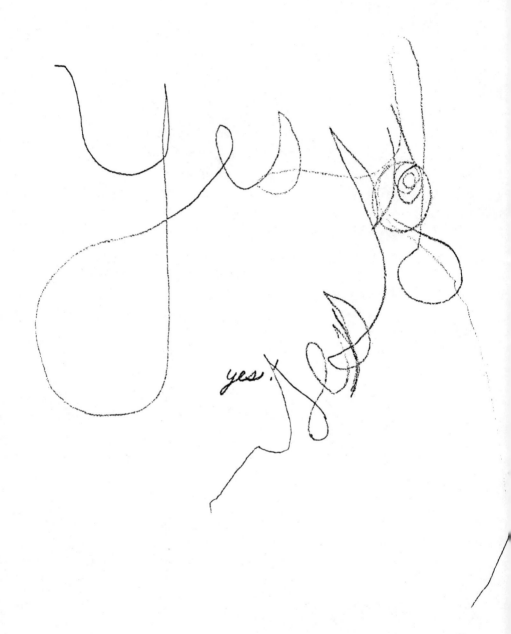

Figure 3: The third sheet of Jill's automatic writing, where she writes "yes" several times in large, sometimes overlapping script. The small clean "yes" toward the bottom is her normal adult writing, done later.

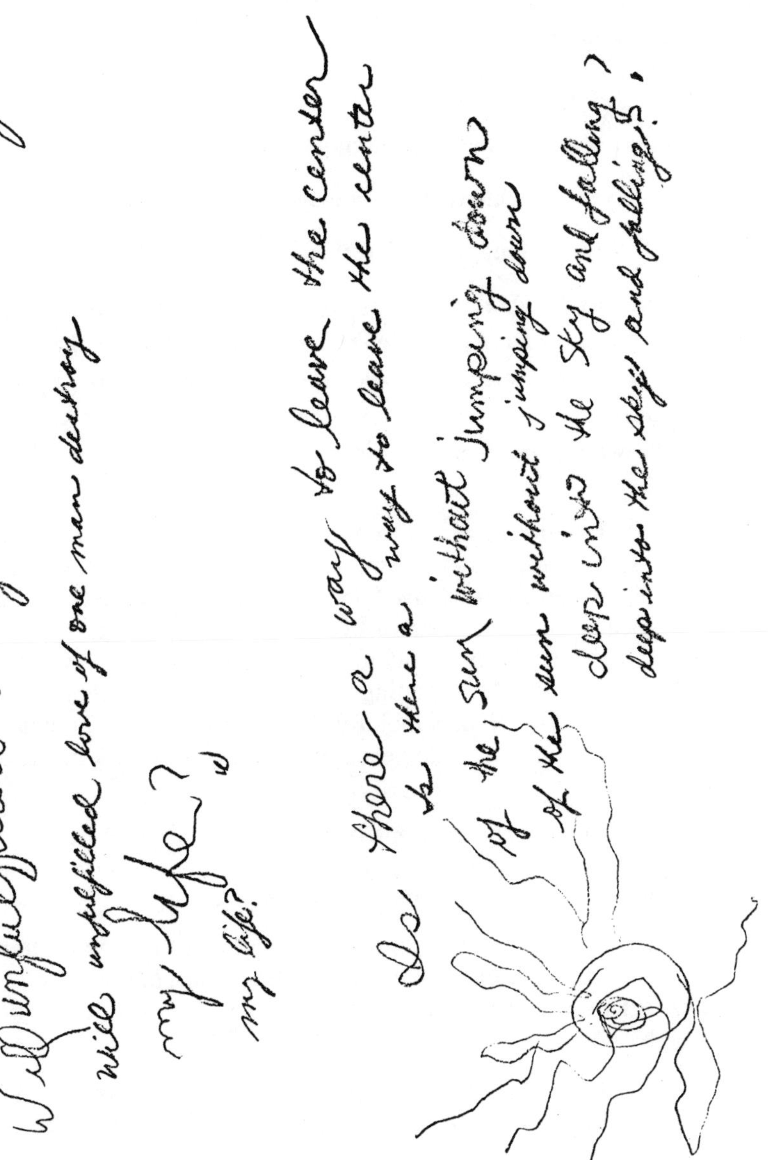

Will unfulfilled love of one man destroy

my life?
my life:

Will unfulfilled love of one man destroy

Do there a way to leave the center
Is there a way to leave the center

of the sun without jumping down
of the sun without jumping down

deep into the sky and falling?
deep into the skys and fallings:

Figure 4: The fourth sheet of Jill's automatic writing. The larger script is automatic, the smaller, repeating the same words, is her normal adult writing done later for comparison.

[The senior author reveals the fourth sheet of paper with her automatic writing—Figure 4.]

I wrote that too?

[She reads with deep feelings and some tears.]

"Will the unfulfilled love of the new destroy my life?
Is there a way to leave the center of the sun without jumping down deep into the fire and falling?"

E: Does it mean something to you?

J: In a deep way, but not in a lollipop way.

E: I have a very ridiculous question to ask you: What color is your hair?

J: Blond. Rinsed Blond. My natural color has some blond in it.

E: Because my daughter was asking me about a blond-haired girl and I did not know a blond-haired girl! [Referring jokingly to the fact that Erickson is color blind] And Pete Thompson, who I've know for many years . . .
[The senior author goes on for a few minutes about blond hair thus starting a casual conversation distracting from the psychological work at hand.]

E: Reading aloud is different than reading silently so she had to ask for specific permission to read aloud. It's another aspect of her dissociation. Now I made no effort to find out what she meant. When she said this was "strange" writing, that means it is foreign to her consciousness. You have to be aware of the possible double-meaning words like "sun" that could be "son." You always look for those possibilities. I may have my ideas about what it means but I'm not going to ask her to betray it.

R: The fact that she speaks of the possibility of her life being destroyed suggests that you are right in believing that the issues are delicate and so your caution is justified.

E: Yet she *is* trying to betray something to me even though I don't feel I'm entitled to it at this early stage of the game. So I let her betray something to me but I choose what it will be: her blond hair.

R: You utilized her premature impulse to betray by side-tracking the betrayal to the relatively innocent issue of her artificial blond hair.

E: Then from betrayal I further deflect the conversation to my daughter, my life, and finally my friend Peter which takes her far away from the hot material indeed. For psychotherapy you take learnings out of context and use them in new ways.

Source Amnesia

E: By the way, what do you know about that? [Referring to the tapestry on the office wall]

J: Is it something pre-Columbian? I don't?

E: What makes you think it is pre-Columbian?

J: I saw the design on there. The design? The design looks like a, I don't know? I really don't know. The faces though look like it somewhat. I could be wrong but I don't know—it's attractive—but I don't know too much about it.

E: Was it I who told you that was pre-Columbian?

J: Who, you?

E: Yes.

J: Well, I never asked you about it, that I know of. Why? Were you supposed to have? [Pause] Were you supposed to have told me something about it?

E: Not supposed to—I did!

J: You did, really!

> R: Here J is demonstrating a source amnesia: She knows about the pre-Columbian symbols you spoke to her of earlier while she was in trance, but she does not know the source of this knowledge.

Age Regression via Visual Hallucination of Many Self-Images

Indirect Associative Focusing to Facilitate Certain Direction in Trance Induction

After hearing an interesting case history for a half an hour about the adoption history of two little girls, their struggle for acceptance, and the many lives they lived in different homes, Jill becomes fixated in her attention and her eyes blink as if she were going into trance. Her eyes finally close. A few minutes later her hand begins to levitate and float about spontaneously. She is evidently in close rapport because she smiles and sobs at appropriate places.

E: And J
in your lifetime
you really have been
many different little girls.
And one of the things you can do, Jill, you can do it with your eyes open,
you can do it with your eyes closed. Line up
a whole line
of girls. Have each of them in some significantly meaningful state.

> R: You are again using indirect associative focusing when you tell this interesting case about little girls to begin the process of activating her own personal associations and memories of her own childhood. She is entirely absorbed in your story; her attention is focused and fixated so she naturally begins to manifest the initial signs of trance.
>
> Here you make a smooth transition from your case history to your first overt directive to facilitate J's current trance experience.
>
> E: Yes, and if she has any doubt within her about being able to see these little girls, you depotentiate it by giving her the choice of having her eyes open or closed. I then use the words "significantly meaningful" to help her reach personally meaningful material.

The Objective Observer

E: As for you, Jill, you can be an objective intelligence off to one side,
delighted to look at those little girls, that long line of little girls. And you
can describe them as freely as you wish.

> R: Here you give her consciousness the task of being an objective observer. Perhaps this is the best place for consciousness in this initial, uncovering stage of therapy. You allow the unconscious to do the uncovering via a series of images of girls that consciousness can simply receive. Consciousness is thus placed in a receptive mode (the ideal mode for trance), where it is not likely to direct or interfere with images emerging automatically from the unconscious.
>
> The phrase "freely as you wish" then gives a positive and

reinforcing orientation to your permissive suggestion to describe her experience.

Catharsis Balanced with Positive Affect and the Objective Observer: Implication

E: **You can be pleased, amused. You can empathize with the little girls, but you will be a detached intelligence.**

R: Telling her she can be "pleased" and "amused" facilitates the experience with a positive affect. Allowing her to "empathize" permits emotional flow and a possible catharsis while still protecting her with the objective observer.

E: "Pleased" and "amused" evoke different aspects of the spectrum of her inner life. You can be amused by a bad girl and pleased with a good girl. So she has a tremendous amount of freedom to explore all these possibilities in her past—and all this by implication.

Now being that detached intelligence you need not know that you are Jill. You are something separate. But a knowing something. You need not know that those little girls are a succession of Jills. And I would like to have you enjoy that experience tremendously.

Covering Many Possibilities of Response to Depotentiate Doubts

E: **You see those girls as if they were tangible hallucinations or you can see them in your mind's eye or you can see them not knowing that they are mental images. You see them and think that they are flesh and blood.**

R: You now cover a number of possible ways she can see the images: as hallucinations, as images in the mind's eye, or a total belief in their reality out there as flesh and blood.

E: Yes, you also depotentiate her doubts by giving her many possible modes of response.

Not Knowing to Depotentiate Left-Hemispheric Functioning?

E: **And you need not know that each is related to the other. But I would like to have you perform this task very completely, and you can do it while in a trance state or you can be fully awake and recall the experience as an extremely vivid dream that you can relate to me and to Dr. Rossi. And you** can feel free to discuss that little girl or that slightly bigger girl or that much bigger girl. That is something that you can do in a manner far better than you know. In a manner that will be a pleasure for you to learn that you can do it so well. Now let your hands come to rest on your thighs and just rest comfortably.

R: I wonder if not needing to know the images are related together is a way of dismissing or depotentiating left-hemispheric functioning?

E: That could well be. As I read this transcript I'm amazed how long experience has taught me to cover many possibilities of reponse whenever I'm exploring a patient's inner life.

R: Yes, you enumerate many possibilities of response, from constructing the images while in trance to recalling them later as a dream.

Voice Locus as a Cue for Visual Hallucinations

E: And feel very, very comfortable, and whenever you want to start, you line those girls up [At this point the senior author shifts his body 45 degrees away from J so he is now oriented to an imaginary wall in that direction] against that   nice white wall. [J opens her eyes and blinks with a blank look] And you are looking, is there enough wall there for you to see all of them? [J looks up in the new direction Erickson has oriented himself to. She now stares with dilated pupils with her eye focus shifting about. She is apparently hallucinating with her eyes open.]

J: It isn't just a wall.

R: This is an interesting use of voice locus and body reorientation as a cue for the direction where she may experience a visual hallucination.

Dangling Phrases to Facilitate Self-Expression

E: I know.
I can say it's a wall, but you can say it's a—

J: Porch, it's a gate. But it is white and some of the paint is splintering. There is a little girl standing behind it, but it is like a gate porch fence kind of. And there is a big tree with gray bark that crumbles off when you put your fingernail on it, and she is doing it. She is watching it fall down and the sun feels very warm. She is wearing a dress that is patched from old sheets, or new sheets. It has patches on it. She likes the design of the patches better than her dress because it feels fuzzy under her finger and it has a red flower on it. And she is thinking, she is thinking the tree is her backyard tree. It is a Sunday and her father is coming with ice cream, but she knows it really isn't true.

E: But it is nice to think so.

J: She has a little calico cotton dog, a red background with little white flowers and its nose part is orange. It is like a patch dog made of more patches. She loves it. And she feels that now she is feeling it and she is hugging it.

R: You use an incomplete dangling phrase here for her to finish.

E: Yes, dangling phrases give her an opportunity to express herself.

R: You always let the patient fill in the blanks whenever possible. In this way the therapist is always seeking out the patient's frames of reference and association rather than intruding his ideas on the patient.

E: Yes, therapy should always be designed to fit the patient and not the patient fit the therapy. Her vivid description of how as a child she crumbles the gray bark "when you put your fingernail on it" is one of those ingenuously personal details that tends to ratify trance.

Body, Head, and Eye Orientation as Cues to Visual Hallucinations

J: And she is watching someone walk up the dirt way. It is not paved. It's got stones, and he kicked one stone and she liked it. And because he kicked the stone she liked him. And she is waving to him now. And she knows that she wants to push the fence, but she is going to have to walk around, more than push it right there, to where there is an opening. And she is going up to him. She wants to hug him.

R: As she spoke these words her body, head, and wide-open eyes oriented in the direction where she was apparently hallucinating someone kicking stones. As she talks about the fence, she looks up as if it's taller than herself.

415

Evoking a Complex

J: She feels she doesn't have a father. She would like the man to be her father. I can feel that she does.

E: She doesn't know that there are other little girls standing there a little bit older.

J: And she has a father, but she is not sure of him because she is walking down the sidewalk and there is a man coming along supposed to be her father. She feels like she is pretending, really, but she wants that pretending to be real. So she is going to pretend real hard and she is going to go over to him though she doesn't know him, and she feels like she is brave, you know.

> R: Jill is obviously incorporating elements of your case about the adopted girls here. It's almost as if your preinduction case history is now functioning as an implanted complex (Huston, Shakow, and Erickson, 1934).

> E: She is using some material I offered, and what she uses is a function of her personality, not mine. Her using this detail indicates how, like most children, she has had fantasies about being adopted. My preinduction story evokes that complex within her.

Many Levels of Simultaneous Functioning in Trance

J: I can feel it what she is feeling, I can see it in her face, but she is also very happy and waving-like. And she goes and says I have a new house. She is not at the fence anymore. She is not in the same place at all. She is in a neighborhood where there are regular homes. There are some fences and a gate, but it is different, she is just different.
And she goes up to him and she says, "Can I walk with you and hold your hand?" Then she knows that, that he is going to be, he is really going to be her father. And they walk into a house and it has some steps in the front, reddish-colored steps.

> E: When she says, "I can feel it, what she is feeling," it indicates that she is functioning on many levels simultaneously here.

> R: The detached observer facilitates these multiple levels of functioning.

416

Two-State Dissociative Regression to Facilitate Objective Perception and Left-Hemispheric Functioning

E: Does she know about the first little girl?

[Pause]

J: No, I don't think so.   No.

E: Well, you have seen the first little girl, the second little girl.

J: Yeah, but—

E: There are a lot of them.

J: But she doesn't   I don't think she realizes that there was another little girl standing near fences, but they were different, they feel different. Now she is in school. She really does live in that house. And she goes to school, there is also another little girl that was at a party. They are both somehow. One is at school, one is at a party.

R: You are now reinforcing the dissociation between the images of the two girls when you ask if the second knows about the first little girl.

E: Yes. This is another example of what I called a "two-state dissociative regression" (Erickson, 1965a). You can see things better in such a dissociative state. Dissociation helps you realize different experiential states. If these different experiential states do not know each other, the observation of them can be all the more objective.

R: The objective observer and such two-state dissociative regressions could thus be means of facilitating the left hemisphere's objective perception of the many dimensions of the total personality. Since Jill falls so easily into right-hemispheric experience, her psychological problems may stem from a relative weakness of her left-hemispheric functioning; her ego identity and stability may be too fluid. The objective perception you are facilitating here may be a means of strengthening her left-hemispheric functioning.

Facilitating the Objective Observer: Resolving Childhood Problems

E: I want to make clear to your intelligence that you will become those

little girls and that they really are all the same little girl at different times. But you can see any other girl that you wish.

J: There is a little little girl, she looks like someone I know. She is going up to these high school girls. She is very little. She is only about two or three, wearing a diaper.
She lives right near the high school and there are lots of steps because she lives above a store, but she goes, she likes to go out the door and walk down these steps. Sometimes she has to crawl down, and she likes to go over and see what is going on.
She has chubby little legs and one curl across the top of her head. She is pulling a little dog. Not a real dog. And she smiles at this big high school girl, really pretty girl who is with her boyfriend.
And they seem to be talking about dancing or something like that. She knows what dancing is, though she is little.

> R: The objective intelligence can recognize that all the images are of the same person even though each image (or ego state related to a specific age) remains dissociated from all others.
>
> E: The objective observer that sees and describes current realities can also alter and change earlier childhood realities.
>
> R: This is really amazing! The mind is a self-improving system that can change past distortions and traumatic experiences from the more adult point view. I have described a class of "healing dreams" wherein this appears to be one of the constructive functions of dream experience. (Rossi 1972a).

Facilitating the Objective Observer: Language Cues of Interacting Age Levels

E: Find all those girls named Jill and look at little Jill and little bigger Jill and a little bit bigger Jill and a bigger Jill. Because they really don't know each other. Of course there will be other boys and other girls. But little Jill . . .
[Pause]
And each little Jill   has her own time, and each of them, they won't really see each other. They won't even know that they are all there. Your intelligence can see them and understand them.
[Pause]

J: There is another girl. She is just four. No, she is not even four, she is

418

almost four. She loves the boulevard because there is so much going on. The girl that takes care of her is looking all over for her. She is delighted to get down those stairs and down the street, and there is a big movie show. She is walking by it. Then there is another boy. She turns the corner and there is a huge park, it looks so big with grass in the middle, and this lady that everyone calls Crazy Mama is picking up papers. She has a white scarf on a huge behind and a big big arm and a white apron and a brown blouse. And she has a stick that she picks up papers with. This little girl is watching her, fascinated, because they say she ate her father and put him in a pot and cooked him. Could it be true? Then there is another girl who lives in that building, but she is older. She is five and a half. And she is very sad because she is moving away and she doesn't know where except that it is far, it is very far.

[J now gives a long and detailed account of moving from one part of the country to another and her perception of a few more age levels.

Throughout this period her eyes are alternately opened and closed. When they are open, she is apparently hallucinating visually as she looks about describing the scene as she sees it. She concludes with the following.]

J: She is about ten and she is in the fourth grade and she knows all her work so well that they are skipping her into the next grade. She is very proud. She doesn't have pretty dresses like the other ones. The shoes have patches on them, but she doesn't mind it. She likes the designs on the patch. It doesn't matter. But she is doing very well. She has two spelling books because she is doing the next grade work and her work, and they are skipping her. She is proud when she gets up and knows all the right answers. And they are moving again. [Pause]

R: You're again suggesting that each girl will not recognize the others even though the objective intelligence can relate them as one. Why?

E: There can be a freer recognition and recovery of many self-images if they do not have to recognize each other. The adult does not like to recall the experience of wet diapers of the infant or the running nose of the child.

R: So the objective observer that relates them is detached even from her adult self.

E: In this section we also witness the shifting levels of her vocabulary and perceptions. Words like "boulevard," "delighted," "huge," and "fascinated" belong to the adult. Yet they are used to describe childhood images in a childlike way, as when she speaks of Crazy Mama's "huge behind" and her question "could it be true?" that she put her father in a pot and ate him. The detached, objective observer can recover childhood perceptions with an adult's understanding. This is a valid characteristic of trance. The detached observer is a center pole and fixed reality about which the patient can explore many childhood experiences in adult words. Memory is not all of one piece; it's always fragments of adult and child interacting.

Posthypnotic Suggestion for Time Distortion Yielding Long Rest and Recovery

E: **Would you like to rest?**

J: **I am very tired.**

E: **All right.**
Just close your eyes and rest.
Very comfortably.
Rest.
And have a long rest. A rest that seems hours long. Hours long with hours of comfort.
[Pause]
And as the comfort builds up in your body that supports that intelligence, and looks at that larger number of little girls each named Jill, but a different Jill each time, feeling different, doing different, thinking different, and really different, yet always Jill. And soon this intelligence will renew its curious, fascinating looking at that long line of girls all Jill. None of which can see the other, all of which have only faint memories, partial memories of smaller Jills, and only partial ideas of what the bigger Jill is like that this intelligence can look in curiosity and interest and enjoy describing each one of those Jills. A feeling so rested now, as if you had eight hours of sound and restful sleep.
[Long pause]
It is going to be a pleasure to open your eyes and start talking about those girls.

> E: I use time distortion here to allow her to adjust to the awake state, yet allowing her to retain all the memories of the different Jill states.

R: You are giving her a posthypnotic suggestion for hours of time distortion. We will see after she awakens just how effective the suggestion has been.

Confusion of Trance and Dream

J: I felt like I fell asleep. But up here, I think I know different. Is there a Kleenex?
Thank you.
[She yawns deeply]
I felt like I fell asleep and had some dreams. Did I really fall asleep? Did I? I don't think—I feel like I fell asleep, really fell asleep.
I was dreaming about when I was much younger.

E: It was a nice restful sleep.

J: I know. That was not polite.
I didn't come here to fall asleep in a chair. My body feels like it was sleeping. I was dreaming about—

R: She begins by describing a dissociation between *feeling* and *thinking* in her evaluation of her trance. She then confuses the trance with dream experience.

Trance Reinduction via Suggestion of Dream: Language Cues to Visual Hallucinations

E: But the dream is continuing.
[J closes her eyes momentarily and appears to lapse back into trance. She then opens her eyes and continues.]

J: I was dreaming about when I was much younger. It seems so vivid. It *almost* seems like I can see myself standing over there.

E: Sitting there and growing.

J: When I was a little girl. Of course exactly this one plaid dress that I wore I *can* see myself right over there. I wore it until no one could wear it. I *really* can see myself standing over there and going home. We lived on a street called X Avenue. The best part of the place was my father had put like a gate with a fence and a trellis with flowers all over it. I loved that. The house was OK, but it was small. But that part when you walked into the house through the trellis, you felt like you were entering somewhere.

E: And you can see yourself.

J: That's the strange thing. I can see myself right over there. Standing doing that. I can almost reach over there and touch that trellis.

> R: You reinduce trance by simply suggesting the dream continue.
>
> E: Yes, we witness the rapid transition from the more awake state, when she uses the past tense to say "I was dreaming," to the trance state, when she next uses the present tense, "It seems so vivid."
>
> R: The rapid development of visual hallucinations with her eyes open is also indicated by her linguistic transition from "It *almost* seems like I can see myself standing over there" to "*I can* see myself right over there." to "I *really* can see myself standing over there . . ." She then admits her perplexity when she says it's a "strange thing" that she can see herself over there and almost reach over and touch the trellis she obviously is hallucinating.

Two-State Dissociative Regression

E: And I'd like to have you discover something missing. There are two of you there, one taller than the other. Only the taller one doesn't know that the smaller one is there,
but you can see it.

J: The taller one is—there is one in this plaid dress, me in the plaid dress going in from school. And there is another girl wearing an older outfit, she is in high school coming back to see this house because she lived there once. But she is wearing a pongee pink plaid skirt, in fact she made it herself. She learned to sew so she could make them. Very pretty and she washes them and takes care of them herself so they are always very fresh. She is going to see that house. She is not sad, just nostalgic because she is looking to see if there are still marigolds growing there because she lived there once. And she loved these flowers that grew there. That is what she is coming to look for. This other girl that is walking from school, she feels like stopping here and asking her if the flowers are still growing there. She would even like to ask if she could come in that house again and look around.

> R: In the first sentence she begins with a phrase describing the taller and older girl and then shifts to the younger in the plaid dress. In the second sentence she returns to the older girl in high school coming back to see her former house where she will see

her younger self. Within a moment she thus creates a situation wherein her younger and older self-images could be plausibly interacting. You suggested that the taller girl not know the smaller one is there, but by the end of this section it's apparent that the taller is seeing the smaller. So you must now try to reinforce the two-state dissociative regression.

Reinforcing Two-State Dissociative Regression: Creative Rationalizing in Trance

E: The smaller girl doesn't know the larger girl is there.

J: She doesn't see anyone else. She is just walking right into the house. But the taller girl thinks that she is having a dream or something because she thought she saw this girl to talk to. But she was looking at the trellis, and she looked and there was really nobody there. She had a strange feeling, as though it were a memory. Or, could someone run in that fast? I think she feels like she—I don't know, like she is dreaming.

[The senior author continues suggesting older self-images until Jill has received significant periods of childhood, adolescence, and adulthood, into her current marriage. Particularly prominent are a series of memories about moving from the eastern seaboard of the U.S. where she was born, to the west, where she now lives.]

R: You now reverse your earlier suggestion and have the smaller girl not know the larger girl is there. Jill responds immediately to this reversal by rationalizing "but the taller thinks that she is having a dream or something because she thought she saw this girl . . . there was really nobody there."

Awakening with Distraction to Facilitate Amnesia

E: And now let's draw a curtain and leave all that's happened behind the curtain. You shut your eyes. And everything that happened will be behind the curtain of yesterday, and today you will open your eyes into today, ready to begin a new work. And so sleep for what seems like a few hours of very restful sleep. And by the time your left hand gets down to your thigh, it will seem as if hours of restful sleep had passed and you can then awaken.

J: Excuse me. Oh, what a yawn [J stretches and obviously awakens].

E: Now there are some things I would like to introduce here.

[Erickson now distracts J with some interesting anecdotes about his family and the process of memory in psychological development, how different personality types remember via intellectual versus emotional associations, body associations, etc.]

Testing for Amnesia: Open-Ended Questions and Implications

E: Now, what work shall we do today?

J: Um?

E: What work shall we do today?

J: Whatever you would like. I guess I feel a little sleepy.

R: Plane trip make you sleepy?

J: But actually I am not tired. I don't feel like I would go to sleep.

> R: After distracting her with your stories for about five minutes, you test for amnesia with an open-ended question, "Now what work shall we do today?"—with a certain tone and manner that actually implies no trance work has been done yet today. When she says she feels a "little sleepy" with possible reference to trance, you dismiss it by questioning whether it was the plane trip here that made her sleepy. This question tends to reorient her to the earlier part of the day, when she came to Phoenix by plane, and implies that she just arrived and has not yet done any trance work.

A Successful Posthypnotic Suggestion: Ratifying Trance by Time Distortion

E: Carefully, without looking, what time is it?

J: About five?

E: Five what?

J: I mean, probably about five o'clock. I woke up.

J: My body feels morningish. But I know it's not because I wouldn't be here at five in the morning.

E: What time did you arrive in Phoenix?

J: I think I woke up at five this morning. Anyway. I forgot. What time did I arrive? ABout eleven-thirty? Eleven-twenty?

E: How long did it take you to get here?

424

J: About twenty minutes.

E: Now it is five o'clock? What have you been doing?

J: I don't know exactly. We were talking.

E: About what?

J: Well, just now you mentioned something about personality types, right?

E: Yes.

J: Genetic structure.

E: Do you want to look at your watch?

J: I have been somewhere else. I really have been somewhere else, haven't I?

R: It is only two o'clock. How come you estimated five?

J: It's not like five in the morning, but it seems like five in the evening. But it was only two? I really must have been somewhere else.

> R: Your questions about time established that she has experienced a form of lengthening or expanding subjective time that is very characteristic of trance (Cooper and Erickson, 1959.) Three hours of time distortion is more than usual, however, and indicates that she is successfully experiencing your earlier posthypnotic suggestion to have "a rest that seems hours long."

Indirectly Assessing Amnesia

E: This time data is very important.

R: Yes, really!

E: And she had no idea that this would occur, nor did you.

R: That's right. It was a spontaneous thing.

· J: What does that mean?

E: It happened that I personally knew it would happen.

J: Really?

E: Yes. It feels like five A.M., you think it was five P.M.

425

E: Many of my remarks in this section are beginning to lay out opportunities for her to break through her amnesia. But none of these hints helps. Rather than telling the patient outright about the time distortion, as is frequently done in experimental procedures, I prefer the indirect approach of assessing just how strong it is.

Confusion of Time and Place Ratifying Trance

J: Confusion.

E: You are really not tired. But you feel you have been away.

J: A lot of confusion.

R: This sort of confusion she experiences on awakening is another criterion of deep trance involvement.

Questions Indirectly Assessing Hypnotic Amnesia: Rationalizing Trance Associations to Maintain Amnesia

E: Now, where is the place you think you must have been some other place, east? west? south? north?

J: How's that?

E: You say that you feel as if you have been some other place.

J: Yes.

E: Was that east, west, south, or north?

J: East and west both. I don't know why. Why east and west?

E: That's right.

J: I don't feel like east and west. Why was I east and west?

R: Does it make any kind of sense?

J: No, it just feels in my shoulders like I was east and west. Figure that one out, I can't.

E: Now let's make mention of something else. How high is a fence?

J: Depends.

E: How high is a fence? How high do you feel a fence is?

J: First I feel it is high. Really high. Yeah. Why would I feel that way? When I sit down, maybe it is that high. Because I am sitting it must feel high.

E: Trees have bark. How does it feel?

J: Dusty and crumbly. Do you ever like to do that? Do you?

R: Oh, yeah, I love that. Especially in a big redwood forest. Is redwood bark dusty and crumbly? I thought grayish bark is dusty and crumbly. [The senior author provides further trance associations, to no avail. J remains amnesic for her trance experience.]

R: You ask her a series of questions to indirectly assess her amnesia and give her an opportunity to break it down?

E: Yes. Since her trance memories were concerned with the moves from the east to the west coast, my question about directions might have enabled her to build an associative bridge to her trance experience.

R: She acknowledges the relevance of east and west, but she does not know why. She is thus sensing something about the relevance of your question, but the trance experience remains amnesic.

E: Since that did not break down her amnesia, I hint about the fence that was so high in her hallucinations that she had to look up.

R: Her response that it is "really high" again indicates that some trance associations must be leaking through, but still the basic amnesia is not broken. In fact she goes astray when she tries to rationalize that a fence is high when she sits down! Although she acknowledges the trance associations you supply, she rationalizes them away. I wonder if the same process takes place in everyday life, when we may have current intentions about some matter that our right hemiphere knows about but our left hemiphere tends to rationalize away.

E: I make yet another effort by mentioning "trees have bark" as a way of building an associative bridge to her trance memories of the gray bark she crumbled in her fingernails as a child.

R: I join in with more associations about grayish bark, but she cannot use them. Her amnesia remains intact.

[This session now ends. J was seen for a few more sessions during which she learned to utilize her spontaneous trances for artistic work and self development.]

Case 13   Hypnotherapy in Organic Spinal Cord Damage: New Identity Resolving Suicidal Depression*

Some years ago a young woman in a wheelchair approached the senior author and declared that she was profoundly distressed—in fact, suicidally depressed. Her reason was that an accidental injury in her early twenties had left her with a transverse myelitis: she was lacking in all sensations from the waist down, and she was incontinent of bladder and bowel. Her purpose in seeing the senior author was that she wanted to secure a philosophy of life by which to live; the incontinence of bladder and bowel and confinement to a wheelchair were more than she felt she could endure. She had heard the senior author lecture on hypnosis and had reached the conclusion that perhaps by hypnosis some miraculous change in her personal attitudes could be affected. She explained further that as a small child she had been extremely interested in cooking, baking, sewing, playing with dolls, and fantasizing about the home, husband, and children she would have when she grew up. At the age of twenty she had fallen in love and made plans to marry upon completion of college. She had set to work filling a hope chest with hand-sewn linens and designing her own wedding dress. All she had ever wanted was a husband, a home, children, and grandchildren. Her love for her own grandmothers was a strong factor in her life, and she shared much emotional identification with them.

The unfortunate accident resulting in the transverse myelitis put an end to all her dreams and expectations. After some ten years of stormy difficulties and complications, she became able to use a wheelchair and to return to her university studies. Even with this improvement in her situation she saw no future for herself in the academic world, and became progressively depressed with increasing suicidal ideation. She had finally reached a point at which she felt some definite decision had to be made. Therefore she wished the author to induce a "very deep hypnotic trance and discuss possibilities and potentialities for me. Don't speak too softly or gently of encouragement because I will listen with all my intelligence, and if you try to soft-pedal my situation or mislead or misinform me, I will take it that you see no genuine hope for my happiness in the future. I want to be fair with you. I have given you an

---

*Previously unpublished paper by the senior author and reedited for this volume by the junior author.

enormous problem, that of deciding whether I shall live with some philosophy which will make life worthwhile, or whether I had better call it quits and cease to be a dependent, incontinent, ill-smelling wheelchair occupant for life.

"I would like to return next Saturday for your answer, because I know you will need time to think about the problem.

"But now you can hypnotize me. I have read just enough about hypnosis to know that you can't give me posthypnotic suggestions to prevent my suicidal intentions if there is no hope for me. Hence I shall attend carefully to you for the exact meaning or implications of what you say. So please, just train me to be a good subject."

Initial Trance Training: Two Simultaneous Trains of Thought

Her request was abided by and, probably because of her deep motivation, a very deep somnambulistic trance state was elicited. She was tested with great care for her ability to manifest the phenomena of deep hypnosis. Depersonalization, dissociation, time distortion, and hypermnesia of the happy past were either avoided or the suggestions were worded so carefully that there could not be even a seeming attempt to change her views and attitudes.

One suggestion of a therapeutic character that did come to mind was a well-known song of the old variety, which she was asked to hallucinate, visually and auditorily, with an orchestra and singer. The song was the one about the toebone being connected with the footbone, the footbone with the heelbone, the heelbone with the anklebone, and so on. To mislead and confuse her in any speculations that she might spontaneously make, she was asked to be annoyed by hallucinating at the same time another orchestra and singer interfering with the first singer and orchestra. This second group was performing the song "Doing What Comes Naturally." My rationalization to her for this apparently involved maneuver was that I wanted her to be able to entertain simultaneously two different trains of thought, and I could think of no less objectionable way of teaching her that she could entertain mentally and evaluatively compare different sets of thought. The harmless popular songs were as innocuous a way of accomplishing this and of giving such instruction as I could think of.

Unsuspectingly the patient accepted my explanation and became interested rather than annoyed at "listening to two different orchestras and two different and rather silly songs at the same time." In reply I commented that it would be quite a problem to discover if she were listening to me with one ear and to the songs with the other ear. (This was another distraction.)

She proved to be a most unusually capable hypnotic subject and fortunately manifested complete trust in me upon arousing. She was particularly adept in experiencing hypnotic amnesia. Apparently her intention to carefully scrutinize my statements with extreme care while she was in trance had the effect of relegating any understandings and memories achieved during trance to the unconscious mind.

Facilitating a Yes Set with Personal Truisms

During the next few days an informative history was obtained from an intimate friend of the patient. From such information came various items of fact that could be utilized to help the patient give attention and credence to the author's statements. By this means a validity could be attached to the therapist's statements attested by the patient's own personal knowledge, rather than a validity achieved by the taking of a formal history. This is a much more effective method and may be used to elicit unwitting but helpful cooperation from the patient.

> R: Since this was a particularly difficult patient who placed many restrictions on you, it was particularly important to achieve a yes set by gathering and expressing information that had a particular force of truth for her (personal truisms). What were some of the items of information you gathered, and how did you use them?

Formulating the Therapeutic Plan

The next Saturday afternoon, beginning at 1:00 P.M. and ending at 5:00 P.M., was spent with this patient. At first she was watchful and wary, but she soon concluded that the author was fully honest in his intentions of direct, open, and straightforward handling of her problem and his task.

An outline and analysis of her problem was made into a typewritten account. She was shown a separate copy of this material with certain phrases and sentences omitted, and a carbon copy of the account she held in her hands was left lying carelessly on top of the desk. The full copy of all the proposed procedures I planned without omissions was carefully locked up in the desk drawer. The edited material had been worded to omit any use of such words as "suggestions of a therapeutic character," "rationalization," and "unsuspecting" as parts of the general analysis of her character. In other words the purpose was to convince her that her wishes were being met exactly as she demanded and that I was seeking only her ratification of my understanding of her wishes. She read the typewritten material carefully, agreed that the material I had attributed to her in my quotations adequately summarized her thoughts and desires, and agreed that if I wished, I could proceed. Then she interrupted, however, to ask what I intended to do with my typewritten account, to which the reply was given that if she decided the philosophy of life I offered was worthwhile, I might like to publish an account of my work with her, but that if she found it unsatisfactory, I would most certainly want to discard it—what else! This, she stated, seemed most reasonable (she did not realize that the flippancy of the "what else" was an effective stop to that line of inquiry).

Two-Level Communication

While she was still in the waking state, the explanation was then given that she could and should awaken from the trance state "any time that was necessary." Deliberately the words "as considered by her" were not added. The implication was there for her unconscious mind; for her conscious mind the instruction implied any time that was *considered by her* to be necessary. If I had verablized "as considered by her," it would be accepted by her unconscious mind also, and a careful process of unconscious evaluation would be required. I wished, however, to limit her unconscious only to the words used. The unconscious is literal and tends to accept only what is said. This the patient could not appreciate, and hence she accepted in good faith exactly what was said uncritically, at both conscious and unconscious levels.

A Double Bind Utilizing the Patient's Inquisitiveness

Then she was told that she would be given—perhaps systematically, perhaps randomly—a whole series of odds and ends of valid, curious, and interesting information, and that her task would be to take out of all this the meaning most satisfactory to her. (Thus there was no hint that the order of presentation of ideas might be deliberate in significance and arranged in an order to effect certain results.) Again she agreed thoughtfully but without being given much time for reflection.

Then she was told that these same explanations would be repeated to her in the deep trance state, perhaps not in the full totality of the words said but in their essence, and that her unconscious mind could check her unconscious understandings against her conscious ones. Thus, by an incomplete wording of the instructions and by the request that she check her unconscious understandings against her conscious understandings, she was given again and intentionally the illusion of understanding totally and fully at both levels of awareness. She could not recognize the "double bind" placed upon her to make her conscious understandings about the procedure also her unconscious understandings.

> R: This is an ingenious use of the double bind between the conscious and unconscious. It is particularly effective for her precisely because she was so interested in knowing at all levels what you were doing. You thus utilized this inquisitiveness to effect the double bind. The procedure might not function as a double bind for someone less inquisitive, because the inner dynamic or energy for carrying it out would be lacking. This is

431

an excellent example of how double binds are dependent upon a patient's individual characteristics for their effectiveness.

A "Listening Without Interruption" Set

A deep, somnambulistic trance state was then elicited, and she was asked to be patient and considerate of any ambiguity or fumbling in meaning of what the author said. (This was a delaying technique to ensure full consideration.)

The first step of the procedure was to ask her to hallucinate as before the two orchestras and singers, thus setting the stage for the systematic evaluation of ideas and understandings. Once the stage was set, the orchestras and singers were to be removed, and then she was to let nothing interfere with her task. What the patient did not realize was that her task was the evaluation of the *total communication to be offered to her* and that there could be no hasty interruption or coming to a halt. She was thus unwittingly, and deliberately commited in an unrecognizable fashion to a prolonged state of receptiveness to a great variety of ideas.

R: The preparatory work of listening to orchestras and singers established a set to receive total, complete communication without interruption, because when we listen to music we usually do follow it to the end. You thus indirectly established a "listening without interruption set." This approach might not work at all with a music critic, however, who was used to interrupting the music within his own mind to appraise it critically. Here again you are being careful to utilize the individual characteristics of your patient rather than use the same blanket approach for everyone.

Accepting the Patient's Frame of Reference: Utilizing Negativity to Open a Yes Set for an Exchange of Values

Thus, with brutal frankness but with utter simple casualness, she was told that not only was she handicapped by her accident, but unfortunately she could not really be called either a pretty girl or even just fairly good-looking. The simple fact, it was stated, was that she was definitely plain-featured, that as a rule men are attracted by looks primarily, but that it was fortunate that she did have good intelligence and a charming personality even though she was confined to a wheelchair.

E: Such a brutal beginning, with such negative statements only partially balanced by a final qualified favorable statement, could have no other effect than to convince her of my utter sincerity of purpose. Whether I was right or wrong, I could not be accused of trying to win her over to my views, to secure her compliance by favorable and pleasing words. Her evaluation of what I said was much more important than the content of what I actually said. Such brutal frankness also showed my fearlessness in confronting desperate issues. This was the first step in the orientation of her hopes for a fearless, nonsuicidal solution of her problems.

R: You were careful to take cognizance of and then utilize her own negativity so that she could accept your words. I'm sure that she came to you at least in part because you too are confined to a wheelchair, and you too must have experienced some of her bitter emotions. She is desperately looking for an identification with you that will enable her to find a nonsuicidal resolution of her problems. Your brutal fearlessness meets her conscious needs and opens a yes set for further therapeutic identification with you. In openly accepting her mental frames of reference you are making it possible for her to eventually accept yours. This establishes the I-thou interaction that permits a genuine rapport and exchange of values.

Poetry, Parables, Puns, and Metaphor: Evoking Transformative Ideodynamic Processes

The senior author continued: "But men are such curious creatures that they will be attracted to and marry just anything so long as it is female. Imagine any man in his right mind marrying an Ubangi duck-billed woman, *but they do it*. And can you imagine even necking with a Burmese giraffe-necked woman, but their husbands love them. And think of that historically happy, contented bean-pole Jack Sprat and his lard-tub wife. What she ever saw in him or he in her heaven only knows, but *love is blind, so all authorities say*. [An important communication, not recognizable as such.] And please don't ever tell Mr. Hippopotamus that Miss Hippopotamus does not have a lovely smile. [There was no way to ensure, only to hope that the patient in the deep trance might grasp the triple pun so pertinent to her in her condition "hip-pot-mus (mess)." On other occasions even more obscure puns have been readily picked up in the trance state by other patients. This patient resented her hips bitterly, she spoke of the commode as the "pot" and of the area of her hips as being a "mess." Calling a spade a spade, especially in the patient's own language, however unrecognized at the time, often expedites therapy by convincing the patient that the therapist is unafraid of his task and recognizes it clearly.] And of course, could there ever be a love more divine than that of the starry-eyed Hottentot youth fantasizing in erotic reverie the beauty of the steatopygous, the hideous, fatty-tumored buttocks of the maiden of his dreams? Thank goodness, the

433

Gaussian Curve, *the curve of natural distribution exists* [somewhere in that curve she has to fit], and that 'for every Rachel there is a Reuben, and for every Reuben, there is a Rachel' [an old childish song paraphrased]. 'East is East and West is West and never the twain shall meet' was not spoken of male and female."

> E: From the hideous and negative beginning of the last section a markedly positive ending comes in this section. There is admixture of a happy childhood game, of the poetry of youth, the aim of adulthood, all combined by poetic nuances that could not be disputed. She could not find any single thing to dispute. She was caught in a flowing stream of ideas journeying a rough emotional passage but ending pleasantly.

> R: Poetry, parables, puns, and metaphor (love is blind) all flow together in a way that actually utilizes her negative views about herself. The puns tend to evoke unconscious processes of search, and the poetry, parables, and metaphor open dimensions of mind that point to something beyond the limited views of her conscious mind. She is a highly gifted person seeking a philosophy of life, and you meet this need by first grounding your words in her negative "realities" and then point beyond them with your poetic metaphors and parables. Your rich use of the words "curious," "imagine," "love," "heaven," "lovely," "hope," "divine," "starry-eyed," "fantasy," "erotice reverie," "beauty," "dreams" all tend to evoke nonrational ideodynamic processes (of the right hemisphere) that can be potent transformers of the fixed and limited negative views she has of her life situation.

More Poetry, Parables, Puns, and Metaphor: Evoking Inner Search and Unconscious Processes of Therapeutic Transformation

Then quickly, making a sudden change in tone of voice and of ideas before the patient could possibly assess the values of the individual ideas presented, I told the patient with a warning intonation, "And don't ever forget the little child standing tiptoe, with bated breath, with shining expectancy in its eyes, its every movement and *lack of movement* [how could the patient from this type of phrasing consciously apprehend the hidden thought 'paralyzed from the waist down?] showing delight, confidence, surety, and certainty that the gift being offered to him is the *long-wanted* ['long-wanted' is a pertinent and potent word] present from Santa Claus [a mythical figure, a source that one believes in with unlimited and hopeful faith; recognizing that the patient is asking for a miraculous gift from a hoped-for Santa Claus].

"Eyes of expectancy, confidence of manner, security of being and knowing, just waiting to receive, and thus it goes on, year after year, generation after generation after generation." [What did the patient want but 'generation after generation after generation?' How else could all this be said except in the language of a child, remembering the belief in a Santa Claus, and with the firm convictions, memories, and understandings of childhood tied to adult words? There was no other way for the patient to understand except in terms of intense childish beliefs and emotions with all their attitudes of acceptance. Remember how she liked her grandmothers!]

"Also, consider the foolish businessman with a profitable business and worries, worries, worries until the worry in his head has dug a hole right inside his stomach. He takes his upstairs worries downstairs, and wishes vainly that he could get rid of his downstairs pain that is down in his stomach. Poor fool! He does not remember how at the fraternity house he watched some poor fraternity brother eat apple sauce, putting it 'downstairs in his belly,' and then how he, with 'sweet' innocence, asked 'Was that a worm in the apple sauce you just ate?' laughing at the poor fellow leaping up to go elsewhere to put 'upstairs in his mouth' from 'downstairs in his belly' and hence to put outside of him the imaginary worm from downstairs in his stomach. Whatever it is that is downstairs in that poor fellow [the patient, too, is a 'poor fellow'], he can always get it from downstairs to upstairs.

"Why, I can even take this piece of typewritten paper and turn it toward you or toward me [demonstrating], and since I can read upside-down, we can both be pleased. [A male and a female in juxtaposition, and both pleased. The basic elements being mentioned, apparently irrelevantly, become more challenging in the need to understand them. I was a man, she was a woman, we were in juxtaposition; and we could both be pleased reading the same thing, doing something together, I in my way, she in hers. What was it that she wanted? A husband in juxtaposition, both of them pleased. Yet in no way could the patient become alarmed. Rather, she followed along with only curiosity, the symbolic values escaping from her full realization but becoming a part of a consistent series of partially received symbolisms.]

"Oh, yes, 'doing what comes naturally'!" [Back to the first session, back to the beginning of the second session—but why?]

"Among all peoples, from the most primitive to the most civilized, there is a metaphoric language, all the way from 'and when thyself . . . shall pass among the guests star-scattered on the grass, and . . . reach the spot . . . turn down an empty glass' to 'He doesn't know his head from a hole in the ground.' " [Both the glass and the hole are empty, but what a difference in the emptiness! The patient is to make comparisons and contrasts and "do what comes naturally"; all with a somehow related meaningfulness. All this was certainly not appealing to a conscious mind, but for its inescapable unconscious connotations it was bearing upon things known and unknown, consciously and unconsciously.] "For example, I can ask you right now in the deep trance, Which is your dominant thumb—that is, are you right-thumbed or left-thumbed?—and you don't know, and what's more, you don't know how to find out. [Years of inquiry discloses a few naive students who actually comprehend the question.] Your body knows, but you don't know either consciously or unconsciously, do you? [She shook her head, frowned in perplexity thereby indicating that she did not.] All right, clasp your hands together over your head and, keeping them together, bring them down to your lap. Which thumb is on top? That is your dominant thumb. You have known for years that you were right-handed, but you have never noticed that you are not right-thumbed. You didn't even think of it. It is 'not natural' for your right thumb to be on top.

"I noticed that you were left-thumbed, left-eyed, and left-eared last week, and I made up my mind that you should have free access to what your conscious mind knows about your body but does not know that it knows, and what your body knows freely but that neither your conscious nor your unconscious mind openly knows. *You might as well use well all knowledge that you have, body or mind knowledge, and use all of it well.* What does your body know and know full well, which you know and know full well consciously and unconsciously? Just this little thing! You think that erectile tissue is in the genitals, *just the genitals.* But what does your body know? Just take your finger and thumb and snap your soft nipple and watch it stand right out in protest. It knows that it has erectile tissue. You have had that knowledge without knowing it for a long time. And where else do you have erectile tissue? In New York State you stepped out of doors in thirty degrees below zero and felt your nose harden. Naturally! It has erectile tissue! Why else would it harden? And watch that hot baby slobbering for a kiss from the man she loves and see her upper lip get thick and warm? Erectile tissue in the upper lip! [The use of crude adjectives is deliberate and intentional. The patient needs to accept the ideas. Therefore, to ensure acceptance, she is given something to reject, namely the crude adjectives. In presenting therapeutic understandings a little roughage, as in the diet, is essential. Therapists who insist that everything they present is good and acceptable—and must be accepted because it is always tendered in courteous language and manner—are in error. There is a need to give the patient an earnest, compelling desire to protect and to respect that which is accepted. Therefore, let patients reword the presented ideas to please themselves. Then they become the patient's own ideas!]

"And now we come to that toebone connected to the footbone and all the rest of the *connections*. [A word of more than one meaning, particularly in view of the foregoing material.] Let me word them! The external genitals are connected to the internal genitals, and the internal genitals are connected to the ovaries, and the ovaries are connected with adrenals, and the adrenals are connected with the chromaffin system, and the chromaffin system is connected with the mammaries, and the mammaries are connected with the parathyroids, and the thyroid is connected with the carotid body, and the carotid body is connected with the pituitary body, and the system of all these endocrine glands is connected with all sexual feelings, and all your sexual feelings are connected with all your other feelings, and if you don't believe it, let some man you like touch your bare breasts and you feel the hot, embarrassed feeling in your face and your sexual feelings. Then you'll know that every word I've said is true, and if you don't so believe, try it out, but the deep red flush on your face right now says you know it's so.

"So continue sleeping deeply, review carefully every word I have said to you, try to dispute it, to argue against it. Try your level best to disagree, but the harder you try the more you will realize that I am right.

"And what good will it do for you? You! I mean you? Just stop and think! You enter a house! There stands a baby, dirty of face, tousled of hair, runny-nosed, wet, smelly, dirty, and its face lights up and it toddles to you so happily because it *knows* it's a nice baby and *that you will be glad to like it and that you will want to pick it up.* You know what you will do! So does the baby! *You can't help yourself.* [A negative statement with a positive meaning.] And then you enter another house and there stands a beautiful little child, hair combed, clean, neat, in a state of perfection, but its face says, 'Who, just who on earth would *ever* want to pick me up?' Certainly you don't, you agree with the child, and you want to find the parents and slap them around for mistreating that child, because you don't ever want to be greeted again, ever again, by that child in that manner.

"Now put a look of starry-eyed expectation on your face, clothe yourself in an air of happy confidence. Romance for you is just around the corner [a crucial statement], I don't know which corner [a statement that leaves the question undecidable and hence requiring further consideration], *but it's just around the* corner! Don't ever forget there's a Rachel for every Reuben and a Reuben for every Rachel, and every Jean has her Jock and every Jock has his Jean, *and around the corner is your 'John Anderson, my Jo.'*

"One doubt you will have, but naturally you are wrong! Your body knows, so does your conscious mind, so does your unconscious mind. Only you, the person, don't know. *So I'll answer the ninny that you are!* [She can defend only against the accusation that she is a 'ninny,' but to do so she has to admit that she knows the verity of what the author is about to say.]

"Is there anything more ecstatic than the maiden's first sweet kiss of true love? Could there be a better orgasm? Or the first grasping of the little lips of the baby on your nipple! Or the cupping of your bare breasts by the hand of your love? Have you ever felt the chills run up and down your spine when kissed on the back of your neck?

"Man has but one place to have an orgasm—a woman has many.

"Continue your trance, evaluate these ideas, make no error about their validity.

"At five o'clock I shall roll you down to the car that's picking you up. You will see me the same time next Saturday. Rouse up in the car."

Thus was the interview terminated abruptly. She was wheeled to the waiting car, and the senior author admonished silence to the driver by a finger on his lips.

> R: You continue your poetic approach with an incredibly rich flight of ideas, with particular emphasis on evoking ideodynamic processes of attitude transformation that reach into the childhood of personality (Santa Claus) and extend into her adulthood (husband, home, and children) and beyond (generation after generation). You use a blend of just about every approach to indirect suggestion and the unconscious that you have ever developed, including confusion, interspersed suggestions, and the apposition of opposites (male and female; brutal language with the poetic). You completely overwhelm her so that there is so much cognitive overload that her conscious mind cannot possibly cope with it. She is therefore sent on a furious inner search for meanings and frames of reference that could cope with your barrage. This inner search will naturally evoke unconscious processes of transformation in a therapeutic direction. You then abruptly stop and send her home in silence, lest her conscious mind be given an opportunity to limit and dismiss the process you have set in motion.

The Alternation of Hypnotherapy and Counseling: Termination of Therapy

The next Saturday was one of unusual interest. Advice and discussion was wanted by the patient in relation to advanced graduate work. There was no request for therapy and none was offered. The author was obviously in the role of a qualified professional academic advisor. A postgraduate career was outlined, and her visits were discontinued. (An amnesia, comprehensive in character, seemed present, but no effort was made to check it. Clinical results were the goal, no experimental checkings.)

R: I've noticed the same phenomena where patients will return after a particularly intense hypnotherapeutic session with an apparent amnesia and a need to simply discuss their life situation and plans with a counselor rather than a depth therapist. There seems to be an actual aversion to discussing the results of the previous hypnotherapeutic session. Rather, the patients seem to integrate it on an unconscious level, and the conscious mind now wants to go on to the next thing. Much of my work has this seesaw rhythm, where deep hypnotic work alternates with light counseling on alternate sessions.

A Ten-Year Followup

Within two years she was married. Her husband was a dedicated research man, and his field of interest was the biology and chemistry of the human colon. They have been married happily for over ten years, and there are now four children, all by caesarian operations.

Ten years after the marriage the author happened to be lecturing in the state of her residence. She noted a news story on the author and called him on the telephone, asking him to lunch with her the next day. Before meeting her, three duplicate sets of questions were typed out. The answers were filled in on one set, which was sealed in an envelope. The other two sets were placed in separate envelopes.

Upon meeting her, two questions were introductorily asked: "Why did you invite me to lunch?" Her startled reply was, "I know it's an odd thing to do, but you lectured to our class at the university several times, and I thought I would like to take you to lunch."

"Is there any other reason?"

Embarrassedly she replied, "No, I realize that I am presumptuous, since I didn't really know you, or you me, but I hope you don't mind."

The author replied, "Here is a sealed envelope. Put it in your handbag. Then you sit at this table, read the questions in this unsealed envelope (handing her one), and answer them, please, on the paper with a pencil. Use 'yes' or 'no' as much as possible."

She looked bewilderedly at the author, read the questions, flushed very deeply, and said, "If it were anybody except you, I would either slap your face or ask the waiter to call a policeman. But for some reason deep down in me, I don't know what it is, I'll be glad to do it."

The author said, "While you are doing so, I will sit at another table with my back toward you and write what I think your answers are going to be. Then I will want to know how well our answers agree." Again she flushed deeply, saying, "I just don't understand, but it is all right."

Accordingly, the two sets of questions were answered and the questions and answers are in the following summarizing table.

Question	Her answer	Author's answer	Sealed envelope answer
How often do you and your husband make love a week?	3-4	3-4?	3-4?
Do you have orgasms—yes or no?	yes	yes	yes
Right side 1, or 1 and 2, or both*	yes, all	1 & 1 and 1 & 2	1 & 1 and 1 & 2 yes, all
Left side 1, or 1 and 2, or both	yes	1 & 1 and 1 & 2	1 & 1 and 1 & 2
Sometimes left 1, right 2, and vice versa	yes	yes	yes
Sometimes right 1, left 2	yes	yes	yes
Explain above two answers in three words as closely as possible	nipple, and nipple and breast, or one or both depending	either and both of nipples and both breasts or singly of each or combinations	either and both of nipples and both of breasts or singly of each or combinations
Neck	sometimes, base	perhaps	perhaps
Lips	upper	upper?	upper?
Earlobes	no	?	?
Nose	no	?	?
Top of head	no	?	?
Back of neck	seldom	?	?
Others	between breasts	between scapulae	between scapulae
Are their other sensory sexual pleasures	yes	none of my business	none of my business
Do you realize that you are always at liberty to have any desired degree of amnesia for this	yes	none of my business	none of my business

---

*One (1) refers to the nipple and two (2) refers to the breast as a whole. This code was established when the original hypnotic work was done years previously.

440

Question	Her answer	Author's answer	Sealed envelope answer
interogation, the past, and any possible role by me—if I had a role			
Do you know that I am most grateful to you even if it is no more than gratitude for the pleasure of knowing you?	I am grateful to you, but I don't see why you are grateful to me	I just hope	I just hope
Will you treat me merely as a friend with interests in common in scientific research if you so desire?	yes	I hope so	I hope so

(In the author's understanding of human nature it was considered best to terminate the questionnaire at this point. Much more information was wanted, but one cannot risk a clinical success for the possibility of a partial academic clarification.)

She was asked to take the sealed envelope out of her handbag and compare the answers there with those she had written.

She did so with many astonished glances at the author. Finally the author said, "The answers I just wrote down agree with the sealed envelope sheet, which is marked three and which I marked last night. I have envelope number two. Yours is number one."

After a long pause she asked, "What does this mean? I know you are not psychic. But I have obviously an amnesia or you could not have such reliable information about me of such intimate and detailed character. Was I your patient at one time?"

"What do you think?"

"Obviously! Let me see if I can remember. I have a feeling that you gave me something very nice, and then stepped out of the picture so I couldn't thank you. If I remember, do I have to keep on remembering?"

"No, you don't have to remember. I have now learned that some ideas I had were right, and I'm so very glad they were."

"Will you publish it? And if I read it, will I remember?"

"I will try to write into it hidden instructions for you to forget all identities involved, if indeed you are involved. You know and I know there are others like you, and you don't know how many I know. But I will say this. I check to some extent on each one I have treated. I check when possible on those I haven't treated. Perhaps someone learned spontaneously and taught me how to teach others. Maybe others learned spontaneously and convinced me I should make inquiries whenever possible. You are a possibility. My account will be scientifically reliable, the disguise used will serve only to hide identities from anyone actually involved, and I am quite confident, adequately so.''

R: This case history, the assumptions and presumptions, their validity and applicability, leave much to be desired. There is no doubt that the patient was truly benefitted. This is well established beyond all doubt and after the passage of many years. How much credit should be given the senior author is a serious question. That he at least deserves credit for initiating recovery is obvious, but did such recovery derive from the natural capacities of the body to heal itself when once oriented, or did the psychological processes themselves as employed serve to initiate new neural pathways of response and thus to awaken otherwise unrealizable potentialities? In brief, this report poses serious questions concerning the interplay of psycho-neuro-physiological relationships and the possible methodologies for their activation.

Case 14 Psychological Shock and Surprise to Transform Identity*

Meg was twenty-four years old. She had completed high school and secretarial training and had worked satisfactorily three years for a physician and one year for a business firm. She was the oldest child in a closely knit family consisting of her siblings, her long-widowed mother, and two spinster aunts. She contributed all her earnings unnecessarily to the family, and her personal expenditures were rigidly limited as well as rigidly supervised.

At the age of twenty-one she met a young Army private at church, and each felt a strong attraction for the other. Their meetings were confined to the church, the mother's home, or, if they went elsewhere, it was with the chaperonage of either one or both spinster aunts. Despite these difficulties a proposal of marriage was made and accepted with full family approval, all within six months, since the young man was completing his term of service and was returning to his home two thousand miles away. He wished to take Meg home as his bride, but she declared she needed until June, six months in the future, to get ready. As June approached, her letters contained more and more pleas for a December wedding, until the young man finally consented. But the

*Previously unpublished paper written by the senior author and edited for publication here by the junior author.

December wedding was postponed until June, and this went on for three years.

During the third year Meg left her position with the physician and took one with a business firm, seeking out another physician to whom she offered vague, unrealistic complaints. He was straightforward and kindly, but impatient with her complaints and frankly discredited them. Meg returned a few weeks later, complaining of hearing voices that talked to her during the day and awakened her at night. As she told her story, she would lapse into brief silences of a minute or two in which she would stare silently into space. The physician, a general practitioner, was alarmed and tried to refer her to a psychiatrist—the nearest one was more than 150 miles distant—but she refused to go. When he tried to interest her family, he was asked to care for her himself. He tried to do so but recognized his lack of competence. Finally, after months of laborious effort, he persuaded the family to bring Meg to the senior author. She was accompanied on the train by her mother, both aunts, and two grown siblings.

The interview with Meg was most informative. The auditory hallucinations she declared to have experienced for six months were psychiatrically unconvincing. Her sudden lapses of staring into space seemed to be more a pose than a symptom.

Two hours were required to elicit the above history and the additional facts that she was afraid to leave home, that her fiancé would not consent to live in Arizona, that she could not give up the hope of marriage, and that medical help would have to correct all these matters.

Additionally, she insisted on the validity of her auditory hallucinations and insisted that she could not travel by bus, train, airplane, or automobile except in the company of her family. She dropped the pose of staring into distance during the latter part of the interview. She also despairingly expressed an absolute conviction that she was past all medical help.

Trance Induction and Posthypnotic Suggestions

The next visit was made with the same entourage as the first visit. The senior author peremptorily refused to hear her complaints unless she "went to sleep and talked with her unconscious mind but without telling anything she did not want to tell." By carefully worded, reassuring suggestions a medium-to-deep trance was induced in about thirty minutes. This trance was used to give her emphatic posthypnotic suggestions to the effect that, in return for the senior author's listening to all of her fears and her accounts of her hallucinations for the rest of the session, she would listen attentively to many things he would have to say on the occasion of her next visit; that until then she would be almost painfully curious about what he might have to say. Many repetitions

443

were made of this instruction in slightly varying terms to ensure full understanding.

She aroused from the trance and launched into an extensive account of her auditory hallucinations and a brief account of the impossibility of leaving home, the even lesser possibility of leaving Arizona, and of her need to have four or five members of her family with her just to come for her interviews with the senior author. Again the senior author reached the conclusion that the psychiatric portrayal she offered of herself was no more than a symptomatic screen to conceal her actual problem.

Three weeks passed before she was seen again, this time with only four members of her family accompanying her. She was obviously eager, expectant, curious, yet fearful of what the senior author might have to say, and she tried to forestall him by declaring that she had some "new worries."

> R: You utilized her present behavior in a subtle and ingenious manner. Her major behavior was wanting to present her complaints about the difficulties of her life situation. During this second session you blocked her complaints just long enough to induce a trance. You then utilized her need for further complaint by making it a condition for listening attentively to what you would say on the next visit. She did complain to you for the rest of this session, so now she was bound to listen to you on the next. You heighten her *expecting* by telling her "she would be almost painfully curious" about what you would say and then let that expectancy build for three weeks!
>
> E: Yes, I tied her up.

Direct Suggestions While Depotentiating Resistance

She was told firmly to close her eyes and to listen, even to "go to sleep" if she wished, but listen she must. As she closed her eyes the author began a series of instructions: (1) She must move out of the maternal home and room with some other girls, doing this within the week. This was to be explained to her family as medical orders. (The family physician had agreed to confirm this, and he was indeed consulted.) (2) She was to bank her paycheck and pay her own bills. (3) She was not to receive any member of her family as a visitor in her new quarters. (Her spinster aunts patrolled that street nightly for several hours at a time for several weeks.) (4) She was not to visit her home nor to make telephone calls to her family nor to receive them. (5) Her contact with her family was to be limited to brief greetings of not more than three minutes at church. (6) She was to attend the theater, eat at restaurants, go roller skating with her fellow roomers. (The family physician supplied much helpful information, including the actual possibility of two pros-

444

pective roommates for her.) (7) She was to invite her roommates as a lark to go for a bus ride across town and back. (8) She was to come entirely alone on her next trip in two weeks to see the author. (9) One of the preceding instructions—one and only one—she could modify and thus violate it, but not too much, and this would comfort her and enable her to obey all other instructions completely and the modified one satisfactorily.

Over and over these instructions were repeated until she developed a trance state from which she was aroused at the end of the session. The instructions were then again repeated, and she was given another appointment in two weeks' time.

> E: The purpose of the permission to violate and modify one of the instructions was psychologically to compel the acceptance of all the other instructions. Thus, by legitimately violating one, she could meet, at least in part, the author's authoritative instructions.

> R: When you give direct suggestions, you are careful to provide her with some choices she can reject. You have spoken of this as the patient's right to success and failure (Erickson, 1965). Allowing the patient to reject some suggestions in effect depotentiates resistance so the others can be carried out.

> E: When you allow the patient to violate some of your suggestions, they are now indebted to you to carry out the others.

She was definitely triumphant about her accomplishments and was promptly interrupted when she tried to offer an explanation of her mother's presence. (It was better for her to feel guilt toward the senior author than toward her family.) A trance state was immediately induced.

She was instructed in a medium-to-deep trance to execute the following tasks: (1) To travel in a private automobile with friends across the state line (which she had never crossed, although it was but a few miles from her home) and to dine with those friends in some restaurant at least fifty miles from home. (2) To travel by automobile with friends to a specified city, making a round trip of over two hundred miles all in one day. (3) To consider seriously moving from her home town to Phoenix, securing a new job, and living on her savings until the new position was secured. (4) To spend the next half-hour crying, trembling, shivering, dreading, fearing all these tasks, at the same time realizing that one task a week would have to be done and that in the fourth week she would have to come to Phoenix alone, prepared to stay a week while she searched for employment and living quarters, and kept an appointment with the senior author.

During the previous visit and the present one no mention had been made of "the voices." However, as this last series of suggestions was completed, she tremulously spoke: "The voices——" only to be interrupted by the sharply voiced declaration, "Neither of us have ever really believed in those voices. You made Dr. X believe in them, but I didn't. Now, you do everything I have told you to do or Dr. X and I will make you do right away what you are most afraid of. If you are obedient, we will let you build your strength."

E: What else could a girl completely dominated all her life do but yield obediently? This lifelong submission made possible the therapy employed.

R: I've noticed that when you do give direction suggestions, it's usually to a personality who has been trained by previous life experience to accept them. Thus you are again utilizing the patient's own personality needs to ensure the acceptance of your suggestions.

Breaking Family Dependence

A month later she entered the office to report that all tasks were completed. It had taken her one day to find living quarters and one additional day to secure employment beginning the next Monday. (She had wasted three days of the week forcing herself to come to Phoenix.) Then, with utter intensity, she asked when she could visit her home. Entirely casually she was informed, "There is a bus leaving for your home town this afternoon. You will be able to make a surprise visit to your mother tonight in time for dinner. You can stay there overnight, go to church in the morning, and leave on the last bus in the afternoon, which will arrive in Phoenix at 10:00 P.M. Thus you will have a delightful weekend visit at home. This would be a good idea every week or two or three."

She sat silently, contemplatively staring at the author for the next fifteen minutes. Then in a subdued voice, asked, "May I give my mother my new address?" No injunction about this had been even offered her, and her request was interpreted as her own significant desire to begin the end of her family's domination and to cut the bonds of her dependency. She was answered, "Your mother knows my address and telephone number. Just give me your address and telephone number, and in case of any emergency your mother can easily get in touch with you through me." She nodded her head agreeably, stated the information, and departed without completing her allotted time, of which about one-half hour remained.

R: She was now living in your town in Phoenix and only visiting her mother and aunts. You were now functioning as a surrogate parent during this transition period while she was separating from her family.

Trance to Bypass Conscious Limitations

The following Monday noon, during her lunch hour, she appeared to report a "lovely time," to ask for another appointment, and to make payment for the previous appointment.

She was informed that the next appointment would be a most unusual one for her. She was reminded that while she could swim, such activity had always occurred only with other girls and at the Y.W.C.A. A look of horrified dread appeared on her face. The senior author continued, "You always wear clothes that are high-necked, the hems of your dresses are always below the knee, and you wear long sleeves even in summertime. Swimming suits can be very scanty and noticeable in mixed company at a swimming pool." An expression of agonized horror appeared on her face. "But I am not going to ask any such thing of you." She sighed with intense relief. "All I wish is merely that you keep your next appointment wearing the outfit called short shorts." Her gasp of horror was interrupted: "Now close your eyes, sleep deeply, very deeply, now listen! Your next visit here will be kept by you wearing an outfit called short shorts. If it makes you feel more comfortable to do so, you may carry one of your regular dresses in a shopping bag to put on before leaving the office. Arouse now, knowing full well what you are going to do despite the most awful fears that you can manufacture. But bear in mind that this marriage that you want and yet have postponed two to six months at a time for four years is now coming closer and closer. It is now late June and I want a Christmas card from you and your husband this year. Such a Christmas card you are going to send. You will enjoy sending it and you will equally gladly show me the last few letters your fiancé has written to you as soon as you arouse. Now awaken."

As she aroused, the play of emotional expression on her face was most varied, ranging from fear, dread, and deep embarrassment to a look of hopeful anticipation. She was told to let the senior author see a few of her most recent letters from her fiancé. She hesitantly opened her handbag and hastily explained, "I can tell you what he says in every letter—that if I don't marry him this summer, he will find another girl. So I have promised him I will marry him in September."

She was most startled by the senior author's statement, "Yes, that's entirely right. You will be married to him in September, well married."

She appeared for the next interview wearing short shorts of the most extreme sort. She was most embarrassed but became bewildered by the author's apparent oversight of them, his discussion of her past deceptions of hearing voices, of staring into space, of telling her fiancé that she would marry him in a certain month and then changing it, and a discussion, apparently without purpose or point, about the unpredictability of human history, human events, and the unpredictability of the acts and decisions of the individual human being, some of which would occur unexpectedly soon. She was finally given an appointment for the first of July and dismissed. She walked out too bewildered to ask permission to change into her dress.

R: Your apparently irrelevant discussion of the unpredictability of human events is actually a preparation for the shock and surprise you will use in the next session, but she does not know that yet. This discussion serves as a foundation for what will follow. Her previous life had been too predictable. Your discussion of life's unpredictability is thus introducing a new therapeutic frame of reference and at the same time it probably sets many unconscious searches in motion for whatever relevances it can possibly have. Her unconscious knows by now that nothing you do is really irrelevant. A high degree of expectancy and desire is thus aroused for the crucial shock of the next session.

Shock and Surprise to Depotentiate the Old and Transform Identity

She entered the office on July 1 only to find it well-chaperoned. She was asked, "This is July, isn't it, and didn't you promise to marry your fiancé this month?" Her reply was a hesitant "Yes" and then an urgent, "But I promise you I will marry him in September."

Slowly, impressively, she was told, "Since you are so unsure as you have conclusively shown over the past four years, you are today going to prove that you are competent to marry this month, and marry this month you will! I told you that in September you would be married, well married. Now we shall see if there is any reason that you should not be married; we shall learn if you are lacking in any way to justify your marriage postponements."

"Now stand up and, one by one, take off your clothes, naming each article as you place it neatly on the chair."

She looked helplessly at the placid, composed face of the chaperone, then blushingly stood up, hesitated, then took off her shoes, more hesitantly her stockings, then, with many lingering movements, her dress and finally her slip.

"Won't this be enough?" she asked pleadingly, looking first at the author, then looking pleadingly at the chaperone, but no response was made.

Awkwardly, clumsily, she removed her bra, hesitated a moment, then removed her panties and stood in the nude facing the senior author defiantly. Thereupon he turned to the chaperone and remarked, "She looks all right to me. Does she look all right to you?" The chaperone nodded her head.

The author then turned to the patient and stated, "I want to be sure you know and can name all parts of your body. I do not want to point to or touch any part of your body nor does the chaperone. If necessary I can do it, but please don't make it necessary. Just don't try to skip over anything with a name. As you name each part, touch it with one or the other hand, since you must use your right hand to touch your left elbow. Now start from the shoulders and work downward progressively, then turn your back to us and do the same as well as you can. Now go ahead, and no oversights."

With her face suffused with blushes, she did a creditable job. She was commended for this, whereupon her blushes disappeared, and in a most casual, matter-of-fact manner she proceeded to dress.

As she was doing so, she was asked if she thought she would be married by July 15. Her simple answer was, "That would be too soon. I've got to quit my job. I hate to do that without notice, but my boss will understand, and then I've got to travel up north and meet Joe's family and bring him down home, and I've got to tell my family what kind of wedding I want. I saw the kind they gave my sister and I don't want anything like that. But they are going to do it my way or I'm coming to Phoenix and have nobody there except the witnesses. And I better send Joe a telegram right away."

Slightly over two weeks later she brought Joe into the office, explained that she wanted premarital counseling for each of them separately and then for both together. This was done to her satisfaction. A long-distance telephone call assured the senior author that after much struggling the mother and the spinster aunts capitulated and allowed her to have a wedding at which she alone chose the guests instead of the wedding being made a community affair.

E: The way she took over her own marriage plans indicates a radical transformation in her view of herself and reality.

R: Yes, the way her blushes disappeared after she had undressed and then in a matter-of-fact manner proceeded to dress indicate a creative movement of self-transformation. She then proceeds to discuss her immediate plans and forthcoming marriage in a most practical and appropriate fashion.

Followup: First, Second, Third, and Seventh Years

The specified Christmas card arrived, and the next year a birth announcement as well as a Christmas card was received. Three such birth announcements were received, and then no further word was received until about seven years after the wedding. The patient then again sought out the author. She brought her three children with her to display proudly, and then she explained about her marital discord because her husband, in moving with her to Arizona, was finding difficulty in his new occupational adjustment and blaming himself unreasonably. She asked for an appointment for her husband, and at that interview no serious difficulties were found.

Case 15   Experiential Life Review in the Transformation of Identity

This patient made a long-distance telephone call to state that she had been referred by a friend, that she would like an appointment in two weeks' time on a Thursday afternoon, that she would call the office the preceding Wednesday to ascertain the hour, that her name was Miss X. With this statement she terminated the conversation. On Wednesday she called the office, asked the hour of her appointment, and refused to speak to the senior author. The next day at the appointed time Miss X arrived, a woman who appeared to be in her early thirties, haggard and worn, her face tear-stained.

Her story in summary was that she was an adopted child in a family with four older children, the youngest of whom was twelve years her senior. For some unknown reason when she was still a small child her adoptive mother had become pathologically suspicious and inquisitive and had subjected her to interminable inquisitions to learn "if the child had been a bad girl." The adoptive father was cold and undemonstrative, leaving all the children entirely to their mother's care. The four older children had graduated from college, and though they lived not too far away, made only infrequent calls at the parental home, these being extremely brief. Because of this the mother had many times interrogated her about what she had done or said that made the other children avoid the parental home.

The patient had tried to protect herself by absorption in her high school studies, always pleading homework to avoid her mother's repetitious interrogations concerning whether she was a "good girl," whether she had done "bad things," and whether she had "bad thoughts." She won high school honors, but her only social life was rigidly chaperoned by her mother. She entered college but was forced to attend the college in her home town and to live at home. By absorbing

---

*Previously unpublished paper written by the senior author and reedited here for publication by the junior author.

herself in studies, going to summer school and taking special courses to fill in vacation and free time, she escaped much but not all of her mother's pathological questioning. She was forced to take an M.A. degree because "you do not seem to be mature enough to be allowed to try to earn your living, and there is no knowing what bad thing will happen to you away from home."

With the awarding of her M.A. degree, in a state of utterly intense fear, the girl asserted that her age of twenty-two gave her the legal right to leave home. There followed an exceedingly traumatic emotional episode that the father terminated coldly and decisively with the statement, "If you do not want to live with your mother and me in appreciation of all that we have done for you and all the protection we have given you, you may leave. But do not let it be said that we turned you away with no provision. Tomorrow in the bank I will place five thousand dollars to your credit. Take your clothes and leave, and whatever misfortune befalls you is upon your head." The mother's parting words were, "I know you've done something bad. Be brave and tell me."

Weeping, the girl left. She went to another city, secured employment, and then tried to establish relationships with her foster siblings. They rejected her with the explanation, "Mother will descend on us if we are with you, and we have enough trouble with her as it it." They also informed her that each of them had been treated in the same way. That their father had paid off each of them similarly, and only a sense of filial duty made them make their brief calls at the parental home. However, they had been bombarded with letters and telegrams from their mother demanding reports on "my last erring child."

Reluctantly the girl cut all ties, moved to another city where she worked successfully as a secretary, but found herself unable to develop any social life. She became increasingly depressed, unsuccessfully sought happiness in expensive vacations, and finally sought psychiatric aid. The psychiatrist told her he was psychoanalytically trained in the Freudian school. Misunderstandings developed at once, since the question of sex arose in the therapeutic sessions. She desperately sought another and then another psychiatrist. Always the question of sex arose. She began to equate the words sex and psychiatry.

By a desperate effort she could present a good appearance in seeking employment. She applied for a position as a civilian employee connected with the U.S. Army. At first she adjusted well, but as the months went by she became progressively depressed. She sought refuge in studying languages and became fluent in three foreign languages, but even more depressed.

An army psychiatrist recommended her return to the United States for psychiatric treatment. She asked instead for a transfer elsewhere in Europe to a new assignment where her linguistic ability would be of service. This was secured by her twice. The third request was for a transfer somewhere to the Far East. There she was given a teaching position. She tried to learn another language and to lose herself in her work, but her depression became worse. Another army psychiatrist then became insistent that she return to the United States for therapy, and finally she reluctantly did so.

She began the rounds of the psychiatrists she had seen before and rejected them again for the same reason. She sought new psychiatrists but sooner or later the topic of sex arose. Then she learned of hypnosis. A former patient of the senior author's recommended him to her, and she hastily made the telephone call before she "weakened."

What she wanted, she declared, was hypnosis, hypnosis that would blot forever from her mind all thought of "questions" and "sex." And would the author without further delay please settle down to hypnotizing her and meeting her needs?

Since this was her opening request at the very first appointment, a laborious explanation was given to her to the effect that she was asking the author to work completely blindly, and that, considering her tearful appearance, he did not want to work blindly lest unintentionally he might say or do something harmful to her, or do something awkwardly or clumsily, and thus distress her emotionally. Her response was an outburst of uncontrollable sobbing that lasted some minutes.

Advantage was taken of this to explain, "You see, even though I tried to speak gently and intelligently to you, I accidentally broke down your emotional control. So let us work in such fashion that you keep your emotional control; and whatever little you need to say to me, at least say that little, but try to point me in the right direction. In the first place, in order to speak intelligently I need to know the extent of your education—that's all, the extent, not where or how. It is possible that your employment experience, not where or for whom, just knowing the kind of employment experience would enable me to do my task better."

Bit by bit, with intermingled sobbing, the above history was obtained without specific dates, places, or names. Avoidance of asking for specific items of fact aided greatly in securing her cooperation.

She was instructed that the data given above were sufficient to begin work and that no questions would be asked her unless she so indicated a desire. Then she could give whatever additional information she desired. It was also explained that therapy would necessarily cover a number of hour-long periods, spaced in accord with her ability to learn since, as she knew, learning was a task requiring effort. Hypnotherapy would require earnest effort, not passive submission, even as it would require intelligent effort on the author's part. (This emphasis upon the word "intelligent" was to permit the author some freedom of action, and her own history of using her studies as an escape suggested that continued use be made of it.) She agreed, and another long, laborious explanation was given of hypnosis as a learning process, something similar to acquiring "the feel of a new language." This figure of speech was most appealing to her.

No effort will be made to report the separate interviews, since the procedure, rather than the events of specific hours, are of primary interest.

Indirect Induction with Early Learning Set

A wholly indirect hypnotic therapeutic approach was employed. She was asked to choose which of three paperweights looked the most interesting. She chose an agate geode. She was asked to sit comfortably, hands in her lap, to fix her gaze upon the polished surface, to enjoy the various colors, to sit entirely still, to hold her head still, to hold her ears still, and to give herself over to an enjoyment of the colors in the layers of agate, not really being obligated to pay attention to what the senior author was saying. After several varied repetitions of this instruction, her face took on a rather fixed, rigid expression. She was then asked to think through the problem of learning a language—not German, French, Italian, but a much more complex language, the English language as learned by a baby. In a slow, gentle, almost murmuring fashion the senior author described a baby lying in bed, hearing sounds, not knowing what they meant, the progressive articulation of sounds by the infant, its slow physical growth, the change in its features, its hands and feet, new movements, new sounds, bathing, eating, elimination, sleeping, its struggles in crying, its delight in cooing, reaching for things, and so on. Slowly a general comprehensive foundation was laid for extensive thinking by her about the physical growth of a child, its learning of phonetics, eating, elimination, activity, speech, locomotion, and all the rest during the first five years. Initially this was presented as a discussion apparently to illustrate some point to be made by the senior author, but unnoticeably the tenor of the comments shifted slightly. Then stronger and more direct suggestions were made that she lose herself in a wondering but intellectual appraisal of the multitudinous learnings she herself had experienced in the first five or six years of her life.

Evoking Early Repressions with Catharsis

Shortly, within ten minutes, it was obvious that she was in a profound trance and was now oblivious of the agate as well as the rest of her surroundings. Upon a request by the author she plunged into a systematic survey of the memories of her early childhood. This was governed and directed by the therapist by intruding such statements as: "And in that first year what a wealth of fundamental learning, from diapers to pretty things and sounds and colors and noises;" or, "And then you come to the second year, creeping and walking and falling and using the

453

toilet like a *good little baby* and saying little sentences"; and, "Of course, there comes the third year and language is growing, words, so many, the parts of your body, the little hole in your tummy, and you even know the color of your hair."

For each of the first six years this was done, bringing in each year some reference to elimination, *stressing the "goodness" of toilet habits*, body curiosity, the goodness of food, of sleeping, washing, learning all manner of things, and of almost "feeling" herself doing all of these things. This was accomplished in about three hours of utterly concentrated work by the patient.

On the day that it was intended to progress to the next period, the patient entered the office jerkily, her face flushed, and her expression one of furious anger. Explosively she declared, "I'm so mad at you I could slap your face. I just can't think of a name to call you that's bad enough."

"Why not call me a stinking bastard of an S.O.B., since that is probably the best you can do," was the simple, direct reply.

"I will," she shouted and did so, only to burst into a distressed, embarrassed laugh, saying apologetically, "I don't know what made me say that, but in a funny way it makes me feel better."

She was asked, "Since it made you feel better, do you want to repeat the statements, perhaps with improvement?"

"Oh, no, I want to tell you something I don't want to tell you. For two days now I've had a normal bowel movement and my stomach hasn't hurt when I eat, and I'm embarrassed to death to say this to you. I'd have died before rather than tell you. I don't know what you did to me, but something is happening and I don't want to cry either. And that damn psychiatrist in Europe who said that awful obsession I had about the bathtub being filled with bloody water when I shaved my legs showing suicidal tendencies was all wrong. Some day when I ask you, will you tell me what that silly nonsense was? But not right now! But now can we go ahead and let me look at the paperweight?"

Two-Level Communication

In accord with her request, as she spontaneously developed a trance, she was softly instructed to make a comprehensive search of all her *real* childhood memories and *personal* experiences from six to ten. ("Real" and "personal" were words intended to restrict her to self-experiences rather than experiences with others—in particular, with her mother.) Very few suggestions were offered to her, usually, "Did you leave out anything belonging to you at seven?" Vague mention was made of "big girls, you can see when they are big," and "women are like big girls, only different." References to elimination were made more guardedly, "One keeps in good regular body health," and speculations were offered about "little learnings that grow up into the language of life."

It should be borne in mind that the patient was doing this survey as an adult, viewing in vivid, feeling detail a wealth of experiential learnings. Thus, even guarded general suggestions could be freely translated by the subject into more complete, adequate detail. As was later learned, the "little learnings that grow up into the language of life" was translated by her in one of her trance states to refer to genital explorations and stimulation. When first heard, it had "only a poetic sound, and then slowly I gave it a sex meaning, but I don't remember when."

> R: This is an unusually clear example of two-level communication. It took time to develop because an extensive unconscious search was required, and she does not "remember when" precisely because it was an unconscious elaboration that slowly filtered into her conscious mind.

Body Language as an Expression of Ideodynamic Processes

The tenth through the fourteenth years were covered with unexpected rapidity and ease. The senior author had expected tension and difficulty and was extremely guarded and cautious in his emphasis upon the *real,* the *actual,* the *personal* experience belonging to the self and not involving others—"one learns a language not by one's hearing of it but by feeling it in one's own mouth and thoughts, and sensing its untranslatable nuances, and the beauty of a German guttural is a beauty that belongs to a German, however bad it sounds to the untutored ear, and the beauty of self-experience belongs to the self, and all others may vainly call it bad."

As she seemed to be reaching the fourteenth year, she was asked to "take time out just to go back to the very beginning, to fill in overlooked self-learnings, to correct omissions, to note misunderstandings and partial realizations, and to view them well from the simple, rightful dignity of a fourteen-year-old, truly fourteen." That a risk was being taken in that she might not have begun menstruation until after the age of fourteen was fully appreciated, but the hope was entertained that such an error would be detected by observation and study of the emotional play on her face, which had increased progressively from the age of six. From the age of ten to fourteen the play of facial suggestions portrayed the change from a ten-year-old girl's face to that of a fourteen-year-old young adult.

The patient's initial history emphasized the importance of the avoidance of direct questions. However important a clinical and academic matter her thinking was to the senior author, it was serving a more important therapeutic purpose for the patient, which was the paramount purpose of the work.

Alternating Periods of Deep Hypnotherapy and Counseling

Following this review of the ages of ten to fourteen, she entered the office saying, "Can we just talk a while without working?" Upon assent she continued, "Well, I've moved to a nice place, I've got a job, I'm not depressed. I actually am beginning to like me a lot. I'm not especially beautiful; I couldn't stop a clock if I tried. But I've got a nice figure. My mother would die if she had heard that wolf whistle I got the other day. That's the first one I really remember. And believe it or not I'm sorry for my mother. She is sick. It must be a painful sickness for her too, and my father is sick but not as sick as my mother. That five thousand dollars was really all he could give me. And they didn't try to make me sick. They just mistakenly did wrong things with good intentions. Well, mother wanted to keep me a virgin and she succeeded. But I'm going to take some credit for that myself. And that poor psychiatrist in Europe who thought I was suicidal because of my terrible obsession about a bathtub full of bloody water and a razor in my hand. What else could he think? I was taking a bath and I suddenly realized it was about time for my period and I was shaving my legs and I wondered what it would be like to shave my pubic hair, and then that horrible phrase my mother everlastingly dinned in my ears about being a good girl, and thoughts of masturbation, and then I couldn't think any more except of bloody water and the razor. It was awful then. I feel sorry for me then. Sounds funny to say it that way, but I do, I mean it. And I mean I feel sorry for my parents. I don't love them. They are just two people who tried to do me a kindness once, tried hard but failed. And it meant so much to them!

"Another thing! I come to your office, I sit for awhile, I go away, I do nothing. You said hypnosis was learning. I haven't learned any hypnosis. All that's happened to me is I feel different, I think different, I am different. I didn't mind telling you about my bowel movements. A couple of times before, I got up enough courage to go to a doctor, but I was too scared to let him do an examination. When I took the physical to go overseas, I got hold of sleeping pills so I could stand it. They quieted me down but didn't put me to sleep.

"Do you suppose I need to see you? I know your answer is yes, and I agree. I wish I knew why the answer is yes."

"You could ask," she was told.

"Oh, I know that, but I'm not asking. I wonder why, but I certainly am not going to interfere with you, but I can't help feeling curious. Do you know what you are going to do next?"

"Oh, yes."

"Well, that's good. I knew you did. Will it be all right to spend the rest of the time talking?"

The rest of that interview was spent with a highly intelligent, widely read, well-traveled woman who was obviously starved for an opportunity for social expression.

At the next interview, as soon as she had developed a trance she was told, "Well, let's complete the high school days and college years." This was done apparently easily, but frequently sudden manifestations of extreme physical tension would be present.

At the next meeting she remarked casually, "The day we talked and that's all and I sort of reviewed things, do you have anything to say about that?"

With slow, soft-voiced, forceful emphasis she was given the reply, "Yes, I have, a great deal, more than you want to hear."

With an expression of utter fury she leaped from her chair and shouted, "You stinking bastard, you are trying to tell me I was too glib, too smooth, too casual, too intellectual, you stinking bastard."

To this reply was made, "Right, quite right. Sit down, look at the paperweight, then quietly, silently, with deadly hatred and bitterness and gall and venom, tear the hell out of 'a good girl' " (these last words said mockingly).

There occurred a fascinating, almost silent display of emotions—grimacing, writhing, twisting, clenching of fists, spasmodic breathing, clenching of teeth, and moaning—in fact, every manifestation of violent distressing emotions. Toward the end of the hour she began to relax and was finally dismissed with instructions to return to her apartment, feeling tired and sleepy, and to go to bed and "finish the task." In a self-absorbed manner she left the office, not noticing her perspiration-drenched dress.

Hyperamnesia in Reviewing Life History

At the next interview her facial expression and manner were one of bewildered respect. Instead of speaking casually her manner was alert and attentive. She addressed herself formally to the author and repeatedly said "sir." She was asked how she felt.

Her reply was, "Dr. Erickson, it is difficult to start. I have a vague, unclear memory of summarizing my feelings the other day, but, sir, I don't remember what I said. I only remember that what I said was partly right. But since then there have been changes in me. I feel as if I had been dreadfully sick, just dreadfully sick, but that now I am over it but in that weak stage when one is convalescing. Yet, I'm not physically weak, sir, it's just that I am well but haven't got all of my strength back. I began feeling this way when I awakened the afternoon of my last visit here. The bed was all torn to pieces. I had torn the pillowcases. I was drenched with perspiration. I was still in my dress and it was a mess. But before I got up and straightened up the bed and undressed and took a bath, I just lay back in bed and I literally reviewed my life history. I've never told you the real details. It's pretty horrible and painful, but all that is in the past. I almost felt like a stranger looking at all those things—the things I feel deeply that happened to me and that made me suffer so much. It was all real, it all belonged to me, but it all feels differently to me now, sir. It all belongs to the past.

"As I lay there on the bed, I started with my childhood. It is hard to believe the detail in which I remembered things—even the little things I did as a baby creeping on the floor. They were terribly vivid to me. And I went right along, year by year. Things that I thought were forever forgotten stood out in detail, vivid startling detail. That little boy I kissed in the first grade—I could actually feel his lips on mine. A child's feelings are so different, so warm, so wonderful, so innocent. Each year of my life I felt, one by one. I don't know how long I spent lying on the bed. It was pretty horrible when I could hear what my mother was saying to me when I was eight years old. I didn't know then. I thought she meant I should be a good girl and wash my hands, that it was time to eat. Things like that. But while I remembered what I thought and felt then, I knew and understood as if I were an onlooker and at the same time I felt myself right in the midst of it, that mother was saying that to me, grown-up me as well as to eight-year-old me.

"Each year it got worse. I tried to lose myself in my studies but I never did. I kept telling myself I was oblivious to everything and I believed it, but I wasn't. High school was a nightmare, and some of the boys touched my breasts when they would walk past, and everything my mother said became alive. I had just one date in college, and it was awful. Now I know he just asked, but I felt so awful unclean. I prayed and prayed and thought God had deserted me.

"Then that awful scene at home and then the running from myself, one job after another. Everywhere I ran I found myself. I knew I was going crazy. I followed myself all over Europe, to Japan and the Phillipines. I was getting worse and the psychiatrist knew it and I knew it and I wouldn't believe it.

"Then I was crying in that women's lounge, I was so desperate, and that patient of yours told me to see you. I knew it wouldn't do any good, it was hopeless. I couldn't do anything. But I wanted you to do something, so I didn't let you say "no." So I came.

Genuine Age Regression with an Adult Observer

"When I got that fear, I began remembering what happened in the office. I didn't know until then that I was in a trance in your office. I looked at that paperweight, and the next thing I knew *I was a little baby crawling on the floor at home. And I was also a grown-up person watching me.* I never thought about that until these memories came to me.

"I did the whole thing over again. I watched me grow up. I heard my mother talk to me. The big me could hear you. The little me could hear mother—seeing, feeling, being little. I went all the way through all the things that happened in the office. I watched me that day when I talked things over with you. I felt proud of me as I listened to me talk to you. Was I in a trance then? I was really so proud of all I had accomplished, and then the next time I walked in your office I had a feeling that I was going to say something important, and then I felt as if you had hit me with a horrible club. I saw everything stripped raw and bare. I knew that all you had done was just to uncover a horrible job I had to do. I knew I was the only one that could do it, and I hated you. I couldn't see how you did it, but all of a sudden I was right in the middle of the most turbulent and terribly deadly, hateful emotions. I wanted to die, but I couldn't. I got tired.

"Then I heard you send me back to my room, and I kept thinking how tired I was and how good the bed would feel. I didn't see me come into the room or flop on the bed because the next thing I watched was what I did on the bed. I watched me go crazy with fear and desperation. Then I just reviewed everything.

All I can say now, Dr. Erickson, is that the job is done. The past is past, it belongs to me, it doesn't hurt, and I don't want to tell such unhappiness. But I probably will need some mature thinking and advice on how to plan my future."

CHAPTER TEN

Creating Identity: Beyond Utilization Therapy?

Up to this point we have emphasized that hypnotherapy involves the utilization of the patient's own life experiences and that the indirect forms of suggestion are the means of evoking those experiences for therapeutic change. What happens, however, when the patient has been severely deprived in some basic life experiences? Can the therapist supply them vicariously in some way? Sensitive therapists have long recognized their role as surrogate parents who do, in fact, help their patients experience life patterns and relationships that have been missed.

In this final chapter we will present some of the senior author's approaches to supplying a patient with a personal relationship in a manner that anchors her within a more secure inner reality around which she can create a new identity for herself. This is the case of a young woman who so lacked the experience of being mothered that she gravely doubted her own ability to be one. Through a series of age regressions the senior author visited her in the guise of the February Man: A kindly granduncle type who became a secure friend and confidant. A series of such experiences enabled her to develop a new sense of confidence and identity about herself that led her eventually to a rewarding experience of motherhood with her own children.

The senior author has actually played the role of the February Man with a number of patients throughout his career. So complex are some of the details of his work in these situations, however, that he never quite completed any of his manuscripts about them. The following case is thus a synthesis of several of the senior author's original manuscripts together with commentaries on them by the junior author.

The reader is invited to explore with us some of the approaches and issues involved in the work of the February Man. There is much about this work that is beyond our own understanding. The use of indirect suggestions to integrate hypnotic and real-life memories to create a self-consistent internal reality is an art that does not entirely lend itself to rational analysis. We do try, however, fully realizing we have fallen short and are in need of the reader's creativity to fill some of the gaps and to carry the work further.

Case 16   The February Man

Initial Interview: A Lonely Childhood

At midterm of her first pregnancy the wife of a young doctor on our hospital staff approached the senior author for psychiatric help. Her problem was that although happily married and pleased with her pregnancy, she was fearful that her own unhappy childhood experiences would reflect themselves in her handling of her child. She stated that she had "studied too much psychology" since it made her aware of the possible inadvertant unfortunate handling of a child, with resulting psychological traumatization.

She explained that she had been a most unwanted child. Her mother never had any time for her. Her care rested in the hands of her mother's unhappy spinster older sister who, in return for a home, acted as nursemaid, housekeeper, and general factotum. Her preschool days had been spent almost exclusively in her nursery, and she was left to devise her own games and entertainment. Occasionally, when her mother gave a social tea, she would be trotted out briefly for exhibition and told what a sweet, pretty little girl she was and then dismissed. Otherwise, her mother, between social engagements, looked in upon her in the nursery briefly and casually. She had been sent to a special nursery school and later to various private schools for her grade school and high school education. During the summers she was sent to special camps to "further" her education. During these years her "mother took time out from her round of pressing social engagements and trips abroad" to see her daughter as often as was "humanly possible." Essentially she and her mother had remained strangers.

As for the father, he, too, was a busy man, greatly absorbed in his business enterprises and traveling much of the time. He did have a genuine affection for his daughter, however, and had frequently found time to take her, even as a small child, out to dinner, to the circus, to amusement parks, and to other memorably delightful places. He also had bought her toys and presents befitting her needs, in contrast to the "horribly expensive" dolls with which her mother showered her, but with which her aunt would not let her play because they were "beautiful" and "valuable." She had received only "the best of everything" from her mother, but her father had always given her "many little things that were really nice." At the age of eighteen she had rebelled against "finishing" school and, to her mother's intense distress and resentment, had insisted on attending a state university. Her mother's chief argu-

461

ment was the debt the daughter owed her for "practically ruining" her figure in order to give birth to her. The father, greatly dominated by his wife but much in love with her, had secretly abetted his daughter in her decision and had encouraged and aided in every possible way, but without trying to overindulge her.

Her university adjustments had been good scholastically, but she felt that she had made insufficient use of her social opportunities. Early in her senior year she had met an intern, five years older than she, with whom she fell in love. She had married him a year later. This had distressed her mother, since the intern lacked "social position," but the father had privately expressed his approval.

Because of this history she now wondered what kind of mother she would be. Her psychological reading had convinced her that her rejection by her mother and her emotional starvation as a child would in some way adversely affect the handling of her own baby. She wanted to know if, through hypnosis, her unconscious could be explored and either her anxieties relieved or she could be made aware of her deficiencies and thus make corrections. She asked the senior author to consider her problem at length and to give her another appointment when he felt he might be able to meet her needs.

She was told that before this could be done, it would be necessary for her to relate at length all her anxieties, fears, and forebodings. In so doing she was to give as comprehensive a picture of their nature, variety, and development as possible. It was explained that the primary purpose of this report was to make certain that the senior author appreciated as fully as possible her feelings and thoughts before any attempts were made to ascertain causes and remedies. From this additional material, of course, he privately hoped to learn more details of her life history that he could use to facilitate the hypnotherapeutic work.

Second Interview: A Spontaneous Catharsis

At the next interview the patient was exceedingly fearful, anxious, and tearful. She expressed disconnected fears of hurting, neglecting, and resenting her child. She feared feeling tied down by it, of being overly anxious, of giving overcompensatory attention to it, of making it a hideous burden in her life instead of a pleasure, of losing her husband's love, of never loving the child, and so on.

She elaborated upon these ideas poorly but in relationship to every possible stage of the child's eventual development.

She wept throughout the interview, and while intellectually she regarded her fears as groundless, she declared that their "strong obsessional character" was causing insomnia, anorexia, and severe depressive reactions that terrified her.

If she tried to read or to listen to the radio, the printed page or the program would be obscured by vivid, compelling memories of her own childhood unhappiness. She recognized that all her fears were abnormally exaggerated, but she felt helpless to do anything about them.

Except for innumerable anxieties little actual history was obtained. She asked tearfully if the writer thought he could help her, since she felt she was breaking down more rapidly than ever. She was assured that before her next appointment a therapeutic plan would be worked out for her.

Third Interview: The Interpolated Trance; Age Regression and Amnesia.

At the next interview she was assured that an elaborate program had been worked out and that the results would undoubtedly be most satisfying to her. What the plan was could not be disclosed to her yet, but through hypnosis her unconscious would acquire adequate understanding. All that she needed to know consciously was that hypnosis would be employed and that the task could be begun immediately if she wished. She acquiesced eagerly. In this session approximately five hours were spent training her adequately as a hypnotic subject. Particular emphasis was placed upon age regression. Her intelligence and excellence as a subject made possible the elaborate training considered necessary for the planned procedure.

During the training slowly and cautiously she was regressed in time repeatedly to some safe past situation into which, in some fashion, the writer could enter directly or indirectly, without distorting the regression situation. Thus the first regression was to the first interview with her. In having her relive that interview, it became easily possible to introduce a new element not actually belonging to the situation but that could easily fit into it. In accord with her revivification of that interview the writer merely remarked, "Do you mind if I interrupt and introduce a thought that just came to my mind? It just occured to me that you could easily be a good hypnotic subject, and I wonder if you would mind closing your eyes and sleeping hypnotically for a few moments, and then arousing and continuing from where I interrupted?" Thus an interpolated trance was introduced into that reliving of the first interview, in which no hypnosis had occurred.

> R: The first trance has the effect of dissociating the patient away from the surrounding reality into her internal environment. When you then interpolate a second trance into the first, it effects an even deeper regression into herself. The basic purpose of the interpolated trance is to get the patient further removed from outer consensual reality. It's particularly useful for age regression.
>
> E: Yes, I don't have to help her withdraw from the outer

environment with the interpolated trance. When she gets back to reality, it will be much more difficult for her to recover that interpolated trance for which she has an amnesia even in the trance state.

R: So an interpolated trance is another way of effecting a deeper hypnotic amnesia.

E: In future trances she's going to have an amnesia for the interpolated trance, but she would have to go through it to get a complete memory of the first trance in which it took place. I gave her many positive supportive suggestions during the interpolated trance. This served to reinforce all the positive values of that initial interview.

R: It's like a feedback loop, where what comes later reinforces the positive values of what occurred earlier.

E: Yes, and it's reinforcing what happens now by virtue of the "past" that I've transplanted into the initial interview. I work in all directions. In everyday life when strangers meet they may speak casually in a general way until they discover something common in their past: They might have vacationed in the same place or come from the same state or town or gone to the same school. Sometimes they discover to their delight that they have a few acquaintances in common and can now share more intimate details of their lives. They have now created a strong rapport in the present based entirely on experiences from the past.

R: They have created a shared "phenomenal world in common" (Rossi, 1972a). They have built associative bridges that now bind them together in friendship. This is a common everyday process of social relating that you are now utilizing to enhance your rapport with this patient. The interpolated trance is a way of rapidly creating a positive "history" that enhances current relations.

Rapport Protection: Indirect Suggestion and Contingent Possibilities

She was then regressed to an intern's party at which there was a number of the senior author's former medical students. In the process of regression the suggestion was implanted that she might meet him at that party or that someone would mention his name, and undoubtedly this would happen when someone approached her and attracted her attention by gently squeezing her wrist. Then, when this unexpected thing happened, she could make a full response to the wrist pressure and react in accord with whatever situational need developed. Primarily, this was to introduce a physical cue to permit ready induction of a trance state at any time, even during the reliving of past events that had occurred long before meeting the senior author. Various such regressions were induced, aided by special information that had been privately supplied by the husband. These were utilized to condition her for trance induction in any set of psychological circumstances.

E: I was building rapport protection with this procedure. I once regressed a subject at Clark University to ten years of age. While regressed, he explained that he was on an errand to buy a loaf of bread for his mother. We could all see the abject terror on his face because he did not know anyone in that room (where as an adult he was being hypnotized). I spent a wretched four and a half hours trying to get back into rapport with him because he was afraid of me and afraid of everyone else. That taught me that thereafter I'd have a secondary way of establishing rapport with the subject such as touching a wrist. It's an attention-attracting but otherwise meaningless cue. The subject cannot easily incorporate it into the age-regressed pattern of behavior.

R: You did not directly tell her that pressure on her wrist was a cue to enter trance or to pay close attention to what you were suggesting.

E: If I had said it that directly, she could reject it. Therefore I put it in an indirect framework of *contingent possibilities:* She *might* meet me. Someone would approach her; she *could* make a full response to the wrist pressure and react in accord with *whatever situational need developed.* These (the italicized words) are all undefined. There is no demand or threat in all this, and therefore no need for resistance or rejection.

R: We usually don't reject undefined possibilities in everyday life. Rather, possibilities and contingencies usually evoke our sense of wonder, speculation, and expectation. Possibilities actually initiate pressures of *unconscious search* within us that may trip off useful unconscious processes. "Whatever situational need" also covers all possibilities, including whatever suggestions you give her. You give her the most general form of an indirect suggestion here.

E: A most general form that can be filled in by the patient's specific understannding.

Interpolating New Life Experiences: The February Man

She was trained to develop in good fashion extensive regressions that were made to serve merely as a general background and situation for new, interpolated behavioral responses. She was regressed to past situations, and that frame of reference was employed merely as a background into which new hypnotic behavior could be interpolated. When sufficient training had been completed to ensure good responses, she was regressed to childhood at the age of four. The month of February was selected because it was her birthday. She was oriented to the living room of her childhood in the act of merely walking through it. She had often walked through her living room. Since the state of regression was limited to that act, it would constitute only a frame of reference. The walking through could be arrested and new behavior introduced into that setting without altering or falsifying the situation. Thus the new behavior intruded into that situation could be related temporally to the events of that age-regression period.

As she roused somnambulistically in this regressed state, she was greeted by the senior author: "Hello, little girl. Are you your Daddy's girl? I'm a friend of your Daddy's, and I'm waiting for him to come in to talk to me. He told me yesterday that he brought you a present one day and that you liked it very much. I like your Daddy, too. He told me it would soon be your birthday, and I'll bet he brings you an awful nice present." This was followed by silence, and the senior author apparently absentmindedly snapped open and closed his hunting case watch, with no further effort to engage her in conversation or to attract her attention. She first eyed him, then became interested in the watch, whereupon he held it to his ear and stated that it went "tick, tick" very nicely.

E: "Hello, little girl" assigns her a hypnotic role.

R: In that first second when she opens her eyes in somnambulistic trance you immediately reinforce the age regression so there could be no doubt about it. Is she going to see you as Dr. Erickson or as someone she does not know in her past? Your opening remark orients her into the past.

E: And there have been people in her past who have said just such a thing.

R: You then attract her attention appropriately by playing with your watch. This is just about right for a four-year-old; you do not introdue yourself in a direct or demanding way. You behave very much as a visitor to her house might when she was a child.

Wrist Cue as a Nonverbal Signal for Metasuggestions Orienting the Somnambulistic State

After a few moments the suggestion was offered that she might like to snap the case open or to listen to the watch. She nodded her head shyly and extended her hand. Taking hold of her wrist as if to help her, the senior author handed her the watch. She looked at it and played with it. The suggestion was offered that if she listend to it for a little while, it would make her very sleepy. This was followed by the comment that soon the senior author would have to go home, but that some time he would come back, and, if she wished, he would bring his watch so she could open and close it and listen to it.

She nodded her head, and her hand holding the watch was guided to her ear. Her wrist was slowly squeezed, and trance suggestions were given accompanied by suggestions that maybe next summer the senior author would come again, and maybe she would recognize him.

E: I had to get out of her house. I ended that interpolated life experience with the wrist cue in an appropriate way (guiding her hand with the watch to her ear) and suggesting she would get sleepy as she listened to it.

R: Having her go to sleep is fairly appropriate behavior for a four-year-old listening to a watch, and her sleep allowed you to leave. It also enabled you to give her the posthypnotic suggestion about seeing her again next summer *maybe*, and *maybe* she would recognize you. These possibilities are appropriate for her age because a four- to five-year old child might not recognize a friend after a year. But why did you give her the rapport cue by squeezing her wrist as you added these suggestions?

E: Although she was in a somnambulistic trance, further hypnosis would be needed to effect an alteration of that state to induce other phenomena.

R: I see. Even during a somnambulistic state special rapport is needed to effect important suggestions. The wrist cue is an orienting signal for the metasuggestions you will use to guide the somnambulistic state; it tells her important suggestions are coming. I have had the difficulty of working with some subjects who were so obstinate during the somnambulistic state that I could hardly get a word in edgewise. Like self-centered children, such subjects would soon take over the situation and simply live out an inner experience without my being able to relate to them. This may be valuable for cathartic purposes, but it does not permit the therapist to interpolate new experience as you are doing here.

E: You need another hypnotic frame of reference to orient her to important suggestions without verbally defining it as such and without altering my role as a stranger, Daddy's friend.

467

R: Classical age regression has typically been a simple reliving of a past life experience. A catharsis or process of desensitization is relied upon as the therapeutic means of resolving pent-up emotions of life traumas.

E: That does not add anything. Here I'm adding to the past.

R: That's the object of the entire procedure. You regress her to establish a frame of reference into which you can interpolate therapeutic life experiences. You are adding new experiences to her memory bank; you're adding new elements of human relating that she missed in reality.

E: You can add belief to something that does not exist if you repeat it often enough. That's why I had to give her many experiences with me as the February Man. I'm adding reality to a nonexistent thing.

R: It becomes "real" in terms of internal reality. With this approach you can alter a patient's belief system; you cannot really change her past, but you can change her beliefs about her past.

E: You can change beliefs and values. It's not really that we can believe lies; rather, we discover more things. Patients believe their limited reality until they discover more reality.

R: I wonder if we can equate "discover more reality" with creating new consciousness? There is still a basic question here, however. Are you (1) really adding something new to the personality, or are you (2) simply helping her discover and experience a natural, inherent pattern of human relating (the archetypal child-parent relationship) that she very much needed and wanted? Utilization theory would emphasize the second alternative; you are structuring circumstances that allow her to evoke and utilize inherent (species-specific) behavior patterns that must be expressed for normal development. But you are certainly adding a new content within the framework of this inherent pattern.

Continuing Experiences with the February Man: Ratifying the Historical Reality of Age-Regressed Experience

She was then permitted to experience about fifteen minutes of profound hypnotic sleep. This sleep was a passage of time during which my departure and eventual return (as had already been suggested) could take place. Her wrist was then again gently squeezed, and suggestions were offered that she better be in the yard because the flowers were blooming for the first time since her birthday last winter, and perhaps her Daddy's friend might come again. At all events she could really open her eyes very, very wide to see the flowers. She opened her eyes and was apparently enjoying her visual hallucinations when the writer, from behind, addressed her, "Hello, little girl. Do you remember me?" She turned, eyed him carefully, smiled, and said, "You're Daddy's friend." The reply was made, "And I remember your name. It is R." In this way the senior author became established as an actual figure in her past life without impinging upon realities or distorting them, but merely by adding to them by a simple process of temporal association. Thereupon a casual conversation was initiated at a childish level about the red and pink and yellow flowers (she said they were tulips), whereupon she reminded the writer about his watch, and essentially the same course of events ensued as had previously. Many more comparable instances were developed to ensure the possibility of the writer's intrusion into her past without invalidating the regression state. She was given extensive experience with the February Man, a figure that became more and more established in her life history.

> E: I had learned from the initial interviews that her childhood home did have extensive flower gardens with red, pink, and yellow flowers. I would further ratify the historical aspects of the experience by pretending to have an unclear memory of my previous visits with her. How clear does anyone remember an experience of a year ago? Two years ago? Four years ago? I also introduced changing views. As she gets older, she gets a different perspective on things. I'd say, "That first doll you had was really very nice." "Remember your enthusiasm for that first circus?" I might make such remarks to the ten- or twelve-year-old girl about the six-year-old girl.

> R: You built associative bridges between the trance experiences at different age levels that established the historical reality of your visits with her.

Indirect Posthypnotic Suggestion

Finally she was placed in a profound trance and given extensive posthypnotic suggestions to ensure a comprehensive amnesia for all trance events and to ensure continued cooperation. I'd gently squeeze her wrist and say "You have now completed that task. I want you to go into a profound trance at this time. I want you to enjoy resting. I want you to feel fresh after you've awakened, comfortably enjoying the feeling of being wide awake, prepared for a new day's activities."

> E: That latter suggestion, "prepared for a new day's ac-

tivities," implies that she will be ready for more work; we are just beginning.

R: That's how you also imply a posthypnotic amnesia without directly telling her she would not remember. You could then put her back into trance for another experience with the February Man.

Time for Hypnotic Work

In subsequent sessions, usually of several hours' duration, essentially the same procedure was followed.

E: I had to have several hours in order to let her have an experience with the February Man at one age level, rest, and then another experience at another age level. Time is expandable and compressible, but a certain amount of real clock time is still needed for careful work. Initially you really don't know what the patient's capacities are. Time is needed to explore them.

Integrating Hypnotic and Real-Life Memories: Creating a Self-Consistent Internal Reality

A number of hypnotherapeutic sessions now took place following this same pattern. She was regressed to many different periods of her life, usually in a chronologically progressive fashion, taking care not to let the created situation impinge contradictorily upon the actual realities of the past. For example, on one occasion, regressed to a nine-year-old level, she manifested intense astonishment upon opening her eyes and seeing the senior author. Cautious inquiry disclosed that she was visiting a distant relative for the first time and had just arrived the previous night. A few questions elicited enough information to orient the senior author so that he could claim a business friendship with her relative. This laid a foundation very necessary for the subsequent ubiquity of him in her life experience. Aiding in the acceptance of his ubiquity was the fact that both of her parents traveled extensively and often unexpectedly, and that they had innumerable acquaintances and friends. Hence it was easily assumed that the same was true of the senior author as "Daddy's friend." Also of importance was the February Man's knowledge of various cities she had visited and the fact that he, as well as she, had studied psychology, all of which provided a wide background permitting her to accept him unquestioningly. As the procedure continued, the technicalities of securing responsive behavior became minimal, and a dozen regressed states could be developed in an hour's time. These were all utilized to secure a report by her of things and attitudes current to the regression period, as well as an account of expected or anticipated

470

events. Anticipated events served admirably in enabling the senior author to direct regression states to "safe" periods. However, care had to be exercised, since anticipations were not always fulfilled. Frequently, however, the "visit" was devoted to an account of what had happened since the last "visit" that is, the preceding regressed state. She learned to look upon the senior author as a recurrent visitor and as a trusted confidant to whom she could tell all her secrets, woes, and joys and with whom she could share her hopes, fears, doubts, wishes, and plans.

From time to time it became necessary to induce comprehensive amnesias, obliterating various of the senior author's "visits," and to regress her to an earlier age and to go over an already partially covered period of her life more adequately. Thus, some sudden change in her life, not anticipated at an earlier age regression, might have become established before the period of the next age regression, thereby creating a situation at variance with established understandings. On such occasions the last age regression would be abolished by amnesia suggestions, and a new regression to an earlier time would be induced to permit the securing of pertinent data.

> R: You made a very careful and extensive effort to integrate hypnotic and real memories so they were molded into a self-consistent inner reality. This would ensure the permanence of the new attitudes you were facilitating in her. If there were contradictions and a lack of consistency between the hypnotic and real memories, self-corrective processes within the unconscious would have tended to gradually eliminate the hypnotic suggestions as foreign intrusions. This may be why so much hypnotic work in the past has had only temporary or partial effect. Direct suggestions made even while a patient is in a deep somnambulistic state are not programmed within the mind forever in a rigid way. The human mind is a dynamic process that is continually correcting, modifying, and reformulating itself. Inconsistencies are either worked out in a satisfactory manner or are expressed as "problems" (complexes, neuroses, psychosomatic symptoms, etc.). There is thus nothing magical or mysterious about the effectiveness of your approach: It is based on very careful, thorough work integrating real memories with hypnotic experience.

Facilitating Therapeutic Attitudes: A Therapy of Life Perspectives: Dreams and Hypnosis

The consistent and continual rejection she experienced from her mother presented many opportunities to reorganize her emotions and understanding. By this procedure the senior author's role became one of friendship, sympathy, interest, and objectivity, thereby giving him the opportunity to raise questions concerning how she might later evaluate a given experience. Thus, in expressing her grief over breaking a cheap little china doll her father had given her and which she treasured, she could declare that, when she grew up and became a mother and had a little girl who broke her doll, she would know that it wasn't something "awful bad" but that she would know just how her little girl would feel. Similarly, a fall on the dance floor in her teens was regarded by her as an utterly and completely devastating experience. Yet she manifested a readiness to understand the senior author's comment that she should rightly appreciate it as such in the present but that at the same time she could also understand how, in the future, it could really be regarded as a minor and completely unimportant event, perhaps even amusing. Her first adolescent infatuation, her jilting by the boy, and her tremendous need to understand herself in relation to that event were dealt with. Her resolution to leave the finishing school, to enter the university, her choice of studies, her scholastic struggles, and her limited social life were all covered. The meeting with the man who became her husband, her doubts and uncertainties about him, the eventual engagement, and the mother's attitude toward him, toward the marriage, and toward the subsequent pregnancy were all detailed to the senior author in "current" accounts of what was happening to her. Numerous other instances of rejection, neglect, and disappointment by her mother and father were relived and discussed with the February Man. Real happy memories were also relived and integrated with the hypnotic memories to ensure a comprehensive integration of them.

R: Whenever she had a traumatic life situation, she could now discuss them with her father's friend, the February Man. In effect you became a therapist at such times. This is a curious state of affairs, you as her current therapist became a therapist in her past, helping her deal with her difficult life situations as they occurred. I've noticed something similar in dreams. Some patients seem to relive their past in dreams but correct the traumatic aspects of their past with their current adult perspectives (Rossi, 1972a; 1973c). This again points out the self-corrective aspect of the psyche; it is in a continual process of reformulating or resynthesizing itself to achieve a more integrated pattern of functioning. You utilize and facilitate this resynthesizing aspect of psychic functioning with your role as the February Man. You are doing hypnotically what frequently happens naturally during dreams.

E: Yes. [The senior author now recalls such a dream of his

own, when the adult Dr. Erickson observed himself as a child (Erickson, 1965a).] Dreams give us the opportunity to relive past events and appraise them critically from an adult perspective.

R: Dreams are autotherapeutic processes that help the mind correct and integrate itself. I also believe we are synthesizing new phenomenological realities in our dreams that become the basis of new patterns of identity and behavior (Rossi, 1971; 1972 a, b; 1973 a, b, c.).

A Reversal of Realities: Deepening the Therapeutic Frame of Reference

Toward the end of this extensive reorganization of her attitudes about her past, a new memory was recalled: Her secret resolve years ago to have hypnotic anesthesia should she ever marry and become pregnant. As she now again considered this possibility, she received a letter of foreboding from her mother requesting that the term "grandmother" never be used—in essence, rejecting the unborn baby. This letter intensified the patient's anxieties and fears anew.

To deal with these renewed anxieties a variation in our hypnotic procedure was developed. In this variation a blanket amnesia was first induced for all her previous hypnotic work, and she was asked to again relate all her fears and anxieties. In this state, as expected, her account was comparable to her original expression of her problems before hypnotherapy.

A new trance state was then induced in which the blanket amnesia was removed. She was then regressed to a week *before* the arrival of her mother's letter. In this state of hypnosis she was asked to recall fully all the many visits, talks, and discussions over the years she had had with the senior author as Daddy's friend. As she recalled his many visits and their conversations on so many subjects, the suggestion was offered that she ought to consider the present minor worries against that total background. As she began this correlation of her unhappy ideas in the past as she conceived it at the moment, she began to develop amazing insights, understandings, and emotional comfort.

Having reestablished the new attitudes developed in the hypnotic work, the senior author next led her into an age-regression state covering the period just *after* the receipt of the mother's letter. After expressing some sensible views about her mother's problem, she was asked to give the reactions she could develop if she did not include in her thinking "all she knew about her past." She was told that she ought to speculate aloud on how she could really enlarge her reactions into exaggerated fears and anxieties by just "not being comprehensive in her thinking." She was urged to offer "speculative statements" expressing such anxieties. She then proceeded to verbalize them as she thought would be possible if she "did not think intelligently." This speculative account was identical with that which she had originally given just before therapy began and the previous account with the blanket amnesia for all the hypnotherapeutic work. But it was given as a "speculative" account which was decidedly different from the new reality of her emotional life that now included the new frames of reference she had developed with the February Man.

Subsequent regression states were similarly utilized. Her "speculations" about how she could exaggerate her fears always gave accounts similar to the one she gave originally before hypnotherapy. These speculations were always in sharp contrast to her "real attitudes" developed with the help of Daddy's friend, the February Man. She now drew extensively upon her "actual" past history, with all its interpolated experiences with Daddy's friend. During this period a tremendous amount of her past history came out in clear relevance to her entire current problem. As this type of activity continued, she developed insights that were remarkably corrective.

> R: This is an ingenious twist: what was originally a painful reality now becomes the "speculative account," while the new attitudes introduced by hypnosis become the abiding reality. That is, she is now accepting her expanded frame of understanding developed with the February Man as her "real" views, while her previous behavior is now seen merely as a speculative account of how badly things could be if she "did not think intelligently." This procedure may be helping her integrate the February Man frame of reference at an even deeper level. This is particularly the case because she is already in a deep hypnotic state as she experiences this reversal of realities.

Termination: A Final Conscious Integration of All Trance Work

Finally, as she progressed in this regard, the topic of hypnotic anesthesia for the delivery of her child was mentioned increasingly by her while she was in trance. She was reassuringly told that as the months of pregnancy passed, it was absolutely certain that all of her anxieties would be comprehensively and comfortably understood and thus become a resolved experience of the past. In their place would be a realization that in some way she would meet someone who would teach her to understand herself happily. Since she was in an age-regressed state, this was naturally a reference by implication to the senior author as someone she would meet in the future. In so doing she would be

474

trained to become an excellent hypnotic subject and thereby her college resolve for a hypnotic delivery would be fulfilled.

The termination of therapy was accomplished rather simply. She was regressed to the time of preparation for her first visit to the senior author's office. She was assured by him—still in the role of Daddy's friend—that her trip would be fully successful in many more ways than she really expected. The scene was then shifted to the office, and she was much astonished to see the February Man. The senior author was also astonished! She was puzzled at his presence, explained that she had come to see Dr. Erickson. She was assured that she would see Dr. Erickson and that he would meet her wishes fully, but that, for a few minutes, she should sleep most profoundly. During this trance approximately one half-hour was spent instructing her so that after she awakened she would recall from the beginning, in chronological order, every trance experience she had had, together with all insights and understandings that she had developed up to the date shown by the day's newspaper on the desk. At the close of the interview she was told to spend a few delightful days reviewing her memories, making certain that she understood, remembered, and accepted all her past in an adjusted fashion. As for the hypnotic anesthesia, she would be certain of it, but the minor details would be arranged in the next interview.

R: This was a final summation for a final conscious integration of all her therapy. She now finally learns how you played the role of the February Man, how you reversed her realities, and so on. Yet this does not undo the effectiveness of the new attitudes and frames of reference you helped her develop. Why doesn't it? After all your incredibly complex efforts to develop a new frame of reference, integrate it, and deepen it, why do you end the therapy with this complete denouement?

E: Because I may have made some errors. She may have made some errors. Let's make sure we get the whole set of errors corrected.

R: You are not afraid of undoing your therapeutic work because you actually have helped her develop new frames of reference and understandings that have therapeutically altered her emotional life. This case contrasts sharply with those cases in which you like to maintain an amnesia for all hypnotherapeutic work. What is the difference?

E: Some personalities need amnesia, some do not. It's a matter of clinical experience to distinguish them.

R: Those patients whom you judge to have destructive conscious attitudes toward the therapy might do better with an amnesia.

E: This patient was actually left with some amnesia for the negative emotions she experienced in relation to her mother. My final posthypnotic suggestion to her was to "spend a few delightful days reviewing her memories, making certain that she understood, remembered, and accepted all her past in an *adjusted* fashion." This precluded any regression into the catastrophically negative affects and anxieties she was experiencing before therapy.

Training for Obstetrical Analgesia: A Two-Year Followup

At the next session some days later she stated that she had been interested primarily in thinking about her hypnotic delivery. After much discussion with her husband, during which he was primarily the listener, she had decided on an analgesia if it were possible. She explained that she wished to experience childbirth in the same fashion as she had, as a child, sensed the swallowing of a whole cherry or a lump of ice, feeling it pass comfortably and interestingly down the esophagus. In a similar manner she would like to feel labor contractions, to sense the passage of the baby down the birth canal, and to experience a sense of distension of the birth canal. All this she wished to experience without any sense of pain. When questioned about the possibility of an episiotomy, she explained that she wanted the sensation of the cutting without pain and that she wanted to feel in addition the suturing that would be done. When asked if she wished at any time to experience any feeling of pain merely as a measure of sampling it, she explained: "Pain shouldn't have any part in having a baby. It's a wonderful thing, but everybody is taught to believe in pain. I want to have my baby the way I should. I don't want my attention distracted even a single minute by thoughts of pain." Accordingly, as a measure of meeting her wishes, she was taught to develop complete hypnotic anesthesia. (Usually the procedure is to proceed from numbness to analgesia to anesthesia.) Since in this instance an analgesia was the primary goal, anesthesia was induced extensively and then systematically transformed into an analgesia. (That a complete transformation of anesthesia to analgesia could be effected is doubtful, but the patient's wishes could be met in this manner, and whatever anesthesia remained would only supplement the effectiveness of the analgesia.)

When she had been trained sufficiently to meet various clinical tests for analgesia, extensive training was given to her to effect the development of a profound somnambulistic posthypnotic trance with "that degree and type of analgesia you have just learned," so that she could enter into labor without any further contact with the senior author.

Additional instructions were that she would awaken at the completion of labor with a full and immediate memory of the entire experience. Then, when she returned to her room, she would fall into a restful, comfortable sleep of about two hours' duration, and thereafter she would have a most pleasant hospital stay, planning happily for the future.

About seven weeks after the delivery she and her husband and baby daughter visited the senior author. They reported that, as she entered the hospital, she had developed a somnambulistic trance. During the labor and delivery her husband was present. She had talked freely with her husband and the obstetrician and had described to them her labor contractions with interest. She had recognized the performance of the episiotomy, the emergence of the head from the birth canal, the complete delivery of the baby, and the suturing of her episiotomy—all without pain. The expulsion of the placenta caused her to ask if there was a twin because she felt "another one moving down." She was able to laugh at her error when informed it was the placenta. She counted the stitches in the repair of her episiotomy and inquired if the doctor had "cheated" by giving her a local anesthetic because, while she could feel the needle, it was in a numb, painless way that she associated with the numb feeling of her cheek after a local dental anesthetic. She was relieved when informed that there had been no local anesthetic.

She was shown the baby, looked over it carefully, and asked permission to awaken. She had been instructed to be in full rapport with her husband and the obstetrician and to do things as needed to meet the situation. Hence, inexperienced in the situation, she carefully met the need of abiding by the situation by making sure it was in order to awaken. She again looked the baby over. Then, upon telling her husband that she had full memory of the entire experience and that everything had occurred exactly as she desired, she suddenly declared that she was sleepy. Before she left the delivery room, she was sound asleep, and slept for one and a half hours. Her stay in the hospital was most happy.

Two years later she announced to the senior author she was having another baby, and asked that she be given a "refresher course, just to make certain." One session of about three hours in the deep trance sufficed to meet her needs. Much of this time was used to secure an adequate account of her adjustments. They were found to be excellent in all regards.

References

Bakan, P. Hypnotizability, laterality of eye-movements and functional brain asymmetry. *Perceptual and Motor Skills,* 1969, *28,* 927–932.

Bandler, R., and Grinder, J. *Patterns of the hypnotic techniques of Milton H. Erickson, M.D. Vol. 1.* Cupertino Calif.: Meta Publications, 1975.

Barber, T. *Hypnosis: A scientific approach.* New York: Van Nostrand Reinhold, 1969.

Barber, T. Responding to "hypnotic" suggestions: An introspective report. *The American Journal of Clinical Hypnosis,* 1975, *18,* 6–22.

Barber, T., Dalal, A., and Calverley, D. The subjective reports of hypnotic subjects. *American Journal of Clinical Hypnosis,* 1968, *11,* 74–88.

Barber, T., and De Moor, W. A theory of hypnotic induction procedures. *The American Journal of Clinical Hypnosis,* 1972, *15,* 112–135.

Barber, T., Spanos, N., and Chaves, J. *Hypnosis, imagination and human potentialities.* New York: Pergamon, 1974.

Barron, F. *Creative person and creative process.* New York: Holt, Rinehart and Winston, 1969.

Bartlett, F. *Thinking: An experimental and social study.* New York: Basic Books, 1958.

Bateson, G. *Steps to an ecology of mind.* New York: Ballantine, 1972.

Bernheim, H. *Suggestive therapeutics: A treatise on the nature and uses of hypnotism.* New York: Putnam, 1895.

Birdwhistell, R. *Introduction to kinesics.* Louisville, Ky.: University of Louisville Press, 1952.

Birdwhistell, R. *Kinesics and context.* Philadelphia: University of Pennsylvania Press, 1971.

Bogen, J. The other side of the brain: An appositional mind. *Bulletin of the Los Angeles Neurological Societies,* 1969, *34,* 135–162.

Cheek, D., and Le Cron, L. *Clinical hypnotherapy*. New York: Grune and Straton, 1968.

Cooper, L., and Erickson M. *Time distortion in hypnosis*. Baltimore: Williams & Wilkins, 1959.

Diamond, S., and Beaumont, J. *Hemisphere function in the human brain*. New York: Halsted Press, John Wiley and Son, 1974.

Donaldson, M. M. Positive and negative information in matching problems. *British Journal of Psychology*, 1959, *50*, 235–262.

Erickson, M. Possible detrimental effects of experimental hypnosis. *Journal of Abnormal and Social Psychology*, 1932, *27, 321–327*.

Erickson, M. Automatic drawing in the treatment of an obsessional depression. *Psychoanalytic Quarterly*, 1938, *7*, 443-4-6.

Erickson, M. The induction of color blindness by a technique of hypnotic suggestion. *Journal of General Psychology*, 1939, *20*, 61–89.

Erickson, M. Hypnotic psychotherapy. *The Medical Clinics of North America*, 1948, 571–583.

Erickson, M. Deep hypnosis and its induction. In L. M. Le Cron (Ed.), *Experimental hypnosis*. New York: Macmillan, 1952, pp. 70–114.

Erickson, M. Pseudo-orientation in time as a hypnotherapeutic procedure. *Journal of Clinical and Experimental Hypnosis*, 1954, *2*, 261–283.

Erickson, M. Self-exploration in the hypnotic state. *Journal of Clinical and Experimental Hypnosis*, 1955, *3*, 49–57.

Erickson, M. Naturalistic techniques of hypnosis. *American Journal of Clinical Hypnosis*, 1958, *1*, 3–8.

Erickson, M. Further techniques of hypnosis-utilization techniques. *American Journal of Clinical Hypnosis*, 1959, *2*, 3–21.

Erickson, M. Historical note on the hand levitation and other ideomotor techniques. *American Journal of Clinical Hypnosis*, 1961, *3*, 196–199.

Erickson, M. Pantomime techniques in hypnosis and the implications. *American Journal of Clinical Hypnosis*, 1964, *7*, 65–70. (a)

Erickson, M. Initial experiments investigating the nature of hypnosis. *American Journal of Clinical Hypnosis*, 1964, *7*, 152–162. (b)

Erickson, M. A hypnotic technique for resistant patients. *American Journal of Clinical Hypnosis*, 1964, *1*, 8–32. (c)

Erickson, M. A special inquiry with Aldous Huxley into the nature and character of various states of consciousness. *American Journal of Clinical Hypnosis*, 1965, *8*, 14–33. (a)

Erickson, M. The use of symptoms as an integral part of therapy. *American Journal of Clinical Hypnosis*, 1965, *8*, 57–65. (b)

Erickson, M. Experiential knowledge of hypnotic phenomena employed for hypnotherapy. *American Journal of Clinical Hypnosis*, 1966, *8*, 299–309. (a)

Erickson, M. The interspersal hypnotic technique for symptom correction and pain control. *American Journal of Clinical Hypnosis*, 1966, *8*, 198–209. (b)

479

Erickson, M. Further experimental investigation of hypnosis: Hypnotic and nonhypnotic realities. *American Journal of Clinical Hypnosis*, 1967, *10*, 87–135.

Erickson, M. A field investigation by hypnosis of sound loci importance in human behavior. *American Journal of Clinical Hypnosis*, 1973, *16*, 92–109.

Erickson, M. and Erickson, E. Concerning the character of posthypnotic behavior. *Journal of General Psychology*, 1941, *2*, 94–133.

Erickson, M., Haley, J., and Weakland, J. A transcript of a trance induction with commentary. *American Journal of Clinical Hypnosis*, 1959, *2*, 49–84.

Erickson, M., and Rossi, E. Varieties of hypnotic amnesia. *American Journal of Clinical Hypnosis*, 1974, *16*, 225–239.

Erickson, M., and Rossi, E. Varieties of double bind. *American Journal of Clinical Hypnosis*, 1975, *17*, 143–157.

Erickson, M., and Rossi, E. Two-level communication and the microdynamics of trance. *American Journal of Clinical Hypnosis*, 1976, *18*, 153–171.

Erickson, M., and Rossi, E. Autohypnotic experiences of Milton H. Erickson. *American Journal of Clinical Hypnosis*, 1977, *20*, 36–54.

Erickson, M., Rossi, E., and Rossi, S. *Hypnotic Realities*. New York: Irvington Publishers, 1976.

Evans-Wentz, W. *The Tibetan book of the dead*. New York: Oxford University Press, 1960.

Freud, S. Jokes and their relation to the unconscious. In *Standard Edition of the Complete Psychological Works of Sigmund Freud Vol. 8*. Strachey (Ed.) London: Hogarth Press, 1905.

Freud, S. The antithetical meaning of primal words. In *Standard Edition of the Complete Psychological Works of Sigmund Freud Vol. II*. Strachey (Ed.) London: Hogarth Press, 1910.

Galin, D. Implications for psychiatry of left and right cerebral specialization. *Archives of General Psychiatry*, 1974, *31*, 527–583.

Gaito, J. (Ed.) *Macromolecules and behavior* (2nd Ed.) New York: Appleton-Century Crofts, 1972.

Gazzaniga, M. The split brain in man. *Scientific American*, 1967, *217*, 24–29.

Ghiselin, B. (Ed.) *The creative process: A sympsoium*. Berkeley: Menton, 1952.

Gill, M., and Brenman, M. *Hypnosis and related states*. New York: International Universities Press, 1959.

Haley, J. *Strategies of psychotherapy*. New York: Grune and Stratton, 1963.

Haley, J. *Advanced techniques of hypnosis and therapy: Selected papers of Milton H. Erickson, M.D.* New York: Grune and Stratton, 1967.

Haley, J. *Uncommon therapy*. New York: Norton, 1973.

Harding, E. *The parental image: Its injury and reconstruction*. New York: Putnam, 1965.

Hartland, J. *Medical and dental hypnosis*. London: Bailliere, Tindal and Cassell, 1966.

Hilgard, E. *Hypnotic susceptibility*. New York: Harcourt, 1965.

Hilgard, E., and Hilgard, J. *Hypnosis in the relief of pain*. Los Altos, California: Kaufmann, 1975.

Hilgard, J. *Personality and hypnosis*. Chicago: University of Chicago Press, 1970.

Hoppe, K. Split brains and psychoanalysis. *Psychoanalytic Quarterly*, 1977, 46, 220–244.

Huston, P., Shakow, D., and Erickson, M. A study of hypnotically induced complexes by means of the Luria technique, *J. General Psychology*, 1934, *11*, 65–97.

Jaynes, J. *The origin of consciousness in the breakdown of the bicameral mind*. New York: Houghton Mifflin Co., 1976.

Jung, C. G. *Symbols of transformation*. New York: Pantheon Books, 1956.

Jung, C. The transcendent function. In *The structure and function of the psyche, Vol. 8* of *The collected works of C. G. Jung*. Bollingen Series XX, 1960.

Lassner, J. (ed.) *Hypnosis in anesthesiology*. New York: Springer-Verlag, 1964.

Kinsbourne, M., and Smith, (Eds.) *Hemispheric disconnection and cerebral function*. Springfield, Ill.: C. C. Thomas, 1974.

Kroger, W. *Clinical and experimental hypnosis*. Philadelphia: Lippincott, 1963.

Le Cron, L. A hypnotic technique for uncovering unconscious material. *Journal of Clinical and Experimental Hypnosis*, 1954, *2*, 76–79.

Luria, A. *The working brain*. New York: Basic Books, 1973.

McGlashan, T., Evans, F., and Orne, M. The nature of hypnotic analgesia and the placebo response to experimental pain. *Psychosomatic Medicine, 31*, 227–246.

Meares, A. A working hypothesis as to the nature of hypnosis. *American Medical Association Archives of Neurology and Psychiatry*, 1957, *77*, 549–555.

Melzack, R., and Perry, C. Self-regulation of pain: Use of alpha feedback and hypnotic training for control of chronic pain. *Experimental Neurology*, 46, 452–469.

Nichols, D. Language, projection, and computer therapy. *Science*, 1978, *200*, 998–999.

Orne, M. On the social psychology of the psychological experiment: With particular reference to demand characteristics and their implications. *American Psychologist*, 1962, *17*, 776–783.

Ornestein, R. *The psychology of consciousness*. New York: Viking, 1972.

Ornstein, R. (Ed.) *The nature of human consciousness*. San Francisco: Freeman, 1973.

Overlade, D. The production of fassiculations by suggestion. *American Journal of Clinical Hypnosis*, 1976, *19*, 50–56.

Platonov, K. *The word as a physiological and therapeutic factor*. (2nd

Ed.). Moscow: Foreign Languages Publishing House, 1959. (Original in Russian, 1955).

Prokasy, W., and Raskin, D. *Electrodermal activity in psychological research.* New York: Academic Press, 1973.

Rogers, C. *Client-centered therapy.* Boston: Houghton-Mifflin Co., 1951.

Rossi, E. Game and growth: Two dimensions of our psychotherapeutic zeitgeist. *Journal of Humanistic Psychology,* 1967, *8,* 139–154.

Rossi, E. The breakout heuristic: A phenomenology of growth therapy with college students. *Journal of Humanistic Psychology,* 1968, *8,* 6–28.

Rossi, E. Growth, change and transformation in dreams. *Journal of Humanistic Psychology,* 1971, *11,* 147–169.

Rossi, E. *Dreams and the growth of personality: Expanding awareness in psychotherapy.* New York: Pergamon, 1972 (a).

Rossi, E. Self-reflection in dreams. *Psychotherapy,* 1972, *9,* 290–298 (b).

Rossi, E. Dreams in the creation of personality. *Psychological Perspectives,* 1972, *2,* 122–134 (c).

Rossi, E. The dream-protein hypothesis. *American Journal in Psychiatry,* 1973, *130,* 1094–1097 (a).

Rossi, E. Psychological shocks and creative moments in psychotherapy. *American Journal of Clinical Hypnosis,* 1973, *16,* 9–22 (b).

Rossi, E. Psychosynthesis and the new biology of dreams and psychotherapy. *American Journal of Psychotherapy,* 1973, *27,* 34–41 (c).

Rossi, E. The cerebral hemispheres in analytical psychology. *The Journal of Analytical Psychology,* 1977, *22,* 32–51.

Schneck, J. Prehypnotic suggestions. *Perceptual and Motor skills,* 1970, *30,* 826.

Schneck, J. Prehypnotic suggestions in psychotherapy. *American Journal of Clinical Hypnosis,* 1975, *17,* 158–159.

Scheflen, A. *How behavior means.* New York: Aronson, 1974.

Sheehan, P. Hypnosis and manifestations of "imagination." In E. Promm and R. Shor (Eds.) *Hypnosis: Research developments and perspectives.* Chicago: Aldine-Atherton, 1972.

Shevrin, H. Does the average evoked response encode subliminal perception? Yes. A reply to Schwartz and Rem. *Psychophysiology,* 1975, *12,* 395–398.

Shor, R. Hypnosis and the concept of the generalized reality-orientation. *American Journal of Psychotherapy,* 1959, *13,* 582–602.

Smith, M., Chu, J., and Edmonston, W. Cerebral lateralization of haptic perception. *Science.* 1977, *197,* 689–690.

Snyder, E. *Hypnotic poetry.* Philadelphia: University of Pennsylvania Press, 1930.

Sperry, R. Hemisphere disconnection and unity in conscious awareness. *American Psychologist,* 1968, *23,* 723–733.

Spiegel, H. An eye-roll test for hypnotizability. *American Journal of Clinical Hypnosis*, 1972, *15*, 25–28.

Sternberg, S. Memory scanning: New findings and current controversies. *Quarterly Journal of Experimental Psychology*, 1975, *22*, 1–32.

Tart, C. (Ed.) *Altered states of consciousness*. New York: Wiley, 1969.

Tinterow, M. *Foundations of hypnosis*. Springfield, Ill.: C. C. Thomas, 1970.

Watzlawick, P., Beavin, A., and Jackson, D. *Pragmatics of human communication*. New York: Norton, 1967.

Watzlawick, P., Weakland, J., and Fisch, R. *Change*. New York: Norton, 1974.

Weitzenhoffer, A. *Hypnotism: An objective study in suggestibility*. New York: Wiley, 1953.

Weitzenhoffer, A. *General techniques of hypnotism*. New York: Grune and Stratton, 1957.

Weitzenhoffer, A. Unconscious or co-conscious? Reflections upon certain recent trends in medical hypnosis. *American Journal of Clinical Hypnosis*, 1960, *2*, 177–196.

Weitzenhoffer, A. The nature of hypnosis. Parts I and II. *American Journal of Clinical Hypnosis*, 1963, *5*, 295–321; 40–72.

Weizenbaum, J. *Computer power and human reason: from judgment to calculation*. San Francisco: Freeman, 1976.

Woodworth, R. and Schlosberg, H. *Experimental psychology*. New York: Holt and Co., 1954.

Zilburg, G., and Henry, G. *A history of medical psychology*. New York: Norton, 1941.

Index

[Page numbers in regular type refer to illustrations of the material in the induction and commentary sections of the text. Page numbers in *italic* type refer to the more extensive discussions of the topic.]

487